Trauma Certified Registered Nurse (TCRN®) Review

Kendra Menzies Kent, MS, RN, CCRN, CNRN, SCRN, TCRN, is the nursing director of neuroscience programs in the Marcus Neuroscience Institute at Boca Raton Regional Hospital in south Florida. She is a highly experienced critical care trauma nurse and an accomplished instructor, with multiple specialty certifications in critical care and extensive clinical experience in a majority of critical care specialty areas. Ms. Kent provided seminars for Med-Ed in Charlotte, North Carolina, and was a speaker for Health and Sciences Television Network (HSTN) and HSTN videos. Ms. Kent has edited or contributed to *Decision-Making in Medical Surgical Nursing, Evaluation Process: Competency-Based Orientation, Expert 10-Minute Physical Examination Expert Rapid Response, AACN Neuroscience Orientation PowerPoint for Traumatic Brain Injury, Critical Care Essentials,* and *CCRN Review Q&A*. She is the author of *Adult CCRN® Certification Review: Think in Questions, Learn by Rationales* published by Springer Publishing Company.

Trauma Certified Registered Nurse (TCRN®) Review

SECOND EDITION

Kendra Menzies Kent, MS, RN, CCRN, CNRN, SCRN, TCRN

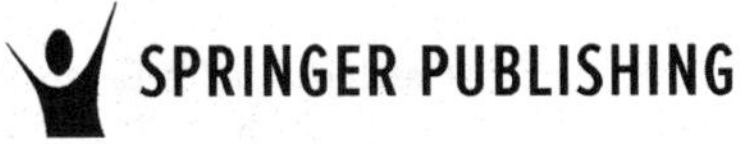

First Springer Publishing edition 2017 (978-0-8261-3194-2).

Springer Publishing Company, LLC
11 West 42nd Street, New York, NY 10036
www.springerpub.com
connect.springerpub.com

Acquisitions Editor: Jaclyn Koshofer
Senior Content Development Editor: Lucia Gunzel
Compositor: diacriTech

ISBN: 978-0-82616-592-3
ebook ISBN: 978-0-82616-593-0
DOI: 10.1891/9780826165930

22 23 24 25 26 / 5 4 3 2 1

The author and the publisher of this Work have made every effort to use sources believed to be reliable to provide information that is accurate and compatible with the standards generally accepted at the time of publication. Because medical science is continually advancing, our knowledge base continues to expand. Therefore, as new information becomes available, changes in procedures become necessary. We recommend that the reader always consult current research and specific institutional policies before performing any clinical procedure or delivering any medication. The author and publisher shall not be liable for any special, consequential, or exemplary damages resulting, in whole or in part, from the readers' use of, or reliance on, the information contained in this book. The publisher has no responsibility for the persistence or accuracy of URLs for external or third-party Internet websites referred to in this publication and does not guarantee that any content on such websites is, or will remain, accurate or appropriate.

Library of Congress Cataloging-in-Publication Data: 2022946227

Publisher's Note: **New and used products purchased from third-party sellers are not guaranteed for quality, authenticity, or access to any included digital components.**

Printed in the United States of America by Hatteras, Inc.

*To my wonderful husband, Robby, and to my parents,
Sid and Judy, for all the love and support they have given me. Mom, I know you are still
looking over me and supporting everything I do!*

Contents

Introduction

Welcome to the journey toward certification. This book was written to help guide you on the pathway of that journey. It is written in a question/answer format to encourage you to think in questions when studying for the examination. When you study, I encourage you to ask yourself, "What questions about this particular topic could appear on the certification exam? What would be a good question?" This prepares you for questions; you are not just attempting to memorize content for the certification examination.

The book provides multiple-choice questions similar to the questions that are found on the Trauma Certified Registered Nurse (TCRN®) examination. These questions allow the nurse to practice taking an examination and assist the nurse in determining areas that require further study prior to taking the TCRN examination. The answers and rationale, including some test-taking skills, are provided for every question, further preparing the nurse for the real examination.

WHY CERTIFICATION?

The most important reason for becoming certified is to do it for yourself. Certification is viewed as a mark of excellence in an area of specialty. It can be seen as an achievement and qualification by peers, physicians, healthcare institutes, and patients/families. Becoming certified takes dedication to trauma nursing and demonstrates a level of competency. The TCRN examination is developed to verify knowledge in trauma nursing.

Reasons to become certified

- Validate your knowledge of trauma to your hospital and peers
- Validate your knowledge of trauma to the patients
- Validate your knowledge of trauma to the physician
- Promote continuing excellence in the nursing profession
- Demonstrate competency
- Promote self-confidence
- Encourage continuing education
- Hospital credentialing
- Monetary benefit (from some hospitals)

TCRN EXAMINATION INFORMATION

The TCRN examination was developed by the Board of Certification for Emergency Nursing (BCEN) and incorporates care of a trauma patient, from prevention and injury to rehabilitation. The examination covers all ages: pediatrics through geriatrics. The examination follows the test plan developed by the BCEN and the test is developed and reviewed by experts in trauma nursing. *The TCRN Application Handbook* can be accessed from the BCEN's website (www.bcencertifications.org). The examination application can be completed online. The TCRN is a 4-year certification for trauma nurses.

EXAMINATION

The TCRN examination includes 150 scored multiple-choice questions, with 25 unscored questions that will not count for or against you. Those 25 questions are included as "tests" for use in future examinations. You will not know which questions count, so complete all 175 questions as if they all do. The test is not arranged per any body system but is randomized. You may have one question on chest trauma and the next one may be on spinal cord injury. The time allowed to complete the examination is 3 hours. To be eligible to take the TCRN examination one must be a licensed RN with 2 years of practice, at an average of 1,000 practice hours per year, across the trauma continuum. *Trauma practice* is defined as providing direct patient care, supervision, education, and advocacy for patients and their families. Additionally, test takers must complete 20 to 30 hours of trauma-specific coursework across the trauma continuum.

The TCRN examination is offered year-round as a computer-based test (CBT) through PSI testing centers. Once BCEN receives the application, applicants may schedule an appointment on the PSI website to sit for the examination. Live remote proctoring is also offered. This is a proctored session using a computer in a secure location of your choice. Immediate test results with score breakdown are available. Following successful completion of the examination, a certificate will be sent in the mail within 3 to 4 weeks.

Renewal of your TCRN certification can be achieved through continuing education (CE) or retaking the examination. The CE requirement is 100 hours. Of the 100 hours of CE, 50 must be from an accredited source and 75 must be within the clinical category. For more details on renewal, see the BCEN website for recertification and an explanation of the CE requirements.

EXAMINATION REVIEW

This TCRN examination review is a blueprint for the examination content. Each major body system is divided into subheadings and topics.

Trauma Certified Registered Nurse examination review

Clinical Practice: Head and Neck **33**

A. Neurologic trauma
   1. Traumatic brain injuries
   2. Spinal injuries

B. Maxillofacial and neck trauma
   1. Facial fractures
   2. Ocular trauma
   3. Neck trauma

Clinical Practice: Trunk **37**

A. Thoracic trauma
   1. Chest wall injuries
   2. Pulmonary injuries
   3. Cardiac injuries
   4. Great vessel injuries

(*continued*)

Trauma Certified Registered Nurse Eexamination review (*continued*)

B. Abdominal trauma **1.** Hollow organ injuries **2.** Solid organ injuries **3.** Diaphragmatic injuries **4.** Retroperitoneal injuries **C.** Genitourinary trauma **D.** Obstetrical trauma (pregnant patients)
Clinical Practice: Extremity and Wound 25 **A.** Musculoskeletal trauma **1.** Vertebral injuries **2.** Pelvic injuries **3.** Compartment syndrome **4.** Amputations **5.** Extremity fractures **6.** Soft-tissue injuries **B.** Surface and burn trauma **1.** Chemical burns **2.** Electrical burns **3.** Thermal burns **4.** Inhalation injuries
Clinical Practice: Special Considerations 25 **A.** Psychosocial issues related to trauma **B.** Shock **1.** Hypovolemic **2.** Obstructive (e.g., tamponade, tension, pneumothorax) **3.** Distributive (e.g., neurogenic, septic) **4.** Cardiogenic **C.** SIRS and MODS
Continuum of Care 15 **A.** Injury prevention **B.** Prehospital care **C.** Patient safety (e.g., fall prevention) **D.** Patient transfer **1.** Intrafacility (within a facility, across departments) **2.** Interfacility (from one facility to another) **E.** Forensic issues **1.** Evidence collection **2.** Chain of custody **F.** End-of-life issues **1.** Organ/tissue donation **2.** Advance directives **3.** Family presence **4.** Palliative care **G.** Rehabilitation (discharge planning)

(*continued*)

Trauma Certified Registered Nurse examination review (*continued*)

Professional Issues	**15**
A. Trauma quality management	
1. Performance improvement	
2. Outcomes follow-up and feedback (e.g., referring facilities, EMS)	
3. Evidence-based practice	
4. Research	
5. Mortality/morbidity reviews	
B. Staff safety (e.g., standard precautions, workplace violence)	
C. Disaster management (e.g., preparedness, mitigation, response, and recovery)	
D. Critical incident stress management	
E. Regulations and standards	
1. HIPAA	
2. EMTALA	
3. Designation/verification (e.g., trauma center/ trauma systems)	
F. Education and outreach for interprofessional trauma teams and the public	
G. Trauma registry (e.g., data collection)	
H. Ethical issues	

EMS, emergency medical services; EMTALA, Emergency Medical Treatment and Active Labor Act; HIPAA, Health Insurance Portability and Accountability Act; MODS, multiple organ dysfunction syndrome; SIRS, systemic inflammatory response syndrome.

The following are testable nursing tasks on the examination:

- **I.** Assessment
  - **A.** Establish mechanism of injury
  - **B.** Assess, intervene, and stabilize patients with immediate life-threatening conditions
  - **C.** Assess pain
  - **D.** Assess for adverse drug and blood reactions
  - **E.** Obtain complete patient history
  - **F.** Obtain a complete physical evaluation
  - **G.** Use Glasgow Coma Scale (GCS) to evaluate patient status
  - **H.** Assist with focused abdominal sonography for trauma (FAST) examination
  - **I.** Calculate burn surface area
  - **J.** Assessment not otherwise specified
- **II.** Analysis
  - **A.** Provide appropriate response to diagnostic test results
  - **B.** Prepare equipment that might be needed by the team
  - **C.** Identify the need for diagnostic tests
  - **D.** Determine the plan of care
  - **E.** Identify desired patient outcomes
  - **F.** Determine the need to transfer to a higher level of care
  - **G.** Determine the need for emotional or psychosocial support
  - **H.** Analysis not otherwise specified
- **III.** Implementation
  - **A.** Incorporate age-specific needs for the patient population served
  - **B.** Respond with decisiveness and clarity to unexpected events
  - **C.** Demonstrate knowledge of pharmacology

D. Assist with or perform the following procedures:
   1. Chest tube insertion
   2. Arterial line insertion
   3. Central line insertion
   4. Compartment syndrome monitoring devices
      a. Abdominal
      b. Extremity
   5. Doppler
   6. End-tidal CO_2
   7. Temperature-control devices (e.g., warming and cooling)
   8. Pelvic stabilizer
   9. Immobilization devices
   10. Tourniquets
   11. Surgical airway insertion
   12. Intraosseous needles
   13. Intracranial pressure (ICP) monitoring devices
   14. Infusers:
      a. Autotransfusion
      b. Fluid
      c. Blood and blood products
   15. Needle decompression
   16. Fluid resuscitation:
      a. Burn fluid resuscitation
      b. Hypertonic solution
      c. Permissive hypotension
      d. Massive transfusion protocol (MTP)
   17. Pericardiocentesis
   18. Bedside open thoracotomy

E. Manage patients who have had the following procedures:
   1. Chest tube insertion
   2. Arterial line insertion
   3. Central line insertion
   4. Compartment syndrome monitoring devices
      a. Abdominal
      b. Extremity
   5. End-tidal CO_2
   6. Temperature-control devices (e.g., warming and cooling)
   7. Pelvic stabilizer
   8. Immobilization devices
   9. Tourniquets
   10. Surgical airway
   11. Intraosseous needles
   12. ICP monitoring devices
   13. Infusers
      a. Fluid
      b. Blood and blood products
   14. Needle decompression
   15. Fluid resuscitation:
      a. Burn fluid resuscitation
      b. Hypertonic solution

c. Permissive hypotension
d. MTP
16. Pericardiocentesis
F. Manage patients' pain relief and sedation by providing:
1. Pharmacologic interventions
2. Nonpharmacologic interventions
G. Manage patient sedation and analgesia
H. Manage tension pneumothorax
I. Manage burn resuscitation
J. Manage increased abdominal pressure
K. Provide complex wound management (e.g., ostomies, drains, wound vacuum-assisted closure [VAC], open abdomen)
L. Implementation not otherwise specified

IV. Evaluation
A. Evaluate patients' response to interventions
B. Monitor patient status and report findings to the team
C. Adapt the plan of care as indicated
D. Evaluation not otherwise specified

V. Continuum of care
A. Monitor or evaluate for opportunities for program or system improvement
B. Ensure proper placement of patients
C. Restore patient to optimal health
D. Collect, analyze, and use data:
1. To improve patient outcomes
2. For benchmarking
3. To decrease incidence of trauma
E. Coordinate the multidisciplinary plan of care
F. Continuum of care not otherwise specified

VI. Professional issues
A. Adhere to regulatory requirements related to:
1. Infectious diseases
2. Hazardous materials
3. Verification/designation
4. Confidentiality
B. Follow standards of practice
C. Involve family in:
1. Patient care
2. Teaching/discharging planning
D. Recognize need for social/protective service consults
E. Provide information to patient and family regarding community resources
F. Address language and cultural barriers
G. Participate in and promote lifelong learning related to new developments and clinical advances
H. Act as an advocate (e.g., for patients, families, and colleagues) related to ethical, legal, and psychosocial issues
I. Provide trauma patients and their families with psychosocial support
J. Assess methods continuously to improve patient outcomes
K. Assist in maintaining the performance improvement programs
L. Participate in multidisciplinary rounds
M. Professional issues not otherwise specified

PREPARATION

Be positive! Avoid any negative thoughts about passing the examination. These can result in a self-fulfilling prophecy. Set the test date and then establish a realistic schedule for preparing for the examination. Set your priorities; study those areas you are less familiar with first. Look at the percentage of questions devoted to each body system and establish timelines based on the percentage of questions pertaining to that topic. Know your best method of study—by yourself or in study groups—and follow that method. Flash cards, practice questions, review courses, study books in outline format, and study books in narrative format are available to assist you. Practice your test questions within a set time limit to familiarize yourself with the time limitations. Allow 2 minutes or less per question (remember, the rule is to answer 50 questions per hour).

When using the practice test questions to study, determine several things when reviewing the answers and rationale. Analyze why you missed the question. Did you just not know the content? Go back and restudy the relevant section. Did you misread the question? Did you misread the answers? Did you miss an important element in the question or scenario? Was there a clue based on age, timeline, or symptoms you missed?

DAY OF THE TEST

Eat a healthy meal and limit the amount of liquids you drink (to avoid the need for breaks) before the examination. Remember, restroom breaks are allowed but the testing time does not stop! Do not try to cram immediately before the test; this will increase your anxiety level. After the examination, make plans to do something special for yourself.

Know how to get to the testing site before the day of your scheduled exam. Plan your route and know how long it will take to get there at the time of day you are scheduled to take the examination. Running late and feeling hurried will increase your anxiety and can poorly affect your test-taking skills. Plus, if you are more than 15 minutes late, they will not let you in to take the examination.

Bring your letter of approval and two forms of identification (one picture ID). You cannot bring anything into the testing room, so leave everything in the car or at home (they will usually have a locker you can put personal items in during the examination).

If you need some assistance with computer-based testing, you are allowed to do a tutorial on the computer before you start your examination. The test time begins once you start the first question of the actual examination. Leaving the testing site without authorization results in an automatic voiding of the test. You will only be allowed 3 hours from the time the test is started.

Results of the examination will be presented onsite at the completion of your examination following a test evaluation.

TEST-TAKING SKILLS

Frequently, the difference between pass and fail depends on test-taking skills. An important reminder: Do not read into the question; take the question and information provided at face value. Answer all questions; do not leave any questions blank. A blank answer will be counted against you. Answering the question, even if it is an "educated" guess, will give you a one out of four chance of being correct.

Key words are important phrases or words used to focus attention on what the question is specifically asking. Examples include *always, earliest, first, on admission, best, least, immediately*, and *initial*.

> **HINT**
>
> **If the question asks for the "best" response, this is an indication that all answers are probably correct and you will have to determine the best answer for that particular scenario.**

Eliminate incorrect options first. Sometimes you will immediately see an answer that is incorrect. Mark through it to narrow down your options and improve your odds. Frequently, you can narrow the choices down to two that are more correct than others.

> **HINT**
>
> **Eliminating incorrect options often gives a 50/50 chance for an educated guess of the correct answer.**

Avoid those answers with words such as *always* or *never*. There is rarely a time in the medical field that you will always or never do a particular action. If three of the four answers are similar, choose the answer that does not sound similar.

Do not change answers unless you are absolutely certain the change is necessary. You can "bookmark" a question that you are not sure about to return to it at the end of the test. Sometimes you will feel more comfortable with the question after you come back to it.

> **HINT**
>
> **First impressions are usually good! Do not take too much time on any one question.**

Do not let it worry you if you do not know all the answers. Take a deep breath and keep going. Rejoice in those answers you know and find easy!

> **HINT**
>
> **You really are not supposed to know all the answers.**

Do not try to establish patterns, such as using "two As in a row" for answers.

If there is a long scenario containing large amounts of data, read the question first, then read the scenario, then reread the question. Sometimes erroneous data will be included that is not required to answer the question. Too much time may be spent trying to comprehend the whole scenario and trying to work through all the information and data can be time-consuming.

> **HINT**
>
> **Do not forget to reread the question to make sure you read it correctly the first time.**

Read all answers before you make a choice; there may be more than one correct answer but one will be the better answer to the question.

> **HINT**
>
> **Do not choose the first option that appears to be correct. Choose the most correct answer.**

Read the question carefully and answer only the question asked. Do not read into the question or think that you require more information/data to answer the question.

> **HINT**
>
> **The question will provide you with all the information needed to answer it correctly.**

Time-frame questions are frequently used on the test. Use the time frame to assist with making the correct choice. Example: Which complication of subarachnoid hemorrhage is seen 7 to 10 days after the bleed?

> **HINT**
>
> **All answers may be correct but only one will occur more often during the time frame provided in the question.**

Questions may be worded using the lead-in, "What is the gold standard?" This is not asking what the most common routine is, but which is the most reliable and accurate.

Scenarios: Read the patient's description word for word. Read the question, then formulate your answer. Read the answer options and choose the one closest to your answer. Reread the question after answering to ensure that you understood the question correctly.

> **HINT**
>
> **Once the question is answered, you are done. Move on to the next question. Do not second-guess yourself.**

Look for answers that facilitate the patient. Facilitative words include *nurture*, *aid*, *support*, *reinforce*, *encourage*, and *assist*.

Pass Guarantee

If you use this resource to prepare for your exam and you do not pass, you may return it for a refund of your full purchase price. To receive a refund, you must return your product along with a copy of your original receipt and exam score report. Product must be returned and received within 180 days of the original purchase date. This excludes tax, shipping, and handling. One offer per person and address. Refunds will be issued within 8 weeks from acceptance and approval. This offer is valid for U.S. residents only. Void where prohibited. To initiate a refund, please contact customer service at CS@springerpub.com.

PART I

Clinical Practice: Head and Neck

Neurological Trauma

1

TRAUMATIC BRAIN INJURY

MECHANISM OF INJURY

Q What is the most common blunt mechanism of injury that causes traumatic brain injury (TBI)?

A Motor vehicle collision (MVC)

An MVC is one of the most common mechanisms of injury that results in TBI. The injury can range from mild to severe TBI. A fall is the most common mechanism of TBI in pediatric patients younger than the age of 12 years. Most adolescent TBI results from an MVC, sports injuries, and assault (Box 1.1).

Box 1.1 Common causes of blunt traumatic brain injury

Motor vehicle collision
Motor pedestrian injury
Fall
Sports-related injury
War injuries
Domestic violence

HINT

A major component of prevention of TBI in MVC is the proper use of seat belts and car seats.

Q What is it called when a moving object impacts a stationary head?

A Acceleration injury

Blunt trauma to the head is described based on the mechanism of injury. The term *acceleration injury* indicates a moving object, such as a baseball bat, impacting the head. Deceleration injury occurs when the head is moving and strikes a stationary object, such as in MVC when the head hits the windshield.

HINT

When you accelerate, you put something into motion. So when an object hits the head, it causes the head to accelerate, or move. This is an acceleration injury.

Q What is it called when a brain injury occurs without any impact to the head itself?

A Indirect injury

An indirect injury occurs when the brain moves in the cranial vault following an acceleration–deceleration without the head impacting an object. A direct injury involves an impact to the head, either through an acceleration, deceleration, or acceleration–deceleration mechanism.

HINT

There are bony protrusions in the skull; when the brain moves against these rough edges, it causes injury, even without a direct impact to the head.

Q Following a gunshot to the head, the bullet is found within the cranial vault. What type of injury is this?

A Penetrating injury

Penetrating injury with a gunshot wound indicates that the bullet entered the cranial vault but did not exit it. The bullet remains in the skull. Perforating injury occurs when the bullet enters and exits the cranium. Penetrating injuries to the brain also include stab wounds through the cranium or penetrating stab wounds to the face, which can enter the cranium. Tangential injury occurs when the bullet glances off the skull; these types of injuries may have a lower mortality rate but can still cause injury.

HINT

In some penetrating injuries to the skull, the bullet is left in the cranium and not retrieved because it is located in one of the eloquent areas of the brain. Retained bullet or skull fragments have not been found to significantly increase infection risk.

Q Following an impact to the head, an injury to the brain occurs on the side opposite the impact. What is this injury called?

A Contrecoup injury

A coup injury occurs in the area of impact and a contrecoup injury is a brain injury that occurs on the opposite side of the impact. Coup–contrecoup injuries are commonly associated with epidural and subdural hematomas (SDHs).

HINT

The mechanism of injury that most commonly causes a coup–contrecoup injury is an impact to the lateral side of the skull ("side-to-side" injury).

Q What type of injury results in diffuse axonal injury (DAI) to the brain?

A Rotational injury

Rotational injury, such as in vehicle rollover, can result in shearing of the brain tissue. This type of injury is called *DAI*. Presence of DAI indicates a poorer functional outcome of the TBI patient.

HINT

Decreased level of consciousness (LOC) that is out of proportion to CT scan findings is indicative of DAI.

Q What type of injury causes chronic traumatic encephalopathy (CTE)?

A Repetitive injuries

Repetitive TBIs that trigger progressive degeneration of brain tissue result in CTE. The injuries frequently are mild traumatic brain injuries (MTBI) related to contact sports injuries.

HINT

CTE may also be found in veterans of war and victims of domestic violence.

Q What patient population is most likely to present with a chronic SDH?

A The elderly

Elderly patients are likely to present with chronic SDH. Other patient populations include alcoholics and dementia patients. Chronic SDHs tend to hemorrhage slowly. These patients have cortical atrophy, which allows for more blood volume to accumulate before an increase in intracranial pressure (ICP) occurs (Table 1.1).

Table 1.1 Classifications of subdural hematoma

Acute SDH	Onset within 24 hours after injury
Subacute SDH	Onset within 24–48 hours after injury
Chronic SDH	Onset days to weeks after injury

SDH, subdural hematoma.

HINT

Chronic SDH patients are frequently misdiagnosed initially as suffering from "old age" or stroke.

Q Secondary injuries include cerebral edema. What is the cerebral edema caused by ischemic or hypoxic insult following a TBI called?

A Cytotoxic edema

Cytotoxic edema causes intracellular swelling and is a result of hypoxia or anoxic injuries. *Vasogenic cerebral edema* refers to swelling or extra fluid in the interstitial space and is a result of trauma to the tissue. TBI will have a combination of both cytotoxic and vasogenic edema. Following a brain trauma, there is a loss of autoregulation in the areas of injury. Cerebral blood flow (CBF) is shunted away from the uninjured areas of the brain to the areas of injury. This causes a "steal phenomenon" and results in hypoxia in uninjured areas of the brain.

HINT

Mannitol is used to treat cerebral edema and pulls fluid from the interstitial space. It is most effective with managing vasogenic edema.

Q What is the anatomical difference in pediatric patients that makes them more likely to experience a brain injury with a trauma?

A Their heads are larger in proportion to their bodies than they are in adults.

The head of a child is larger in proportion to the rest of their body and the stability of the neck and ligaments is not fully developed. This makes the child susceptible to TBI in an MVC.

HINT

Once the child is no longer in a car seat, children typically place the shoulder harness behind them as it does not fit appropriately. This increases the likelihood of TBI.

Q What is the triad of symptoms typically seen in shaken baby syndrome (SBS)?

A Subdural hematoma, retinal hemorrhage, and cerebral edema

SBS is a result of violent shaking of the child. This is also called *abusive head trauma*. The head may or may not have contact with an object, but the movement of the brain contents causes a shearing effect. The result is typically bilateral SDH, cerebral edema, and DAI. The injury is often fatal and can cause lifelong severe neurological disabilities.

HINT

Retinal hemorrhages have a characteristic pattern for SBS and are used frequently to assist with the diagnosis of SBS (Box 1.2).

Box 1.2 Signs of traumatic brian injury caused by child abuse

Injuries that cannot be explained by the reported trauma
Associated long-bone fractures
Associated cervical injuries
Poor hygiene
Bruises at varying stages of healing
Multiple complex skull fractures with reported single-impact history

TRAUMATIC INJURIES

Q What type of fracture is a displaced comminuted fracture of the skull?

A Depressed skull fracture

A depressed skull fracture is a comminuted fracture that is displaced into the meninges and brain tissue. This injury is commonly associated with epidural, subdural, and parenchymal hematomas. A linear skull fracture has a nondisplaced fracture line.

HINT

The displacement of bony pieces into the meninges frequently causes a tearing of the middle meningeal vessels and the development of epidural and SDHs.

Q A patient develops a cerebrospinal fluid (CSF) leak following a blow to the side of the head. What type of fracture does this patient most likely have?

A Basilar skull fracture

Basilar skull fractures may result in CSF leaks from ears (otorrhea) or from the nose (rhinorrhea). The base of the skull is divided into the anterior, middle, and posterior skull base or fossa. Fractures may occur anywhere throughout the skull base, but the anterior fossa is the most common area for basilar skull fractures.

HINT

A blow to the side of the head causes the basilar skull to buckle, resulting in fracture lines along the basilar skull.

Q An area of the brain parenchyma with hemorrhage following TBI is called what?

A Contusion

Contusions are areas of parenchymal hemorrhage that result from acceleration/deceleration and blunt impact. Contusions may initially appear as several small hemorrhaging areas, but these can increase and combine into a larger hematoma. Approximately one third of the contusions will expand in 24 hours.

HINT

Initial CT scan following a TBI may not show the contusion. Frequently, follow-up CT scans are obtained in 24 hours to identify the contusion or determine the increase in size of the contusion.

Q Is an epidural hematoma (EDH) most commonly caused by laceration of an artery or of bridging veins?

A Laceration of an artery

Laceration of an artery is the most common cause of EDH. The most common artery involved in EDH is the middle meningeal artery (MMA). Laceration of veins may also result in bleeding in the epidural space but is less common than arterial involvement. Tearing of bridging veins will hemorrhage into the subdural space (venous sinuses are located in subdural space) causing SDH.

HINT

An EDH typically expands rapidly as a result of being an arterial hemorrhage; SDH may be a slower hemorrhage because of its venous involvement.

Q Tearing of pial veins will cause bleeding following a trauma. Where is the hemorrhage located?

A Subarachnoid space

Tearing of small pial veins causes bleeding into the subarachnoid space and is called *subarachnoid hemorrhage (SAH)*. SAH may also involve blood in the ventricles, but isolated intraventricular hemorrhage (IVH) following trauma is unusual.

HINT

Vasospasms following traumatic SAH are less significant than those that follow aneurysmal rupture.

Q Which two secondary injuries have the greatest effect on neurological outcomes following TBI?

A Hypotension and hypoxia

Secondary injuries are those neurological injuries that occur to the brain after the initial trauma. It has been found that hypotension and hypoxia are the two most important determinants of neurological outcomes (Table 1.2).

Table 1.2 Secondary injuries

Systemic Secondary Injuries	Intracranial Secondary Injuries
Hypotension	Increased ICP
Hypoxia	Cerebral edema
Anemia	Expanding mass lesions (hematomas)
Hypercapnia	Hydrocephalus
Hypocapnia	CNS infections
Hyperthermia	Seizures
Hyperglycemia	Brain ischemia
Electrolyte abnormalities	
Acid–base abnormalities	

CNS, central nervous system; ICP, intracranial pressure.

HINT

Priority of care for managing TBI patients is airway/breathing to improve oxygenation and resuscitation to reestablish perfusion to prevent further neurological injury.

ASSESSMENT/DIAGNOSIS

Q A patient develops bilateral periorbital ecchymosis following traumatic injury to the head. What is the cause of this finding?

A Basilar skull fracture

Patients with basilar skull fracture may develop periorbital ecchymosis (raccoon eyes) and bruising on the mastoid process called *Battle's sign*.

HINT

Raccoon eyes and Battle's sign may not appear immediately following a trauma but typically develop later following the injury.

Q What is the best bedside method for testing drainage from the nose for the presence of CSF?

A Halo test

The halo test is used at the bedside to determine the presence of CSF in drainage from the nose (rhinorrhea) or from the ears (otorrhea). To perform a halo test, dab the drainage onto gauze and look for a yellow ring surrounding the drainage. This is a positive halo and indicates the presence of CSF.

HINT

The halo test is more reliable than testing the drainage for glucose because drainage may contain blood, which also has glucose. A glucose test for CSF has more false positives.

Q What lab test may be used to improve the accuracy of the diagnosis for CSF in drainage?

A Beta-2 transferrin

A halo ring test can cause false positives so the gold standard (most diagnostic) is lab testing the drainage for CSF. Beta-2 transferrin is a variant of transferrin and is used as an endogenous marker for CSF in other bodily fluids.

HINT

Beta-2 transferrin has been called *CSF-specific transferrin* because it is highly specific for CSF.

Q What diagnostic study is considered the gold standard for identifying basilar skull fractures?

A CT scan

High-resolution CT scan of the head is considered the gold standard to identify basilar skull fractures. Differentiation between suture lines and fracture is required to ensure an accurate diagnosis.

HINT

Clinical findings may be used to assist with diagnosis of basilar skull fracture if unable to visualize fracture on head CT scan.

Q Diagnostic CT scan of the brain found air present in the cranium in addition to basilar skull fracture. What is the air in the cranium called?

A Pneumocephalus

Pneumocephalus is a complication of basilar skull fracture and may be identified on brain CT scan. Air enters through the fracture into the cranium. Management of pneumocephalus may be with high oxygen administration.

HINT

Pneumocephalus can become a tension pneumocephalus with a resulting elevation of ICP.

Q An MTBI may be defined by the Glasgow Coma Scale (GCS). What GCS score would indicate minor brain injury?

A GCS score of 13 to 15

MTBI (which used to be called a *concussion*) is often classified as a GCS score between 13 and 15 (Box 1.3). The patient does not have to experience a loss of consciousness to have a TBI. MTBI can be graded on severity (Table 1.3).

Box 1.3 Diagnosis of mild traumatic brain injury

GCS between 13 and 15
Temporary loss of consciousness
Posttraumatic amnesia for less than 24 hours
Transient neurological abnormalities
Transient confusion

GCS, Glasgow Coma Scale.

Table 1.3 Glasgow Coma Scale classification: Severity of traumatic brain injury

GCS 13–15	Mild TBI
GCS 9–12	Moderate TBI
GCS 3–8	Severe TBI

GCS, Glasgow Coma Scale; TBI, traumatic brain injury.

HINT

To be diagnosed as MTBI, neurological abnormalities must not be the result of alcohol, drugs, or caused by other injuries.

▶ HINT

Use of the GCS to determine the severity of neurological injury in intubated and aphasic patients is limited.

Q A patient presents with an altered LOC following a head trauma. What is the best diagnostic procedure to use to identify skull and brain injuries initially?

A Noncontrast CT scan

Noncontrast CT scan is useful in the immediate posttraumatic period to identify intracranial pathology that would indicate the need for immediate surgical management. Noncontrast CT scan is used to identify skull fractures, hematomas, contusions, mass effects, presence of foreign objects, and the presence of cerebral edema (Box 1.4).

Box 1.4 Indications for noncontrast CT scan traumatic brain injury

Loss of consciousness
Posttraumatic amnesia
Vomiting
Age older than 60 years
Presence of headache, drug, or alcohol intoxication
Deficits in short-term memory
GCS <15
Focal neurological deficit
Signs of basilar skull fracture
Posttraumatic seizures
Presence of coagulopathy or currentluse of anticoagulants
Dangerous mechanism of injury (i.e., ejection from vehicle)

GCS, Glasgow Coma Scale.

▶ HINT

Pediatric patients with a GCS less than 15 may be candidates for a noncontrast CT scan.

Q What is the most sensitive indicator of an increased ICP?

A Change in the LOC

A change in LOC is a sensitive indicator for neurological deterioration and an increase in ICP. When performing neurological assessments, it is very important to assess for LOC and symptoms of neurological deterioration (Box 1.5).

Box 1.5 Symptoms of neurological deterioration

Decreased level of alertness
Development of confusion or disorientation
Unequal pupils or change in pupillary response
Dilated pupil(s) or constricted pupils
Vision changes
Vomiting
Seizures
Worsening headache
Changes in respiratory patterns
Cushing's triad

▶ HINT

A change in LOC can include either a change in alertness, a change in orientation, or both.

▶ HINT

Cushing's triad (increased systolic pressure, widened pulse pressure, and bradycardia) are signs of impending herniation but are considered late signs of an increased ICP.

Q What is the most commonly used diagnosis of DAI?

A Clinical diagnosis

Clinical diagnosis reveals a poor neurological status and a decreased LOC that are out of proportion with the injury observed on CT scan. DAI involves microscopic injuries, therefore is not seen as large changes on diagnostic studies such as a CT scan. CT imaging may demonstrate small punctate foci of hemorrhage, but this is not found in all cases of DAI.

▶ HINT

It may be several days before the diagnosis of DAI is made because of the delay in CT presentation of contusions.

Q A patient presents to the ED following a fall off a ladder. The family reports some altered loss of consciousness after the fall. What should be included in the nurse's admission history?

A Duration and severity of altered LOC

A reported altered LOC requires more information from those who observed the injury. This includes the duration of the altered mentation, degree of altered LOC, other neurological symptoms experienced, and mechanism of injury.

▶ HINT

The observer of the traumatic event is a better historian than the person who experienced altered LOC. Patients typically cannot recall the event, deny the loss of consciousness, or are not really aware of how long they were unconscious.

Q What question may the trauma nurse use to evaluate the presence of retrograde amnesia following a TBI?

A "What was the *last* event before your injury that you remember?"

Retrograde amnesia is the loss of memory before the traumatic event. It is commonly determined by asking the patient about the last thing they remember before the traumatic event. Posttraumatic amnesia is the loss of memory from the time of unconsciousness until the first memory after the event. Antegrade amnesia is the inability to create new memory after the event. An example of antegrade amnesia is when a person is unable to remember anything that happened the rest of the day despite being conscious.

▶ HINT

"What is the *first* thing you remember after the event?" is a question used to evaluate posttraumatic amnesia.

Q A rapidly expanding EDH following a severe TBI can result in an uncal herniation. Which pupil will dilate following uncal herniation?

A Ipsilateral

Uncal herniation is a lateral displacement and herniation of brain tissue caused by a unilateral expanding mass. The pupil affected by the herniation is the ipsilateral pupil. It will dilate and become nonreactive. SDH may also be a rapidly expanding mass and can cause uncal herniation with a dilated ipsilateral nonreactive pupil.

▶ HINT

Dilated pupil is caused by the injury or stretch of cranial nerve (CN) III (oculomotor). CNs do not cross (except CN IV), so symptoms are ipsilateral.

Q Which of the hematomas following TBI has the classic presentation of a lucid period followed by rapid loss of consciousness?

A EDH

EDH has a classic presentation of a period of lucidity. The patient may have been unconscious initially, experiences a period of being awake, then loses consciousness again.

▶ HINT

Not all EDHs experience this classical presentation but of all the hematomas, EDH is the one that is most likely to present in this manner.

Q What complication of abdominal trauma can increase ICP and worsen neurological outcomes?

A Abdominal compartment syndrome (ACS)

ACS is a complication of abdominal trauma. It causes an increase in abdominal pressure that results in a decrease in venous drainage from the brain. This elevates the intracerebral blood volume and ICP. Increased pressure in the thoracic cavity can have the same effect as ACS. Multisystem trauma patients with combination abdominal trauma with brain injury should be assessed for the presence of ACS; treatment should be initiated to lower abdominal pressures.

▶ HINT

ACS can be measured and monitored with bladder pressure readings.

Q What is a commonly used assessment tool to measure the deficit in cognitive functioning following a TBI?

A Ranchos Los Amigos Scale

The Ranchos Los Amigos Scale is used to measure a deficit in cognitive function. The tool is frequently used to determine the patient's level of cognitive functioning for rehabilitation capabilities and prognosis following TBI. The scale is divided into eight stages (or 10 stages in the revised version), ranging from appropriate to coma.

▶ HINT

Level VI on the revised score is the point at which the patient requires moderate assistance (vs. maximal assistance) and is the point that benefits greatly from rehabilitation.

MEDICAL/SURGICAL INTERVENTIONS

Q What is the primary management of a depressed skull fracture?

A Surgical debridement

Following a depressed skull fracture, surgical debridement is used to remove the bony pieces that cause damage to the meninges and brain tissue. This is followed later by cranioplasty to replace the portion of the debrided skull.

▶ HINT

The use of cranioplasty to repair the skull defect also serves a cosmetic purpose.

Q What is the prehospital and ED priority of care for severe traumatic brain-injured patients?

A To check airway and breathing

Hypoxia and hypotension are secondary injuries that will worsen neurological outcomes. The prehospital goals are to initiate treatment to prevent secondary injuries. This includes obtaining and maintaining airway and breathing to prevent hypoxia and initiating fluid resuscitation to prevent hypotension and hypoperfusion. Care should also be taken to secure the cervical spine as cervical spine injuries are commonly associated with head trauma.

▶ HINT

Intubation is considered in patients with a GCS score of less than or equal to 8.

Q What are the mean arterial pressure (MAP) and the PaO_2 goals for TBI?

A MAP and PaO_2 greater than 80 mmHg

Systemic hypoxia is an independent predictor of increased morbidity and mortality. A single episode of hypotension (blood pressure [BP] less than 90 mmHg) is associated with worsening outcomes. Maintaining an MAP greater than 80 mmHg in severe traumatic brain-injured patients (GCS score less than 8) will improve brain perfusion. If the GCS score is more than 8, then MAP is maintained greater than 70 mmHg. The oxygenation goal is to maintain PaO_2 between 80 and 120 mmHg and arterial saturation greater than 94% to prevent secondary hypoxic injuries.

▶ HINT

The goal in managing severe TBI is to optimize CBF while minimizing cerebral edema and ICP.

Q An ICP monitor was placed in the trauma ICU to monitor a patient with severe TBI. What should be the goal for the cerebral perfusion pressure (CPP)?

A Maintain CPP greater than 60 mmHg

CPP is a measurement used at the bedside to estimate CBF. The CPP is calculated when the patient has an ICP monitor and the goal is to maintain CPP greater than 60 mmHg to improve CBF (Box 1.6). The ICP should be maintained at less than 20 mmHg. If CPP is less than 60 mmHg following adequate fluid resuscitation, a vasoconstrictor may be administered to increase MAP. CPP more than 70 mmHg is not recommended because of the risk of hyperperfusion and worsening of cerebral edema.

Box 1.6 Calculation of cerebral perfusion pressure

MAP – ICP = CPP

CPP, cerebral perfusion pressure; ICP, intracranial pressure; MAP, mean arterial pressure.

▶ HINT

To improve CPP, increase MAP and reduce the ICP. The focus of interventions is on both sides: the driving force (MAP) and the opposing force (ICP; Box 1.7).

Box 1.7 Indications for intracranial pressure monitoring

- GCS <8
- Abnormal brain CT scan includes:
  - Hemorrhage
  - Contusions
  - Swelling
  - Herniation
  - Compressed basal cisterns
- Normal brain CT scan and two or more of the following:
  - Age older than 40 years
  - Unilateral or bilateral motor posturing
  - Systemic hypotension
- Patient will not be examined for a prolonged period of time.

GCS, Glasgow Coma Scale.

HINT

Infants and young children may tolerate increased pressure better because of open sutures and fontanelles, but they can still experience increased ICP and may require ICP monitoring similar to adults.

Q What is the osmotic diuretic used to treat cerebral edema and lower ICP?

A Mannitol

Mannitol is an osmotic diuretic that is used to increase serum osmolality, creating a pull of fluid from the extravascular to intravascular space. This lowers cerebral edema and ICP. While administering mannitol, care should be taken to avoid hypovolemia (because of the diuresis) and hypotension. Fluid resuscitation may be required to prevent hypovolemia. Serum osmolality and sodium levels need to be obtained at least every 6 hours with hyperosmolar therapy.

HINT

Hold administration of mannitol if serum osmolality is greater than 320 mOsm/L.

Q What is the potential adverse effect of administering hypertonic saline to lower cerebral edema?

A Central pontine myelinolysis (CPM)

Hypertonic saline (3%, 7.5%, 23%) may also be used to increase serum osmolality instead of mannitol (Table 1.4). The highest risk for causing CPM is in hyponatremic patients. If the patient has a normal serum Na^+ (sodium) level, the chance of causing CPM when using 3% saline in appropriate dosages is not common. Monitor serum Na^+ levels while administering hypertonic saline and hold if Na^+ levels are greater than 155 mEq/L (Table 1.5).

Table 1.4 Hyperosmolar therapy

3% saline	100 mL intravenous every 2 hours as needed
Mannitol	0.25–1 g/kg intravenous every 6 hours

Table 1.5 Adverse effects of hyperosmolar therapy

Mannitol	Hypertonic Saline
Rebound phenomenon	Rebound phenomenon
Hyperosmolar state	Central pontine myelinolysis
Dehydration	Hypernatremia
Acute renal failure	Worsening pulmonary edema

HINT

Avoid administering hypertonic saline in patients who are hyponatremic to manage cerebral edema. Mannitol would be the better answer in that situation.

Q Sustained hyperventilation with hypocarbia and respiratory alkalosis can cause what harmful effects in a traumatic brain-injured patient?

A Reduced CBF

$PaCO_2$ is a potent cerebral vasodilator. If the $PaCO_2$ is decreased because hyperventilation and hypocarbia occur, this causes cerebral vasoconstriction, reduced CBF, and a decrease in ICP. Sustained or aggressive hyperventilation is not recommended because of its effect on CBF, even though it can lower ICP. The $PaCO_2$ goal is 35 to 45 mmHg unless resistant to cerebral hypertension, then may hyperventilate to $PaCO_2$ of 30 to 34 mmHg.

HINT

When a patient suddenly loses consciousness because of a rapidly elevating ICP, the trauma nurse may hyperventilate for a short period to lower the ICP until definitive management of the patient can occur.

Q A patient is admitted to the ICU after craniotomy to remove acute SDH. The bone is left out and will be replaced at a later date. What is this called?

A Bone flap or craniectomy

A bone flap is removed during the craniotomy and not replaced to allow for more room for the brain to swell. This is called *decompressive surgery*. Patients still can herniate through the bone flap, causing strangulation of brain tissue, and will still need to be treated for an increase in ICP. A hemicraniectomy may also be performed to allow a greater amount of decompression.

HINT

The trauma nurse should assess the bone flap for tension or any bulging, indicating an increase in ICP.

Q What is the temperature goal when caring for a severe TBI patient?

A Between 36°C and 37°C (96.8°F and 98.6°F)

Elevated body temperatures have adverse effects on TBI patients and normothermia should be maintained. Even though non-brain-injured patients' fever is allowed to increase body temperatures to the range of 38.3°C to 38.5°C (100.94°F and 101.3°F), the brain may begin to experience injury at a temperature greater than 37°C (98.6°F). Fever increases brain metabolism, elevates levels of proinflammatory cytokines, and may increase ICP. Hypothermia has also been found to worsen outcomes in traumatic brain-injured patients and should be avoided unless there is refractory elevated ICP.

HINT

Remember neurological patients are also at risk for central neurogenic fever and can elevate body temperatures rapidly and severely.

Q Which type of intravenous (IV) fluid is most commonly used to maintain fluid volume in a TBI patient?

A Normal saline (NS)

NS is an isotonic crystalloid commonly used to resuscitate and maintain fluid volume in a TBI patient. NS may also be used initially to correct hyponatremia (Na^+ less than 140 mEq/L).

HINT

Avoid dextrose in the IV fluids because hyperglycemia is considered a secondary injury and can worsen neurological outcomes.

Q Sedation and analgesia may be provided to control agitation and pain following TBI. What adverse effect should be monitored closely to prevent secondary brain injuries?

A Hypotension

Analgesia and sedation can lower the ICP and facilitate mechanical ventilation but may cause vasodilation with hypotension and decreased CBF. Hypotension is a secondary injury that may worsen neurological outcomes. Close monitoring of BP is required when administering analgesics and sedatives. Analgesia and sedation may also affect respiratory functions and should be used cautiously to prevent respiratory depression and hypoxia, unless mechanically ventilated.

HINT

Sedation also involves the potential loss of an accurate neurological assessment.

Q What interventional radiology (IR) procedure can be performed to assist with controlling expansion of SDH?

A MMA embolization

MMA embolization can be used to control the bleeding and expansion of the SDH. It may be used before or after craniotomy to evacuate the hematoma.

Q How long should the seizure prophylaxis be continued following a severe TBI?

A For 7 days

Seizure prophylaxis is recommended for 7 days following a severe TBI. If the patient has not had a seizure within 7 days following the trauma, the antiepileptic drug may be discontinued. Seizure prophylaxis is not recommended in mild to moderate traumatic brain-injured patients.

HINT

Continuous EEG monitoring may be used to identify nonconvulsive seizures in TBI patients who do not wake up following the trauma.

Q When would a barbiturate coma be considered following a severe TBI?

A When there is persistent elevation in ICP

Inducing a barbiturate coma is not the first-line treatment to manage an increased ICP but may be used if the ICP is refractory despite tier-one interventions (i.e., osmolar therapy; Box 1.8). Continuous EEG monitoring is frequently used to titrate the barbiturate therapy by burst suppression.

Box 1.8 Potential treatments for refractory increased intracranial pressure

Barbiturate coma
Decompressive craniotomy
Mild hyperventilation ($PaCO_2$ 30–34 mmHg)
Mild hypothermia (33°C–35°C)
Neuromuscular blocking agents

ICP, intracranial pressure.

HINT

Monitor hemodynamics of a patient in a barbiturate coma because of the adverse effect of myocardial depression.

HINT

Corticosteroids are not recommended in managing cerebral edema or increased ICP in TBI patients.

NURSING INTERVENTIONS

Q A gastric tube is required in a patient with TBI. What type of gastric tube should be placed?

A Orogastric tube (OGT)

An OGT is the preferred gastric tube in patients with TBI with a potential risk of having basilar skull fracture. Nasogastric tube placement can result in the tube entering the brain through the cribriform fracture in basilar skull fractures. The cribriform plate is located in the anterior fossa or skull base.

HINT

Never place any nasal tube following facial or head injury because of the risk of brain cannulation.

Q Where is the gauze placed in patients with rhinorrhea?

A Taped under the nose

Frequently, gauze is taped under the nose to absorb the drainage. This allows for the estimation of the amount of CSF drainage that is occurring because of the leak.

HINT

Never pack the nose with gauze in patients with rhinorrhea. This can increase the risk of meningitis.

Q Following a basilar skull fracture with a known CSF leak, at what level should the head of the bed (HOB) be placed?

A Greater than 30 degrees

The HOB should be elevated greater than 30 degrees in patients with a known CSF leak. Conservative treatment is usually recommended for basilar fractures and CSF leaks, which include strict bed rest; elevated HOB; no coughing, sneezing, and straining. Antibiotic prophylaxis is not recommended following a basilar skull fracture and CSF leak.

HINT

Instruct the patient with a CSF leak not to forcefully blow their nose.

Q A patient is being discharged home from the ED following an MTBI sustained while playing football. What is the most appropriate recommendation on when the patient can return to playing football?

A Once the patient is symptom free

Current guidelines recommend a graduated increase in the level of activity for the athlete progressing from the initial stage of "light exercise" toward "full contact" activity, once the athlete is completely symptom free at rest. This is to prevent second-impact syndrome, which can result in death and repetitive injuries.

HINT

Second-impact syndrome can occur with a second impact to the head within hours to weeks of the initial TBI.

Q A patient with a TBI should be placed in what position to assist with lowering the ICP?

A Elevate the HOB

Elevating the HOB by 30 degrees facilitates venous drainage and lowers blood volume in the cranium, thereby lowering the ICP. Laying the HOB flat will increase the ICP. Also maintain the neck in a neutral position to avoid jugular vein constriction.

HINT

Maintain an elevated HOB in TBI patients unless contraindicated by other injuries.

Q A severe traumatic brain-injured patient in the ICU develops a temperature of 39°C (102.2°F). What nursing intervention should be performed to lower the body temperature?

A Apply a cooling blanket

Elevated body temperatures should be managed quickly in brain-injured patients to prevent secondary brain injury. Applying a cooling blanket to lower the body temperature is a nursing intervention that may be used. Other methods to lower the body temperature may include administering antipyretic medications, controlling the room temperature, and intravascular cooling (Box 1.9). The goal is to maintain a normothermic body temperature.

Box 1.9 Other interventions for traumatic brain injury patients

Appropriate and early nutrition
Venous thrombosis prophylaxis
Stress ulcer prophylaxis
Early mobility
Prevent infections
Treat hyperglycemia (>180 mg/dL)
Prevent skin breakdown

HINT

Shivering can also increase metabolism and should be treated if it occurs during cooling of the patient.

COMPLICATIONS

Q Following a depressed skull fracture, the patient develops fever and elevated white blood cell (WBC) counts. What would be the potential complication of the depressed skull fracture?

A Meningitis

CNS infections, such as meningitis, are potential complications following a depressed and basilar skull fracture.

HINT

Signs of an infection are elevated temperature and WBC count; meningitis is the infection associated with depressed skull fracture.

Q Which CN may be injured by a basilar skull fracture when the patient presents with asymmetrical facial expressions?

A Facial (CN VII)

CN injuries can be associated with basilar skull fractures. CN I (olfactory or sense of smell) can be affected if the cribriform plate is fractured. CN II (optic) injury can result in unilateral blindness and dilated pupil. The facial nerve (CN VII) is more commonly damaged with middle fossa and temporal bone injury. This presents with a facial droop (asymmetry of the face).

HINT

CN injuries can occur with skull fractures and facial fractures.

Q A head CT scan of a trauma patient finds intracerebral hemorrhage. What medication therapy would the trauma nurse suspect the patient may be taking?

A Anticoagulation or antiplatelet therapy

Anticoagulation and antiplatelet therapy are the common therapies that result in intracerebral hemorrhage and may occur following any trauma. Reversal of the bleeding complications is considered a priority and may include administering a reversal agent if there is an antidote for the medication. Correct the coagulopathy with prothrombin complex concentrates (PCC) in life-threatening bleeds. Other blood products may include fresh frozen plasma (FFP) and cryoprecipitate.

HINT

If the patient was on antiplatelet therapy, it may be beneficial to administer platelets.

Q Repetitive mild TBIs in contact sports can result in what complication?

A CTE

CTE is a complication of repetitive brain trauma frequently seen with players of contact sports (Box 1.10). This used to be called *punch drunk* in boxing. These repetitive injuries result in deposits of tau proteins in the cortex, causing degeneration and atrophy of the brain similar to that seen in cortical dementia.

Box 1.10 Symptoms of chronic traumatic encephalopathy

Memory loss
Depression
Suicidal thoughts and suicide
Lave tremors as all of the other symptoms
Aggressive behavior

(*continued*)

Box 1.10 Symptoms of chronic traumatic encephalopathy (*continued*)

Tremors

Ataxia (gait abnormality)

Slowed movements

Speech abnormalities

Confusion

HINT

The pathophysiology of CTE is similar to Alzheimer disease and Parkinson disease, but this is a preventable dementia.

Q A patient presents to the clinic with frequent headaches and states he had a concussion about 2 months ago. What is the cause of the headaches?

A Posttraumatic headaches

Posttraumatic headaches develop in about 30% to 40% of patients following MTBI. The headaches may increase during periods of stress, tension, or activity (Box 1.11).

Box 1.11 Complications of mild traumatic brain injury

Headaches

Posttraumatic stress disorder

Fatigue, exhaustion

Sleep disturbances

Posture and balance issues

Memory problems

Seizures

HINT

Management of posttraumatic headache is similar to benign headaches and includes abortive treatments with triptans.

Q What is the brain's ability to reorganize neural pathways called?

A Plasticity

Plasticity is the ability of the brain's neural pathways to reorganize based on stimulation, new experiences, and new learning. Pediatric brains have the greatest plasticity, but adult brains can reorganize neural pathways to learn and improve one's recovery. Engaging in activities helps the brain develop new pathways.

HINT

The brain is most susceptible to plasticity early after a trauma, so rehabilitation begins on admission.

Q How many months following the TBI does the neurological improvement begin to slow down?

A At about 6 months

The greatest improvements following TBI occur within the first 6 months, then begin to slow down with minimal improvement after 1 year.

HINT

Inform the family that it may take up to 1 year after the injury to have an understanding of the degree of physical recovery achieved; however, psychological recovery may take even longer.

SPINAL CORD INJURY

MECHANISM OF INJURY

Q A hyperflexion mechanism of injury may result in rupture of which longitudinal ligament?

A Posterior longitudinal ligament

Hyperflexion injury occurs when the spine is flexed beyond the normal range of motion. An example is a head-on MVC. The head continues forward with sufficient speed and force for the chin to touch the chest. The stretch occurs posteriorly, causing the rupture, or tearing, of the posterior longitudinal ligament. The anterior vertebral body may be involved in a compression or wedge fracture. This injury may result in subluxation and/or disk herniation. A pediatric patient is at high risk for this mechanism of injury because of the laxity of longitudinal ligaments.

HINT

A "lipstick sign" is when the trauma victim has lipstick on her shirt, which can indicate a hyperflexion injury.

Q A patient is diagnosed with cervical injury following a rear-end MVC. What is the most likely mechanism for the spinal injury?

A Hyperextension

Hyperextension injuries occur when the spine is moved into an extreme hyperextension position. The stretch of the spine now occurs anteriorly, so the anterior longitudinal ligament would be the most likely ligament to be injured. The posterior vertebral body is at highest risk for fractures. Subluxation and herniated disks may also occur with this mechanism of injury. Extreme hyperextension can cause compression injury from the ligamentum flavum, resulting in cord contusion and hypoxia.

HINT

Whiplash is commonly caused by hyperextension mechanism of injury.

Q Axial loading or vertical compression mechanisms result in what type of vertebral fracture?

A Burst fractures

Axial loading refers to force applied vertically through the spine, causing increased pressure and vertebral burst fractures. Bone and disk matter are sent in all directions, including into the spinal canal, causing cord injury. This is commonly seen with diving injuries.

HINT

Burst fractures are considered unstable even with intact ligaments because of the risk of bony pieces impinging on or penetrating the spinal cord.

Q Side impact MVC can result in which type of mechanism of injury to the spinal column?

A Rotational

Rotational injuries occur with a twisting motion of the spine. Lateral flexion of the spine, along with axial rotation, is the mechanism for injury that causes rupture of the posterior longitudinal ligament, dislocation of facets, and vertebral compression fractures.

HINT

The most common cause for rotational injury is side-impact MVC with an unrestrained occupant.

Q What type of trauma is most likely to result in a distraction injury to the cervical spine?

A Hangings

Distraction injuries occur when the spine comes to a sudden stop while weight and momentum of the body continue to pull, causing tearing and laceration of the spinal cord.

HINT

Another trauma that has been associated with distraction mechanism of injury is bungee jumping.

Q Following a gunshot wound, the bullet is found to travel near the spinal cord but did not transverse through the cord. The injury to the spinal cord would be caused by what mechanism?

A Concussion

Concussive forces from the velocity of the bullet can cause injury to tissue without direct contact with the tissue. Penetrating cord injuries are caused by gunshot wounds and stab wounds. Gunshot injuries can penetrate the spinal cord and may be of high or low velocity. Low-velocity injuries may not be associated with bony fractures.

HINT

Avoid MRI if bullet fragments are present within the spinal cord or cord canal because the effects of the magnet may dislodge the bullet.

Q Trauma to the spinal column resulting in burst fractures may cause cord injury by compression. Would this be considered a primary or secondary injury?

A Primary injury

Primary injuries are those that occur as a result of the initial traumatic injury. This includes tissue destruction (lacerations, avulsions), compression (bony fragments, hematomas), and ischemia (damage or impingement of spinal arteries). Spinal cord injuries can occur without radiographic evidence of vertebral fractures or dislocations. Secondary injuries are those injuries to the spinal cord that result in further injury and neurological deficits after the initial trauma (Box 1.12).

Box 1.12 Secondary injuries to the spinal cord

Ischemia/hypoperfusion
Vasogenic edema
Release oxygen free radicals
Acid–base imbalances
Inflammation
Hemorrhage/hematomas
Obstruction CSF flow

CSF, cerebrospinal fluid.

HINT

Level of function may be one or two levels above the level of injury as a result of secondary injuries that worsen neurological function.

TRAUMATIC INJURIES

Q Which of the types of odontoid fractures is considered to be a stable fracture?

A Type I

The odontoid process (also called *the dens*) is the bony structure of C2 that comes up anteriorly into the ring of C1 and allows for rotational movement of the neck. Fractures of the odontoid are classified into types I, II, and III, based on where the fracture occurred on the odontoid bone (Table 1.6). This is also used to describe stability and guides the treatment of the fracture. Type I is considered the most stable of the odontoid fractures. Instability of odontoid fractures is caused by cord compression and penetration of bony fragment or ligament disruption between the odontoid process and the anterior aspect of C1.

Table 1.6 Types of odontoid fractures

Type	Description
Type I	Tip of odontoid bone above transverse ligament
Type II	Base of odontoid between transverse ligament and body of axis
Type III	Bone extends into the vertebral body

HINT

Type II odontoid fractures are the most common and are considered the most unstable of the odontoid fractures.

HINT

A less common odontoid fracture is the vertical fracture through the odontoid and axis body.

Q What is the bilateral fracture of the ring of C2 with or without subluxation called?

A Hangman's fracture

Hangman's fracture (also called *traumatic spondylolisthesis*) is the bilateral fracture through the neural arch of C2. This injury may or may not be associated with anterior subluxation. Even though it is called *Hangman's fracture,* it is less likely to be seen with hangings. It is most commonly associated with falls and MVCs. Hanging typically causes fracture-dislocation of C2 and complete disruption of ligaments between C2 and C3. The burst fracture of the ring of C1 is called *Jefferson's fracture.*

HINT

Hangman's fracture is often associated with other spine pathologies, including osteoarthritis, and may be seen in elderly patients.

Q Which type of cervical injury commonly results in death at the scene of an MVC?

A Atlanto–occipital dislocation

Atlanto dislocation (also called *internal decapitation*) is the avulsion of the atlas (C1) from the occiput and is usually fatal or results in prehospital cardiopulmonary arrest. The severe disruption of ligaments allows the cranium to move out of alignment of the spine. There are cases of patients presenting without neurological injury who commonly complain of the sensation that their "head is falling off."

HINT

Atlanto–occipital dislocation is more common in the pediatric population than in adults.

Q What is the instability between C1 and C2 that results in excessive movement between these two joints called?

A Atlantoaxial instability

Atlas (C1) and axis (C2) instability may result from a cervical trauma and commonly involves injury to the transverse ligament or odontoid process. Injury severity varies from subluxation to dislocation.

HINT

Congenital disorders may increase the risk of atlantoaxial instability as a result of ligament laxity. Down syndrome is an example.

Q A patient presents with a total loss of motor and sensory function below the level of injury. What is this type of injury called?

A Complete cord injury

There is some degree of correlation between the level of function and level of radiographic injury, but this is not always consistent. The neurological level of injury (NLI) is the most caudal spinal cord level at which the normal motor/sensory function persists following spinal cord injury.

HINT

An incomplete cord injury may initially appear functionally as a complete cord injury due to inflammation and edema in the cord.

Q Following a traumatic injury, a football player presents with motor impairment that is greater in the upper extremities than the lower extremities following a traumatic injury. What is this incomplete injury called?

A Central cord syndrome

This spinal cord injury occurs in the central portion of the cord and is characterized by greater involvement of the upper extremity than the lower, especially the hands. The upper extremity axons are located in the central portion of the spinal cord and the axons that control the lower extremity movement are located laterally in the cord. This incomplete cord syndrome is frequently caused by a hyperextension injury or a fall and may or may not be associated with a fracture. There is often a gradual return to function with the lower extremities returning first, followed by the upper, and finger movement returns last with the hand being the most common site of residual motor weakness. Urinary retention and sensory abnormalities vary with the severity of injury.

HINT

Key to recognizing this syndrome is weakness in the upper extremities that is greater than weakness in the lower extremities.

Q What is typically spared in a patient with an anterior cord syndrome following a traumatic injury?

A Vibratory sensation and proprioception

Anterior cord syndrome is characterized by immediate onset of complete motor paralysis and loss of pain and temperature with preservation of the posterior column of sensation (includes vibration sense, position sense, deep pressure, two-point discrimination, and light touch). The anterior horn of the spinal cord contains the lower motor neurons (LMN) and signs of LMN involvement include flaccid paralysis, atrophy of muscles, and areflexia. These are frequently associated with anterior cord syndromes. Commonly caused by the occlusion/compression mechanism of injury (i.e., traumatic herniated or dislocated disk, presence of bone fragments, or EDH) or infarcted spinal cord in the areas supplied by the anterior spinal artery.

HINT

This is the worst prognosis of the incomplete injuries, with only 10% to 20% recovery of motor function.

Q In Brown–Sequard syndrome, there is an ipsilateral loss of what function?

A Motor function

Brown–Sequard syndrome is a hemisection of the spinal cord that results in the ipsilateral loss of motor function and contralateral loss of pain and temperature. It is often seen with penetrating injuries but may also be seen with EDHs and a traumatically herniated cervical disk.

HINT

This syndrome has the best prognosis with a 90% recovery of ambulation, sensation, and bowel/bladder function if the injury was caused by compression.

Q When the lumbosacral spinal nerves roots are damaged at level of L1 to L5, the syndrome is called?

A Cauda equina syndrome

Cauda equina syndrome (CES) is caused by damage to the lumbosacral nerve roots within the spinal canal at the level of L1 to L5. The cauda equina (CE) is a bundle of nerves distal to conus medullaris. *Cauda equina* is Latin for *horse's tail* and the nerve roots are called this because of the resemblance. CES results in areflexic bladder and bowel, and lower extremity paralysis. It is a peripheral nerve injury and so is considered to be an LMN lesion. The syndrome causes variable motor and sensory losses. The prognosis of the recovery of motor function is good.

HINT

A common sensory abnormality is called *saddle anesthesia* in which there is a paresthesia in the perineal region.

ASSESSMENT/DIAGNOSIS

Q A lateral plain radiograph can be used to diagnose what type of injury?

A Bony or vertebral fractures

A lateral x-ray is used to visualize bony abnormalities and fractures. Ligament injuries are not identified on plain radiographs unless the spinal column is out of alignment. Flexion/extension x-rays may be obtained on an awake, cooperative patient without distracting injuries. MRI is the more definitive radiographic study used to identify ligament injuries.

HINT

A patient with normal lateral cervical spine x-rays who complains of pain in the neck region should remain in cervical immobilization until flexion/extension views or MRI is obtained.

Q While obtaining lateral radiographs of the cervical spine, what is most likely to interfere with visualization of the lower cervical vertebrae?

A Shoulders

Visualization from the occiput to T1 is required on lateral cervical x-ray to clear the presence of bony fractures. The shoulders frequently interfere with the ability to visualize C7 and the top of T1 in lateral C-spine radiographs. Obtaining a lateral x-ray in the swimmer's view can assist with identifying C7 and T1 vertebral bodies. Swimmer's view with a lateral x-ray involves downward traction on one arm and upward traction on the other with the x-ray beam aimed through the axilla of the abducted arm.

HINT

The trauma nurse can retract downward on both arms equally to pull the shoulders out of the way to improve visualization of the cervical spine.

Q Which radiographic view is used to determine the height and alignment of vertebral bodies?

A Anterior–posterior (AP)

The AP view allows visualization of the vertebral bodies and determination of the height and alignment of the vertebral bodies.

HINT

AP view with open-mouth techniques is the odontoid view and is used to recognize odontoid fractures.

Q Which radiographic study can distinguish between spinal cord hemorrhage and vasogenic edema?

A MRI

An MRI is the gold standard for radiographic study of the spinal cord. It is able to distinguish between ischemic injury, edema, and hemorrhage within the cord.

HINT

MRI is also considered the gold standard for recognizing spinal ligament injuries.

Q What is the purpose of magnetic resonance angiography (MRA) following a blunt trauma to the cervical region?

A To evaluate vertebral and carotid arteries

A complication of a blunt trauma or flexion/extension injury to the neck may result in vertebral or carotid artery injuries. Arterial dissections are injuries associated with cervical fractures and spinal cord injuries.

HINT

Altered mentation or focal neurological changes may indicate vertebral or carotid dissection and stroke.

Q The presence of sacral sparing following a traumatic spinal cord injury indicates what type of injury?

A Incomplete injury

Anal contraction with stimulation or the ability to feel pinprick or touch around the anus is called *anal sparing* and indicates incomplete injury. This is a phenomenon of sensation in the sacral region even though sensation is absent in the thoracic and lumbar areas. Sacral fibers may be more protected from compression injury thus sparing the sacral dermatomes.

HINT

Assessing for sacral sparing assists in differentiating an incomplete injury from a complete injury.

Q Sensory assessment of cervical regions is tested through how many cervical levels?

A C8

There are seven cervical vertebrae and eight paired cervical nerve roots. Sensory assessment of the cervical region is tested through C8. The cervical region is the only portion of the spinal column that has a greater number of paired nerve roots than vertebrae.

HINT

Sensory assessment is performed using dermatome levels in spinal cord–injured patients, whereas motor assessment is performed using myotome levels.

Q Motor evaluation of the patient assesses which spinal cord tract?

A Corticospinal

The corticospinal tract controls voluntary movement assessed with motor evaluation. The spinothalamic tract controls pain and temperature and is assessed by pinprick, light touch, and temperature. The posterior column of the spinal cord is responsible for proprioception and stereognosis. Proprioception is the ability to know where the body and extremities are in space. Stereognosis is the ability to perceive or recognize an object by sense of touch.

HINT

The first part of the word identifies where the spinal tract originates, and the second part identifies where it terminates.

Q What does the Modified Barthel Index (MBI) tool measure?

A Functional outcomes

The MBI is a functional outcome tool that may be used to assess the deficits associated with spinal cord injuries. The Functional Independence Measure (FIM) is another tool recommended to assess the deficits associated with spinal cord injuries.

HINT

Acute spinal cord assessment may be done with American Spinal Injury Association (ASIA) scores, which utilize a motor index score, sensory index score, and functional outcome score.

MEDICAL/SURGICAL INTERVENTIONS

Q What is the primary prehospital intervention utilized to prevent further injury to the spinal cord?

A Immobilization

The initial goal when caring for a trauma patient at the scene is to limit motion of a potentially injured spine and prevent further neurological involvement. A combination of a rigid cervical collar and supportive blocks on a backboard with straps is commonly used to stabilize the spine in the prehospital setting. The "neutral" position with the chin in midline position without hyperextension is recommended for spine immobilization.

HINT

The use of rigid collars and spinal stabilization can increase ICP, the risk of skin breakdown, and aspiration.

Q What is the primary management of a patient with burst fractures of cervical vertebrae?

A Surgical cord decompression

Burst fractures may require surgical removal of bone to achieve cord decompression. Bony pieces may compress the spinal cord and cause neurological injury. This injury requires surgical management; closed reduction with cervical traction is not recommended on burst fractures.

HINT

Immobilization of the spinal column is important to prevent further injury to the spinal cord from bony pieces.

Q What nonsurgical treatment is used on a patient with cervical subluxation and significant narrowing of the spinal column?

A Cervical traction

Cervical facet dislocation or subluxation can cause cord compression and may require closed reduction with cervical traction. Early closed reduction of traumatic cervical fractures with subluxation or narrowing of the spinal canal improves neurological outcomes. A halo vest may be used to stabilize cervical fractures externally, especially odontoid fractures.

▶ HINT

The inability to reduce a subluxation with external traction and weights may indicate a locked facet joint.

Q What is the primary treatment for neurogenic shock?

A Fluid administration

The complication of a neurogenic shock is systemic vasodilation with hypotension. Fluid resuscitation is the treatment of choice to correct the hypotension. If fluids do not improve the BP and perfusion, vasopressors may be initiated. The goal is to maintain the MAP between 85 and 90 mmHg to increase perfusion and improve neurological outcomes. The bradycardia associated with neurogenic shock does not typically require treatment unless symptomatic, then an external pacemaker may be placed.

▶ HINT

Neurogenic shock is classified as a distributive shock (similar to septic shock).

NURSING INTERVENTIONS

Q What respiratory parameter should be closely monitored in a spontaneously breathing acute spinal cord-injured patient?

A Forced vital capacity (FVC) and/or negative inspiratory force (NIF)

Respiratory parameters to monitor in a patient with a spinal cord injury to determine the ability to ventilate include FVC and NIF. The FVC is the forced maximal breath in followed by the maximal breath out. NIF is the ability to generate enough negative pressure in the chest to allow for inspiration. The FVC and NIF are used to evaluate the respiratory muscles and their ability to generate an adequate breath.

▶ HINT

These parameters are commonly used to evaluate a person's ability to breathe spontaneously and effectively.

Q When should a bowel regimen begin following an acute spinal cord injury?

A On admission

When an acute spinal cord-injured patient is admitted, the bowel regimen should be ordered and initiated. A bowel regimen includes a suppository with finger stimulation timed appropriately for a once-a-day bowel movement. Timing of daily suppository for bowel training should be scheduled in acute care to facilitate rehabilitation and daily routines once the patient is discharged. A spinal cord injury above T12 may have reflex or spastic bowel, whereas a spinal cord injury below the T12 level may cause hyporeflexia with a flaccid bowel.

HINT

The bowel regimen should only be discontinued with severe diarrhea.

Q A patient is able to void spontaneously following an acute spinal cord injury. What should the nurse assess for following the void?

A Postvoid residuals

If a patient with spinal cord injury is able to void spontaneously, use a bladder scan to assess for residual postvoiding. If greater than 200 to 300 mL, straight catheterization is recommended even if spontaneously voiding. Bladder training is the removal of the indwelling bladder catheter and intermittent catheterization used in the presence of urinary retention.

HINT

Bladder training is initiated as soon as the patient is on the maintenance fluids or oral intake.

Q What may be used to prevent postural hypotension in a spinal cord-injured patient when getting out of bed?

A Abdominal binder

Postural hypotension is a common complication following a spinal cord injury. Position changing should be performed slowly to avoid syncope or near-syncope. Applying compression hose or leg wraps and abdominal binders to patients with spinal cord injuries prior to getting them out of bed can help prevent orthostatic hypotension.

HINT

Maintain adequate fluid volume to assist with management of orthostatic hypotension.

Q A patient is readmitted from rehabilitation following a cervical spinal cord injury. The patient suddenly develops hypertension with a BP of 210/120 mmHg. What would be the nurse's priority of care?

A Find the source of stimulation and remove it

Priority of care with a hypertensive spinal cord-injured patient resulting from autonomic hyperreflexia (AH) is to find the source of obnoxious stimulation and remove it. The trauma nurse should elevate the HOB to lower the pressure and assess the patient for the cause of the AH (Table 1.7). Once the source is identified and removed, the patient's hypertension should resolve.

Table 1.7 Sources of autonomic hyperreflexia and nursing interventions

Potential Sources	Nursing Interventions
Urinary retention	Bladder scan and intermittent catheterization
Restrictive clothing	Loosen or remove clothing
Pressure sores	Reposition off of pressure scores
Fecal impaction	Remove fecal impaction

▶ HINT

Antihypertensives should not be the priority or first choice to manage the hypertension associated with AH because once the source is removed, the patient will become hypotensive.

COMPLICATIONS

Q At what level of spinal injury is the diaphragm affected, which, if a complete injury, requires ventilatory support?

A Fourth cervical level

The C4 level innervates the diaphragm. A patient with a cervical injury to the spinal cord at the C4 level or higher loses innervation to the diaphragm and usually requires intubation and mechanical ventilation. Cervical injuries at the six or seventh cervical level (C6 and C7) may still require intubation and ventilation, at least during the acute period, as a result of cord edema.

▶ HINT

Airway and breathing are the priorities of care in cervical spinal injuries.

Q The lack of ability to internally regulate temperature following a spinal cord injury is called what?

A Poikilothermia

Loss of thermoregulatory function occurs in cord injuries above the thoracolumbar outflow because of loss of sympathetic nervous system (SNS) stimulation. Poikilothermia is the lack of internal regulation of the body temperature, which occurs after a spinal cord injury. Spinal cord-injured patients are unable to vasoconstrict and shiver to conserve heat or sweat to dissipate heat.

▶ HINT

Nursing interventions for spinal cord-injured patients include controlling the body temperature through external interventions.

Q What is the loss of motor and reflexes below the level of injury called?

A Spinal shock

Spinal shock is the loss of reflexes and motor function below the level of injury. Spinal shock occurs immediately after the injury and typically resolves within 2 to 16 weeks.

▶ HINT

Two of the reflexes routinely assessed in spinal cord-injured patients include the anocutaneous and bulbocavernosus reflexes.

Q During neurogenic shock, what is the most common dysrhythmia?

A Sinus bradycardia

Neurogenic shock is caused by the interruption of descending sympathetic fibers in the thoracic and cervical cord producing vasodilation below the level of injury and hypotension. At the cervical level, complete injury interrupts sympathetic outflow to the heart, but the parasympathetic outflow remains intact via the vagus nerve, causing bradycardia in neurogenic shock.

▶ HINT

Neurogenic shock is associated with symptoms of hypotension and bradycardia, whereas spinal shock is the loss of motor function and reflexes.

Q What is the cause of the hypertensive crisis that can occur in patients following a spinal cord injury?

A AH

A spinal cord injury with lesions above T6 may exhibit signs of AH. AH occurs with an obnoxious stimulation below the level of injury followed by life-threatening hypertension. Some of the potential obnoxious stimuli that causes AH include bladder distension, catheterization, urinary tract infection, testicular torsion, pressure sores, and fecal impaction.

▶ HINT

AH is not an early complication and only occurs after spinal shock has resolved.

Q What electrolyte abnormality may commonly occur in a paraplegic patient as a result of prolonged non-weight-bearing?

A Hypercalcemia

Non-weight-bearing status for a prolonged period of time allows calcium to move from bone to serum, thus increasing calcium levels. This is a long-term complication and may require administration of calcitonin.

▶ HINT

Hypercalcemia can cause vasoconstriction and hypertension.

Q What is the level of innervation needed for spinal cord-injured patients to be able to feed themselves independently?

A C5 through C7

The fifth cervical level innervates the biceps, allowing for flexion of the elbow, whereas the seventh cervical level innervates the triceps, allowing the elbow to extend. The flexion and extension of the arm allows patients to be able to feed themselves, even if the required utensils need to be strapped to the hands.

HINT

Flexing the wrist and spreading the fingers occurs at the C8 and T1 level of innervation and allows for fine motor control. This allows for greater independent activities of daily living (ADL).

Q What is the level of innervation at which a paraplegic is able to push themself in a wheelchair?

A Level of C6

The level of C6 innervation is considered to be the level at which spinal cord-injured patients are able to perform ADL such as feeding, grooming, dressing, and pushing a wheelchair.

HINT

This is the level of function, not necessarily the actual level of injury.

KNOWLEDGE CHECK: CHAPTER 1

1. A traumatic brain-injured patient with a ventriculostomy is demonstrating an increased intracranial pressure (ICP) reading of 22 mmHg. The priority nursing intervention for the management of this patient should be:

   A. Elevate head of bed (HOB) to 30 to 45 degrees.
   B. Administer D5NS fluids.
   C. Utilize therapeutic hypothermia.
   D. Administer mannitol immediately.

2. A patient was in an automobile collision and struck a tree; the airbag did not deploy; and the driver was not restrained. The patient has a contusion on the forehead from the steering wheel at the site of impact. This injury can best be described as:

   A. Contrecoup injury
   B. Acceleration injury
   C. Subluxation
   D. Coup injury

3. A patient presents with periorbital ecchymosis and drainage from the nares. This patient has a Glasgow Coma Scale (GCS) score of 9. Which of the following would be an appropriate treatment modality for this patient?

   A. Administer prophylactic antibiotics.
   B. Pack nasal passageways.
   C. Place nasal drainage on gauze to assess for a "halo sign" and determine the amount of drainage.
   D. Apply nasal bilevel positive airway pressure (BiPAP) to ensure airway protection.

4. After brain injury, cerebral blood flow (CBF) frequently decreases to an ischemic level. To prevent further neuronal death, CBF of well-oxygenated blood must be restored. Which of the following worsens CBF?

   A. Increasing mean arterial pressure (MAP)
   B. Increasing intracranial pressure (ICP)
   C. Decreasing ICP
   D. Increasing diastolic blood pressure (DBP)

5. A patient's MRI results just revealed an uncal herniation. The nurse will expect the patient to present with:

   A. Ipsilateral pupil dilation and motor weakness
   B. Conscious, lethargic, but oriented
   C. Ipsilateral pupil dilation and contralateral motor weakness
   D. Glasgow Coma Scale (GCS) score of 12

(See answers next page.)

1. A) Elevate head of bed (HOB) to 30 to 45 degrees.

Increasing the HOB angle to 30 to 45 degrees facilitates venous drainage and lowers ICP. Decreasing the HOB does the opposite and increases the ICP by interfering with venous drainage. The fluid order is inappropriate because the goal is euvolemia, and dextrose is not indicated in neurologically impaired patients. Mannitol is frequently used in patients with a sustained increase in ICP greater than 20 mmHg, but the ICP was only 18 mmHg. Mannitol can increase cerebral perfusion, but this is not the first nursing intervention in this situation. Therapeutic hypothermia has not been found to be effective in traumatic brain injury (TBI) patients.

2. D) Coup injury

This is a coup injury because the injury is on the same side of impact, accelerating the brain forward so it hits the opposite side of the skull. A contrecoup injury is when the injury is on the opposite side of impact. An accelerated injury is when a moving object impacts a stationary object; an example of this would be a blow to the head with a baseball bat. A subluxation is the displacement of the bone from the joint (similar to dislocation).

3. C) Place nasal drainage on gauze to assess for a "halo sign" and determine the amount of drainage.

Periorbital ecchymosis indicates presence of basilar skull fracture. Gauze is placed under the nose to absorb drainage and assess for presence of a halo ring around the drainage, indicating a cerebrospinal fluid (CSF) leak. The frequency of changing the gauze can assist with determining the amount of drainage. Nasal packing is inappropriate and contraindicated due to increased risk of central nervous system (CNS) infections. Prophylactic antibiotics are not indicated. Nasal BiPAP should be avoided due to risk of forcing air up into the cranium. BiPAP does not protect an airway.

4. B) Increasing intracranial pressure (ICP)

An increased ICP would worsen CBF due to the increase in resistance to perfusion. CBF can be increased by raising the MAP, or by lowering the ICP. Increasing systolic blood pressure (SBP) and DBP increases MAP, thereby increasing CBF.

5. C) Ipsilateral pupil dilation and contralateral motor weakness

Ipsilateral pupil dilation and contralateral motor weakness occur with uncal herniation. This lateral herniation compresses cranial nerve (CN) III leading to dilation of the pupil on the ipsilateral side (cranial nerve injury results in ipsilateral symptoms). These patients usually have a severely decreased level of consciousness (LOC) and would not be oriented or have a GCS score of 12.

6. Which of the following is a presenting symptom of a midbrain injury following a trauma?

   A. Myoclonic activity
   B. Respiratory insufficiency
   C. Cushing's triad
   D. Pinpoint pupils

7. The patient was involved in a rollover vehicle trauma. CT of the brain is normal, pupils are equal and brisk, but the patient has an altered level of consciousness (LOC) and a low Glasgow Coma Scale (GCS) score. This is characteristic of:

   A. Diffuse axonal injury
   B. Traumatic subdural hematoma
   C. Epidural hematoma
   D. Subarachnoid hemorrhage

8. After a brain injury with an increased intracranial pressure (ICP) and herniation, a central nervous system (CNS) ischemic response can be activated called *Cushing's triad*. Which of the following describes Cushing's triad?

   A. Increased diastolic pressure, widened pulse pressure, bradycardia
   B. Increased systolic pressure, widened pulse pressure, bradycardia
   C. Increased systolic pressure, widened pulse pressure, tachycardia
   D. Increased diastolic pressure, widened pulse pressure, tachycardia

9. A 45-year-old patient with an old spinal cord injury who is paraplegic presents with restlessness, anxiety, and is complaining of a pounding headache with a pain rating of 8/10. Blood pressure (BP) is 170/94 mmHg, heart rate is 60 beats per minute, and respiratory rate is 18 breaths per minute and regular. On assessment, the nurse notes perfuse forehead diaphoresis. Given the findings, the nurse suspects:

   A. Spinal shock
   B. Autonomic hyperreflexia
   C. Neurogenic shock
   D. Distributive shock

10. A 17-year-old wrestler injured his head. He lost consciousness briefly, regained it but was dizzy, and complained of a headache. He was treated in the ED for a concussion, and education was provided to the patient and caregiver regarding no contact-sport activity until cleared as an outpatient by neurology. The young man played football 2 weeks later, was tackled, and didn't get up. The paramedic team initiated resuscitative measures, but when he arrived in the ED, he had no pulse and was not breathing. What injury should the nurse suspect?

    A. Sudden cardiac arrest
    B. Second-impact syndrome
    C. Concussion
    D. Double-impact injury

(*See answers next page.*)

6. D) Pinpoint pupils

Pinpoint pupils frequently are seen in midbrain and pons injuries. Respiratory function is controlled by the medulla, so insufficiency is usually not seen in midbrain injuries. Myoclonic activity is more commonly seen in anoxic brain injury patients. Cushing's triad symptoms are caused by herniation of the brain typically supratentorial.

7. A) Diffuse axonal injury

A diffuse axonal injury is the tearing or shearing of the axons and is a result of the brain rotating in the skull (occurs with rollover vehicles). CT of the brain is usually negative, but the patient has a poor neurological status. CT of the head would reveal blood in the subdural space if symptoms were the result of a traumatic subdural hematoma. An epidural hematoma is a clot between the dura and the skull; the bleed expands rapidly and increases intracranial pressure (ICP), hemiparesis, and ipsilateral pupillary dilation. A patient with subarachnoid hemorrhage would present with severe headache, declining LOC, and motor deficits.

8. B) Increased systolic pressure, widened pulse pressure, bradycardia

Cushing's triad includes an increased systolic pressure, a widened pulse pressure, bradycardia, and respiratory insufficiency. This response is initiated in an attempt to increase cerebral blood flow (increased systolic and widened pulse pressure) and compression of the medulla (bradycardia). It occurs during herniation and is considered a very late sign of increased ICP.

9. B) Autonomic hyperreflexia

The majority of patients with thoracic (T6) injury and above suffer from autonomic hyperreflexia. The symptoms include hypertension, sweating above the level of injury, piloerection, restlessness, anxiety, bradycardia, pounding headache, and a flushed face. In spinal shock, all reflexes, sensation, and movement are lost below the level of injury, and usually there is no change in vital signs. Neurogenic shock is the impairment of sympathetic pathways, therefore, although the patient is bradycardic, a patient in neurogenic shock is usually hypotensive, not hypertensive. Patients in distributive shock lose autonomic sympathetic function and vasodilation occurs, resulting in hypotension.

10. B) Second-impact syndrome

A patient who sustains an initial concussion may develop some cerebral swelling, initial loss of consciousness, memory impairment, disorientation, dizziness, and headache. The brain's autoregulatory mechanisms compensate for the injury and protect against massive swelling but when the patient sustains a "second impact," the brain loses its ability to autoregulate. In severe cases, this may lead to rapid cerebral edema followed by brain herniation. Death has been reported to occur in a matter of minutes. Cardiac arrest did occur but was not the primary injury. The patient did suffer from a traumatic brain injury when he injured his head with the initial concussion, but second-impact syndrome is more descriptive and fits the injury presentation. Double-impact injury is not a recognized injury.

Maxillofacial Trauma

2

MECHANISM OF INJURY

Q What is the mechanism of injury that can result in naso-orbital-ethmoidal (NOE) injury?

A A direct blow to the nasal region

Following injury to the nasal region, the medial orbital wall can be damaged, causing injury to the ethmoid region. The ethmoid bone is paper thin and is connected to the cribriform plate. Fracture of the ethmoid bone may be associated with a cribriform fracture and an orbital roof fracture.

▶ HINT

A loss of smell is commonly associated with an NOE injury as a result of direct injury to cranial nerve (CN) I (olfactory).

Q What is the mechanism of injury for a "blowout" fracture?

A Direct blow to the orbital globe

Orbital blowout fractures occur when a blunt force is applied directly to the orbital globe. A blowout fracture can cause entrapment, most commonly of the inferior or medial rectus muscle. An isolated orbital blowout fracture is the fracture of the orbital walls without associated fractures of the orbital rims.

▶ HINT

Global entrapment following a blowout fracture causes restriction of eye movement.

Q A penetrating trauma to the roof of the mouth can result in injury to which structure?

A The brain

Penetrating trauma to the roof of the mouth can result in the object entering the brain and causing significant brain trauma. The angle of the penetrating object to the oral cavity or the face can determine whether the brain is involved in the trauma. Lacerations to the floor of the mouth can cause damage to the pharynx, tonsil, submaxillary triangle, or hyoid bone.

Q What is a common mechanism of injury of facial trauma in a front-impact motor vehicle collision?

A Airbag deployment

A common mechanism of injury for maxillofacial trauma includes high-velocity impact, including a motor vehicle collision with airbag deployment.

HINT

Airbag deployment on the passenger side with a child passenger can cause cervical cord injury.

Q Violence or assault is most commonly associated with injuries to which region of the face?

A Midface

Violence or assault is most commonly associated with injuries to the nose, maxillary, zygoma, and frontal bones, which are components of the midface.

HINT

Women are more likely to experience facial fractures than men, following a similar impact to the face, due to thin facial bones.

Q What is a severe injury that can be associated with a significant blow to the face?

A Cervical spine injury

Applying blunt force to the face may cause hyperextension of the neck, resulting in a cervical injury. The care provided by prehospital and ED healthcare clinicians should include cervical stabilization until cervical injury has been ruled out.

HINT

A blow to the back of the head can cause the neck to hyperflex, causing cervical injuries and the possibility of the face impacting an object, resulting in facial fractures.

Q What is the most prominent clinical sign of an optic nerve laceration?

A Immediate-onset blindness

Common mechanisms of injury that result in blindness include penetrating trauma to the eye and sudden acceleration or deceleration movement of the head. Other symptoms of eye injuries include diplopia, or blurred vision. Traumatic injuries to the eye can result in delayed or immediate blindness in the involved eye (Table 2.1).

Table 2.1 Trauma-induced blindness

Immediate or Early-Onset Blindness	Delayed or Late-Onset Blindness
Vitreous hemorrhage (posterior portion)	Retinal detachment
Prolapse globe contents	Hemorrhage
Intraocular foreign body	Glaucoma
Optic nerve laceration	Blindness
Occipital lobe hemorrhage	Cortical blindness

HINT

Diplopia can result from orbital fractures with extraocular entrapment from "blowout" fracture.

TRAUMATIC INJURIES

Q What injury asociated with facial trauma is considered life-threatening?

A Airway obstruction

Injuries associated with facial trauma include cervical spinal injuries, airway obstruction, and brain injury. Airway obstruction is a potentially life-threatening associated injury. Facial trauma is not considered a priority of care unless it involves an airway obstruction.

HINT

Injuries that affect the airway and breathing are the most common life-threatening injuries.

Q What is a significant complication that can occur with scalp lacerations?

A Bleeding

Scalp and facial lacerations can result in extensive blood loss as a result of dense vasculature and therefore may become life-threatening from hemorrhage. Facial and scalp lacerations can injure the temporal artery, leading to an arterial hemorrhage.

Q What type of LeFort fracture results in isolated movement of the maxilla?

A LeFort I fracture

The level of facial mobility following a trauma defines the type of LeFort fracture present. Isolated maxilla movement is a LeFort I fracture and is commonly called a *free floating maxilla*. LeFort I fracture is caused by a horizontal fracture through the maxillary body, causing a detachment of the entire maxilla at the level of the nasal floor. This fracture results from a horizontal or downward force applied to the anterior face.

HINT

To assess for a LeFort I fracture, the maxilla is held with the thumb and forefinger, and a gentle attempt is made to move the maxilla gently as not to cause further separation and injury.

Q What injury is classified as a LeFort II fracture?

A Separation of the midface

A LeFort II fracture is a separation of the midface in a pyramidal shape. The fracture pattern is a result of a horizontal impact to the upper midface. A LeFort II fracture is a LeFort I fracture plus an extension of the fracture through the orbital rim, medial orbital wall, ethmoid sinuses, and nose. It is associated with a sinus roof or cribriform fracture and cerebrospinal fluid (CSF) leak.

▶ HINT

A LeFort II fracture line is similar to the shape and size of an oxygen face mask.

Q What injury is classified as a LeFort III fracture?

A Total craniofacial separation

A LeFort III fracture is a total craniofacial separation. This is commonly called a *craniofacial disjuncture.* The impact of a LeFort III fracture is a downward oblique impact that separates the facial skeleton from the skull base. The floor, roof, and lateral and medial walls of the orbit can be injured in a LeFort III fracture.

▶ HINT

Gently rocking the maxilla produces movement of the entire midface, independent of the skull.

Q What is a severe eye injury that can occur following a sudden acceleration/deceleration of the head?

A Optic nerve avulsion

A sudden deceleration/acceleration force to the head or eye region can result in the avulsion or laceration of the optic nerve. The symptoms include a sudden-onset blindness immediately following the injury. An example of a deceleration injury is a motor vehicle collision in which the victim's moving head impacts the windshield.

▶ HINT

Traumatic brain injuries to the occipital region can result in visual losses, typically in the same visual fields bilaterally, but do not cause a total unilateral blindness.

Q What is the term for an accumulation of blood in the anterior chamber of the eye?

A Hyphema

A hyphema is an accumulation of blood that disperses in layers within the anterior chamber of the eye. The amount of visual impairment is related to the amount of occlusion from the hemorrhage. A severe or complete loss of vision is caused by obscuring the entire anterior chamber of the eye with blood. Associated symptoms may include a deep aching eye pain and increased intraocular pressures.

▶ HINT

The mechanism of injury for hyphema is a direct blow to the globe of the eye.

Q What type of eye injury causes a decrease in intraocular pressure following a facial trauma?

A Perforated globe

Traumatic injury to the eye can cause globe rupture, which results in a lowering of intraocular pressure. A normal intraocular pressure is about 15 mmHg. A low pressure is less than 10 mmHg and indicates a globe rupture. A high intraocular pressure may be caused by retrobulbar hemorrhage.

HINT

A direct blow to the globe can result in a hyphema, or accumulation of blood within the anterior chamber of the globe.

ASSESSMENT/DIAGNOSIS

Q A facial fracture that results in loss of sensation may involve damage to which CN?
A CN V (trigeminal)

CN assessment following facial trauma is important when assessing for complications (Table 2.2). CN V (trigeminal) is responsible for sensation across the forehead, cheek, and jaw. An injury to the peripheral portion of the CN can cause loss of sensation.

Table 2.2 Commonly injured cranial nerves

Cranial Nerves	Assessment
CN II	Visual acuity
CN III, IV, VI	Extraocular eye movement
CN V	Sensory; determined by light touch or pinprick to forehead, cheek, and jaw
CN VII	Symmetry of facial expressions

CN, cranial nerve.

HINT

CN assessment is important following facial trauma. CNs II to VII are the most commonly injured following a facial trauma.

Q What is the trauma nurse looking for while palpating the face and skull during the assessment?
A Bony depression

Assessment following trauma involving the head and neck looks for underlying skull deformities or depression under the area of the scalp, or facial laceration that would indicate bony fractures. Laceration of the scalp may be explored with a finger or blunt instrument to determine the depth of the laceration.

HINT

Displacement of the inner table (thinner wall) of the frontal sinus can result in dural involvement.

Q A trauma patient presenting with epistaxis and nasal discoloration is most likely to have sustained what type of injury?

A Nasal fracture

Edema, epistaxis, deformity, nasal obstruction, pain, and discoloration are signs of a nasal fracture. The recognition of a nasal fracture leads the trauma nurse to assess for complications of nasal fractures, including obstruction of nasal passages with clots.

▶ HINT

Following facial trauma, overt nasal deformity may not be immediately noticeable because of facial edema.

Q When looking at the patient's profile, the nose appears to have an abnormal "pug" appearance. What is the most likely injury?

A NOE injury

Injury of the NOE region results in the patient's profile having the appearance of a depression or a "pug" nose. The frontal view of injury to the NOE region appears to be widened and flattened, creating the illusion of the eyes being farther apart (called *telecanthus*).

▶ HINT

Telecanthus is a result of the disruption of the medial canthal ligaments.

Q What is the primary finding of a blowout orbital fracture with entrapment?

A Restricted eye movement

Following an orbital blowout fracture, the bony pieces impinge on the extraocular muscles, causing restricted eye movement. This is frequently called *entrapment*. Following orbital trauma, the trauma nurse should evaluate vision, eye movement, pupil size and reaction, lid appearance, cornea, and conjunctiva.

▶ HINT

Orbital blowout fractures may have the presence of enophthalmos (globe recedes posteriorly).

Q A patient with pain on opening the mouth with limited jaw movement may have what type of facial injury?

A Mandibular fracture

Mandibular fractures result in a limited ability to open the mouth and produce significant pain on opening the mouth or clenching the jaws. A malocclusion or deviation of the jaw indicates either mandibular or maxillary injury. Another sign of mandibular or mental nerve injury is numbness over a portion of the mandibular body. During the assessment of a mandibular fracture, the temporomandibular joint is palpated bilaterally as the patient opens and closes the mouth.

HINT

In mandibular fractures, airway obstruction can occur because the tongue is secured to the muscle attached to the mandible and a fracture can cause loss of tongue control.

Q What should the trauma nurse assess on a patient with lower facial trauma?

A Inside of the mouth

Following lower facial trauma, the inside of the mouth should be assessed for breaks in the skin, ecchymosis, clots, exposed bone, or bone fragments. Severe injuries of the mandible are characterized by fragmentation of bone and teeth, and disruption of adjacent soft tissue. Hematomas present in the mouth, soft-tissue injuries in the oral cavity, or blood accumulating in the hypopharynx can cause upper airway obstruction.

HINT

As a result of facial injuries, large amounts of blood can be swallowed, so signs of bleeding may not be apparent until the patient vomits blood.

Q Following a traumatic injury to the face, the patient presents with stridor. What would be the trauma nurse's concern about the patient?

A Partial airway obstruction

Stridor, drooling, and cyanosis are some potential signs of partial airway obstruction. Following a traumatic injury to the face, airway obstruction may be caused by swelling, hematoma, bleeding, or laryngeal obstruction. Injury to the vagus or hypoglossal nerve with facial trauma can cause vocal cord or hemi-tongue paralysis, contributing to airway obstruction.

HINT

Blood or vomit aspiration following facial trauma can cause laryngospasm contributing to upper airway obstruction.

Q In the ICU, the trauma patient develops a "beach ball" appearance of the face. What is the most likely LeFort classification of the facial fracture?

A LeFort III

A LeFort III fracture involves a total craniofacial separation and commonly develops massive swelling, which results in a "beach ball" face. Upper airway obstruction can occur, and intubation may be required early, or an emergency cricothyroidotomy may be necessary if a complicated obstruction occurs.

Q When the patient's nose and chin are against the x-ray plate, what is the radiographic view called?

A Water's view

A Water's view x-ray is taken with the nose and chin against the x-ray plate. It is used to identify injuries to maxillofacial bones; maxillary sinus; nasal bones; frontal processes of the maxilla, zygoma, and zygomatic arch; and coronoid process of the mandible, orbit, ethmoid, and frontal sinuses. Caldwell's view involves placing the forehead and nose against the x-ray plate; it provides a different angle used to evaluate structures similar to those seen in Water's view. A lateral facial x-ray is used to identify nasal bones; frontal sinus; and multiple, small maxillofacial floors.

HINT

CT scans commonly have replaced plain films and are considered the gold standard to evaluate facial trauma.

Q What is used to identify the presence of corneal abrasions?

A Fluorescein staining

Identification of surface eye injuries, such as corneal abrasion, is determined with fluorescein staining and examination with Wood's light or a slit lamp. The area of abrasion will appear as green under fluorescent illumination (Box 2.1).

Box 2.1 Signs of serious eye injury

- Sudden decrease in vision or blurred vision
- Photophobia
- Diplopia
- Abnormal papillary reaction
- Proptosis
- Eye pain
- Eye redness or ecchymosis
- Hyphema

HINT

Fluorescein strips are recommended for staining to prevent contamination and eye infections associated with drops.

HINT

Diplopia can be unilateral or bilateral depending on the mechanism of injury.

MEDICAL/SURGICAL INTERVENTIONS

Q What is the initial management of intraoral arterial bleeding from penetrating trauma?

A Secure airway and pack the throat

In penetrating injuries, bleeding in the intraoral or pharyngeal tissue may be caused by injury to the carotid artery, internal jugular vein, and/or their branches. With intraoral injuries, secure the airway and pack the throat to control pharyngeal bleeding. Continued blood loss may require an emergent angiography. Deep tongue lacerations may cause injury to the lingual artery and require suturing of the arterial laceration.

HINT

Blood from the oral cavity can be aspirated or swallowed.

Q What is the preferred method for obtaining an airway in a trauma patient with significant injuries?

A Endotracheal intubation

Mask ventilation of a facial trauma may be difficult and advanced airways may be indicated. Securing an airway following facial trauma is best performed with endotracheal intubation, if possible.

HINT

In patients with maxillofacial trauma and airway obstruction, emergency cricothyroidotomy can be performed to temporarily obtain an airway.

Q Following an ocular injury, what is used to reduce eye movement to facilitate healing?

A Eye patch

An eye patch or shield is used to reduce movement of the affected eye. An eye patch is used with retinal injuries to allow healing. Eye patches and shields may also be used to protect the affected eye from light if photophobic. Any impaled objects in the eye should be stabilized and the unaffected eye patched.

HINT

A suspected or open-globe injury should not be covered with a patch because of the resulting pressure on the globe.

NURSING INTERVENTIONS

Q A patient presents to the emergency room bleeding profusely from a scalp laceration. What would be an appropriate nursing intervention to control the blood loss?

A Maintain direct pressure

To limit blood loss, trauma nurses can attempt to control blood loss from facial or scalp wounds with direct pressure or pressure dressings.

HINT

A stapler or stitches may be required on the scalp or facial laceration for quick control of blood loss until formal repair may be done.

Q What is the cosmetic risk of inadequate cleansing of facial wounds?

A Scarring

Cleansing of the debris from facial abrasions is important to prevent the embedding of the debris, called *tattooing*. Contamination of foreign debris can cause deep tissue infections, which destroy the tissue and affect the tissue's ability to reconstruct. When cleaning, only debride dead tissue because compromised tissue may still survive in this highly vascular area. Large foreign bodies imbedded in the scalp and face need to be removed to prevent cellulitis and abscesses.

▶ HINT

Do not shave eyebrows. They can serve as landmarks for approximation of wound edges in the upper face and may not grow back.

Q What is an appropriate nursing intervention to control epistaxis following a nasal fracture?

A Direct pinch pressure

The trauma nurse can attempt to control epistaxis with direct pinch pressure on the nose for about 10 to 30 minutes without release, which is usually sufficient. If this fails to control the bleeding, nasal packing can be used. Posterior epistaxis requires posterior packing or balloon tamponade. Nonsurgical management of nasal fracture may include butterfly stitches placed across the dorsum of the nose or a moldable thermoplast nasal splint applied within 1 week.

▶ HINT

The trauma nurse assessing the function of the nose can occlude one side and have the patient sniff through the other nostril. Compare both sides for the ability to pass air.

Q Which complication of facial injuries would require immediate surgical intervention?

A Airway obstruction

Airway obstruction is a life-threatening complication of facial fractures and requires a surgical airway to be secured.

Q What is the primary intervention for managing ocular chemical injuries?

A Irrigation

Copious, continuous irrigation with a crystalloid solution, such as normal saline, should begin immediately following exposure to chemical solutions to the eye.

▶ HINT

Neutralization with causative agents is not recommended with ocular chemical injuries.

Q What is the recommended position to place the patient in following an ocular injury resulting in an increase intraocular pressure?

A Elevate the head of bed (HOB)

A patient with elevated intraocular pressure should be placed with the HOB elevated to assist in lowering the pressure. If unable to elevate the HOB, place the patient in a reverse Trendelenburg position.

▶ HINT

Instruct the patient to avoid the Valsalva maneuver, coughing, or bending forward following ocular trauma and increased intraocular pressures.

Q When would it be contraindicated to instill eye drops following an ocular trauma?

A With global rupture

Instillation of eye drops may be used to manage pain, infection, or inflammation but is contraindicated in open globe injuries. Corneal injuries are managed with normal saline drops or artificial tears to keep the cornea moist and prevent further injury.

▶ HINT

The eye may be covered with a sterile, moist saline eye patch to prevent corneal drying and injury.

COMPLICATIONS

Q A patient with facial fractures presents to the emergency room with nasal drainage. What is the potential complication in this patient?

A CSF leak

Facial fractures can result in basal skull fractures and dural tears, causing a CSF leak. Signs of dural involvement in facial fractures include pneumocephalus and CSF. CSF may leak from the nose, ears, or from the facial lacerations.

▶ HINT

Pneumocephalus is diagnosed with a noncontrast CT scan and is demonstrated by air in the cranium (not just in the sinuses).

Q What is the most commonly associated injury with a LeFort I fracture?

A Loose or broken teeth

Loose or broken teeth are complications of maxillary fractures. Following a LeFort I fracture, the upper jaw and mouth are inspected for loose, broken, or missing teeth; open sockets; palate defects; and broken or missing dentures.

▶ HINT

A sign of a LeFort I fracture includes malocclusion of teeth.

Q What is a long-term complication of a LeFort II fracture?

A Loss of smell

Damage to the olfactory nerve may cause temporary and permanent loss of smell.

HINT

One of the signs of loss of smell is the inability to taste food.

Q What is a potential complication of an injury damaging the medial canthus of the eyes?

A Disruption of the lacrimal duct

Injury near the medial canthus raises the suspicion of a potential lacrimal duct injury. Disruption of the lacrimal duct leads to epiphora or tear overflow, which is a result of outflow obstruction. Repair of lacrimal duct injury includes cannulation of the lacrimal duct with a silastic tube that remains in place for 3 to 6 months. This is called *dacryocystorhinostomy*.

HINT

Excessive tearing and the appearance of a "pug" nose indicate injury to the medial canthus and lacrimal ducts.

Q A laceration across the cheek presents with clear fluid drainage. What is the most likely injury or complication of the laceration?

A Parotid duct injury

Parotid duct (also called *Stenson's duct*) injuries may occur with wounds to the cheek or submental region. A cheek laceration can cause injury to the parotid ducts, resulting in clear fluid draining from the laceration. Treatment of a parotid duct injury is to temporarily cannulate with a silastic tube or repair with primary reanastomosis, ductal ligation, or placement of an interposition graft. Disruption of a parotid duct without repair may result in a parotid fistula or sialocele (salivary cutaneous fistula; Table 2.3).

Table 2.3 Complications of traumatic facial injury

Traumatic Injury	Complications
Nasal fracture	Epistaxis, occluded nasal passages, hematoma nasal septum, CSF leak, abscesses
Zygomatic fracture	Malunion, enophthalmos, diplopia
Mandibular fracture	Airway obstruction, fragmentation of bone and teeth
Oral cavity injury	Airway obstruction, traumatic brain injury, abscess, hematoma, CN dysfunctions

CN, cranial nerve; CSF, cerebrospinal fluid.

HINT

CN VII (facial nerve) travels through the parotid gland and can be injured in lacerations and penetrating injuries.

Q Which causes greater damage to the eye, an alkali or an acid chemical burn?

A Alkali

Chemical injuries to the eye can be caused by either exposure to an alkali or acid substance. An alkali substance disrupts the cell membrane causing rapid penetration of the substance and extensive, severe tissue injury. Acidic substances do not penetrate the tissue and cause less injury and tissue damage but can still cause corneal damage.

HINT

Signs of chemical injury to the eye include corneal opacification, pain, and eyelid swelling.

Q Following a corneal abrasion, the patient returns to the ED with the complaint of an increasing gray spot in the affected eye. What is the most likely complication?

A Corneal infection

A corneal infection is a potential complication following a corneal abrasion or injury. Corneal abrasions are frequently treated with antibiotics to lower the risk of infection. Symptoms of a corneal infection are increased pain in the affected eye and an enlargement of the gray area on the cornea. Infection can cause a permanent decrease in visual acuity, and incomplete healing can result in recurring attacks of eye pain, tearing, and photophobia.

HINT

If a foreign body is left and not removed, it becomes a nidus of infection.

KNOWLEDGE CHECK: CHAPTER 2

1. On receiving a trauma patient with facial trauma, the airway should be closely inspected and assessed by checking for which of the following:

   A. Alignment of mandible
   B. Blood clot in nasal passageway
   C. Restricted eye movement
   D. Presence of blood or secretions in oral cavity

2. A patient comes into the emergency room with a facial laceration from a piece of glass. The laceration is deep and clear fluid is leaking out of the site. What is the most likely type of injury sustained?

   A. Posterior table fracture with dural injury
   B. Pneumocephalus
   C. Maxillary fracture
   D. Zygomatic fracture

3. Which of the following is the most appropriate antiseptic when cleansing a deep facial laceration?

   A. Normal saline
   B. Antibiotic solution
   C. Hydrogen peroxide
   D. Lidocaine

4. A patient comes in with a nasal injury. Edema is clearly noted, and the patient is experiencing significant epistaxis. The nurse has been applying direct pressure by pinching the nose for the past 25 minutes without control of bleeding. Which of the following interventions is considered the next recommended intervention in this situation?

   A. Cauterization
   B. Balloon tamponade
   C. Packing nasal passageway with gauze
   D. Surgical reduction of the nose

5. In this particular facial fracture, airway assessment is vital because the tongue can lose control and occlude the airway. What type of fracture is this?

   A. Mandibular fracture
   B. Zygomatic fracture
   C. Oral cavity injury
   D. Naso-orbital-ethmoidal (NOE) injury

(See answers next page.)

1. D) Presence of blood or secretions in oral cavity
Vocalization; the presence of secretions, blood, vomit; and noting loose teeth, foreign objects, edema, or tongue obstruction are all part of assessing for a clear airway. Alignment of the mandible is used to determine presence of mandible fracture. Blood clots in the nasal passageway are not as significant as in the oral cavity when assessing airway. Restricted eye movement is a sign of globe entrapment but is not a sign of airway loss.

2. A) Posterior table fracture with dural injury
Clear fluid from the laceration site indicates a posterior table fracture with a dural injury. The dural injury results in cerebrospinal fluid (CSF) leaks. Pneumocephalus is the presence of air or gas within the cranial cavity and is not associated with leaking fluid. It is usually associated with disruption of the skull such as a depressed skull fracture. Maxillary and zygomatic fractures alone do not cause a CSF leak.

3. B) Antibiotic solution
Irrigation of wounds with antibiotic solution is recommended. Irrigation with normal saline to wash out wounds is also recommended but normal saline is not an antiseptic. Hydrogen peroxide would not be an appropriate medication to use when cleansing a deep facial laceration because of potential damage to healthy tissue. The use of hydrogen peroxide is also contraindicated in wounds with possible sinus involvement. Lidocaine is utilized as a local anesthetic for suturing facial lacerations.

4. B) Balloon tamponade
Control epistaxis with direct pinch pressure for up to 30 minutes; if that is ineffective, balloon tamponade may be utilized. Posterior epistaxis requires posterior packing or balloon tamponade. If this fails, nasal packing can be used with ribbon gauze impregnated with petroleum jelly or cauterization may be needed. Surgical reduction is not recommended as early management of nasal fractures.

5. A) Mandibular fracture
Airway obstruction can occur in mandibular fractures because the tongue is secured to muscle attached to the mandible, and a fracture with damage to those securing muscles results in a loss of tongue control. The tongue can fall backward and obstruct the airway. Ensuring patency of the airway is the primary goal of treatment in mandibular fractures. Zygomatic fractures may involve the mandible, but the tongue is not usually involved. Oral cavity injuries can cause airway issues involving the tongue when there are lacerations to the tongue; this is not as common as mandibular fractures. Naso-orbital-ethmoid (NOE) injuries have more sinus involvement and are not associated with tongue injuries.

6. A patient attempted suicide by shooting themself in the mouth with a pistol. Bullet wounds penetrating the pharyngeal area carry a risk of damaging the carotid artery. What is the appropriate order of events to take care of this patient?

   A. Pack the throat to control bleeding, intubate the patient, and send for angiography.
   B. Send for angiography, intubate the patient, and pack the throat to control bleeding.
   C. Intubate the patient, pack the throat to control bleeding, and send for angiography.
   D. Intubate the patient, send for angiography, and pack the throat to control bleeding.

7. A 16-year-old patient got hit in the mouth with a softball. The patient is experiencing epistaxis, swelling, and missing teeth. How would the nurse assess the patient for a possible LeFort type I fracture?

   A. Rock the maxilla back and forth and watch for movement of the midface.
   B. Face separation from the cranium is noted on rocking the maxilla.
   C. Rock the maxilla to assess whether the maxilla is independent from the remainder of the face.
   D. Place two fingers in the lower jaw and assess whether it moves freely.

8. LeFort II fracture is a LeFort I fracture with the addition of which of the following facial fractures?

   A. Mandible
   B. Zygomaticomaxillary complex
   C. Ethmoid sinus
   D. Lateral orbital wall

9. Which of the following is more commonly associated with a LeFort III fracture than a LeFort II fracture?

   A. Loss of consciousness
   B. Cerebrospinal fluid (CSF) leaks
   C. Risk of airway obstruction
   D. Orbital fractures

10. A patient was injured in a collision with another person while playing football. The patient presents with drooling, lethargy, and is noted to have stridor. The patient's face appears elongated. Which of the following is the priority for this patient's obvious facial trauma?

   A. Obtaining a CT scan for a suspected brain injury
   B. Obtaining an airway
   C. Assessing for a cerebrospinal fluid (CSF) leak
   D. Assessing for a subconjunctival hemorrhage

(See answers next page.)

6. C) Intubate the patient, pack the throat to control bleeding, and send for angiography.

The patient's airway is always the first thing that should be considered, therefore securing the airway with intubation is the first intervention. Then, controlling the pharyngeal bleeding by packing the throat to limit blood loss should be the second intervention. The third step is to transport the patient to interventional radiology because the patient may require an emergency angiography to determine the extent and location of the injury and to guide interventions.

7. C) Rock the maxilla to assess whether the maxilla is independent from the remainder of the face.

Assessment for a LeFort type I fracture is performed by gently holding the maxilla with the thumb and forefinger, and carefully attempting to rock the maxilla forward and back. If the maxilla moves independently of the face, then a LeFort type I fracture is present. If there is separation of the midface in a pyramid shape (appearing like an oxygen face mask), then it is a LeFort II fracture. A LeFort III fracture appears as a complete separation of the face from the cranium. This is also called *craniofacial dysfunction*. Placing two fingers in the lower jaw to assess for movement is not a correct technique to assess for LeFort I fractures.

8. C) Ethmoid sinus

A LeFort II fracture is a LeFort I fracture with an extension through the orbital rim, medial orbital wall (not lateral orbital wall), ethmoid sinus, and the nasal bone. The term *zygomaticomaxillary complex* refers to fractures of the frontal, maxillary, temporal, and sphenoid bones, and is not a part of the LeFort II fracture. LeFort II fractures do not include mandible fractures.

9. A) Loss of consciousness

Lefort II and III fractures are at risk for a CSF leak and upper airway obstruction. They both involve some degree of orbital fractures. These patients are more likely to get intubated or have a cricothyroidotomy. A LeFort III patient has a higher associated loss of consciousness with brain injury and increased blood loss, leading to hypovolemia and altered cerebral perfusion.

10. B) Obtaining an airway

All of these are appropriate assessments and interventions, but securing an airway takes priority over a diagnostic study. The patient is drooling, lethargic, and has stridor, there clearly is an upper airway problem. Assessing for a CSF leak is important because it places the patient at high risk for central nervous system (CNS) infection but is not more important than securing the airway. Assessing for a subconjunctival hemorrhage should be done in suspected facial fractures, but again, it's not as important as checking the airway.

Neck Trauma

3

MECHANISM OF INJURY

Q What portion of the neck is the most exposed to a traumatic injury?

A Anterior neck

The neck is well protected posteriorly with the spine and inferiorly with the chest. The most common areas of neck injuries are the anterior and lateral regions. The larynx and trachea are situated anteriorly and are the most exposed to injury.

HINT

The neck is divided into three zones or regions that are used to assist with the assessment of neck injuries (Table 3.1).

Table 3.1 Zones of the neck

Zone 1	Base of the neck, divided by the thoracic inlet inferiorly and cricoid cartilage superiorly
Zone 2	Midportion of neck and region from cricoid cartilage to the angle of the mandible
Zone 3	Superior aspect of neck, bounded by the angle of the mandible and the base of the skull

Q What is it called when a person experiences neck pain without significant injury following sudden flexion–extension of the neck?

A Whiplash

Whiplash occurs when there is a sudden flexion followed by extension of the neck. This commonly occurs with the mechanism of front-end collision and results in neck pain. The pain originates from the stretching of the ligaments and muscles in the neck region.

HINT

Bony involvement or more significant injuries have been ruled out before the diagnosis of whiplash.

TRAUMATIC INJURIES

Q Which is the most anterior structure in the neck that is commonly injured in neck trauma?

A Trachea

The trachea and larynx are located anteriorly, and thus are more commonly involved in injury. The neck is a condensed area with multiple structures that may be involved in the injury. Trauma to the neck can cause airway (trachea), gastrointestinal (esophagus), neurological (spinal cord, phrenic nerve, brachial plexus, and cranial nerves), vascular (carotid artery and jugular vein), glandular (thyroid and parotid), and musculoskeletal injuries.

HINT

Understanding the location of each structure can assist the trauma nurse in identifying the injuries.

Q Which of the zones of injury in the neck region present with the most obvious injuries?

A Zone 2

Zone 2 is the region in which the injuries are more likely to be apparent and less likely to present with occult injuries. The structures in zone 2 are more likely to be symptomatic on admission than the other two zones in the neck region (Table 3.2).

Table 3.2 Structures at risk based on location of injury

Zone 1	Great vessels Trachea Esophagus Lung apices Cervical spine Spinal cord Cervical nerve roots
Zone 2	Carotid and vertebral arteries Jugular veins Pharynx Larynx Trachea Esophagus Cervical spine Spinal cord
Zone 3	Salivary gland Parotid gland Esophagus Trachea Vertebral bodies Carotid arteries Jugular vein Cranial nerves

HINT

Most carotid injuries are associated with zone 2 injuries.

Q Which of the zones of the neck have the highest morbidity and mortality with injury?

A Zone 1

Zone 1 injuries are associated with the highest morbidity and mortality and, in general, have the poorest outcomes. Blunt trauma to the neck region causing a vascular injury is also associated with high morbidity and mortality.

▶ HINT

Penetrating injuries most commonly affect zone 2 because of accessibility.

ASSESSMENT/DIAGNOSIS (TABLE 3.3)

Table 3.3 Signs and symptoms of neck injuries

Laryngeal and tracheal injury	Hoarseness Hemoptysis Stridor Drooling Dyspnea
Esophageal and pharyngeal injury	Dysphagia Bloody saliva Bloody nasogastric aspirate
Carotid injury	Decreased level of consciousness Hemiparesis Deviated gaze Facial droop Thrill or bruit
Jugular vein injury	Hematoma Hypotension
Cranial nerve injury	Facial (CN VII) drooping Glossopharyngeal (CN IX) dysphagia Vagus nerve (CN X) hoarseness Spinal accessory nerve (CN XI) weak shoulder shrug Hypoglossal nerve (CN XII) deviation of tongue

CN, cranial nerve.

Q A patient develops hoarseness and hemoptysis following a blunt neck trauma. What is the most likely injury?

A Laryngeal or tracheal injury

The signs of neck injury are dependent on the region involved in the trauma. Laryngeal and tracheal injuries can present as hoarseness and hemoptysis.

▶ HINT

A penetrating injury to the trachea commonly results in a hissing or sucking sound, with froth or bubbling at the site of injury.

Q What is the recommended diagnostic study for neck injuries?

A CT scan

When bone or soft-tissue injuries are suspected, CT scans are useful in diagnosing the injuries. Clinically subtle signs of larynx injuries are best recognized with a CT scan. CT angiograms (CTA) can detect vascular injuries in the neck region quickly, although a conventional angiogram produces the most definitive result. Conventional angiograms are used preoperatively to determine surgical needs, including whether the injury is intrathoracic.

▶ HINT

CTA in hemodynamically stable patients significantly decreases the rate of negative exploration without an increase in missed injuries.

MEDICAL/SURGICAL INTERVENTIONS

Q What is the priority of care in a neck injury?

A Airway

Airway and hemorrhage are the two most immediate risks following a neck injury. Obtaining an airway is a priority of care for a patient who has sustained a neck injury. Direct injury to the trachea, either penetrating or blunt, can cause a loss of airway. Swelling in the neck region can compress the trachea, also resulting in the loss of airway. In rare cases, emergency cricothyroidotomy may be required to immediately secure an airway. Excessive vigorous attempts at intubation may worsen the patient's status by causing further injury. Awareness of potential laryngeal injury is important before intubation, even when securing an airway in an emergency.

▶ HINT

Patients with rapidly developing hematomas in the neck should have the airway secured.

Q Persistence in difficulty breathing despite intubation and ventilation may indicate what type of injury?

A Pneumothorax

Signs of respiratory distress even after intubation and ventilation suggest the presence of a pneumothorax. Tracheal injury can result in a pneumothorax or tension pneumothorax. The management includes needle decompression and chest tube placement.

▶ HINT

If there is a persistent pneumothorax, suspect a tracheal injury.

Q Which zone of injury in the neck region might require an emergency sternotomy for repair?

A Zone 1

Injuries located in zone 1 of the neck may require a median sternotomy for repair of intrathoracic injuries. This incision may extend to the sternocleidomastoid or subclavicular regions as well. Endovascular interventions with stent placements have been used in some vascular injuries within this zone.

▶ **HINT**

Subluxation or dislocation of the mandible may be required in zone 3 injuries to repair the injury.

NURSING INTERVENTIONS

Q What is the best way to control hemorrhage in the neck region?

A Direct pressure

Bleeding from the neck is best controlled by direct pressure. Impaled objects should be left in place until surgical repair is available. It is not recommended to blindly clamp a transected vessel because of the potential damage that can occur to surrounding structures. When the injury is to the pharynx, direct pressure may not adequately control the hemorrhage and may require cricothyroidotomy and packing.

▶ **HINT**

Intravenous (IV) access should be avoided in the affected side because of the potential disruption of ipsilateral venous circulation.

COMPLICATIONS (BOX 3.1)

Box 3.1 Complications

Hemorrhage/hypovolemic shock
Expanding hematoma
Airway obstruction
Open trachea
Paralysis
Hemoptysis
Hematemesis and aspiration
Air embolus
Arteriovenous fistula
Tracheoinnominate fistula
Esophagocutaneous fistula
Pneumothorax or tension pneumothorax
Infections or sepsis

Q What is the potential risk if a neck wound is probed or locally explored outside of the operating room?

A Hemorrhage

It is not recommended to locally explore or probe a traumatic wound to the neck in the ED or outside of the operating room. This can result in dislodgement of clots, hemorrhage, and air embolus.

▶ HINT

Placing a patient in mild Trendelenburg position may decrease the risk of air embolization with an open wound to the neck.

▶ HINT

Oral secretions are a major source of infection in neck wounds.

KNOWLEDGE CHECK: CHAPTER 3

1. Which of the following zones of the neck presents with the most obvious injuries?

   A. Zone 1
   B. Zone 2
   C. Zone 3
   D. Zone 4

2. Which of the zones of the neck is associated with the greatest morbidity and mortality?

   A. Zone 1
   B. Zone 2
   C. Zone 3
   D. Zone 4

3. Which of the following is a sign of a penetrating injury to the trachea?

   A. Bubbling from the site
   B. Hemiparesis
   C. Facial droop
   D. Dysphagia

4. Which of the following is the priority of care in a patient with a neck injury?

   A. Placement of a feeding tube
   B. Airway protection
   C. Video swallow evaluation
   D. Obtain brain CT scan

5. Which of the following would be the recommended positioning of a patient following a neck injury to decrease risk of air embolization?

   A. Prone
   B. Reverse Trendelenburg
   C. Supine
   D. Trendelenburg

(*See answers next page.*)

1. B) Zone 2

Zone 2 is the region in which the injuries are more likely to be apparent and less likely to present with occult injuries. The structures in zone 2 are more likely to be symptomatic on admission than the other two zones in the neck region. Zone 4 does not exist.

2. A) Zone 1

Zone 1 injuries are associated with the highest morbidity and mortality and, in general, have the poorest outcomes. Blunt trauma to the neck region causing a vascular injury is also associated with high morbidity and mortality.

3. A) Bubbling from the site

A penetrating injury to the trachea commonly results in a hissing or sucking sound, with froth or bubbling at the site of injury. Hemiparesis and facial droop can be a result of carotid injury with a penetrating neck injury. Dysphagia may be present with esophageal injuries.

4. B) Airway protection

Airway and hemorrhage are the two most immediate risks following a neck injury. Obtaining an airway is a priority of care for a patient who has sustained a neck injury. Following esophageal injury, video swallow evaluation and placement of a feeding tube for nutrition may be indicated but is not the priority of care. A brain CT scan can be used to recognize a stroke following a carotid injury, but protecting the airway is still a priority.

5. D) Trendelenburg

Placing a patient in the Trendelenburg position will lower the risk of air embolism traveling to the brain. Prone position is used for bilateral lung injuries to improve oxygenation. Reverse Trendelenburg would increase the risk of air embolism entering the cerebral circulation and causing a stroke. Supine is not the recommended position.

PART II
Clinical Practice: Trunk

Thoracic Trauma

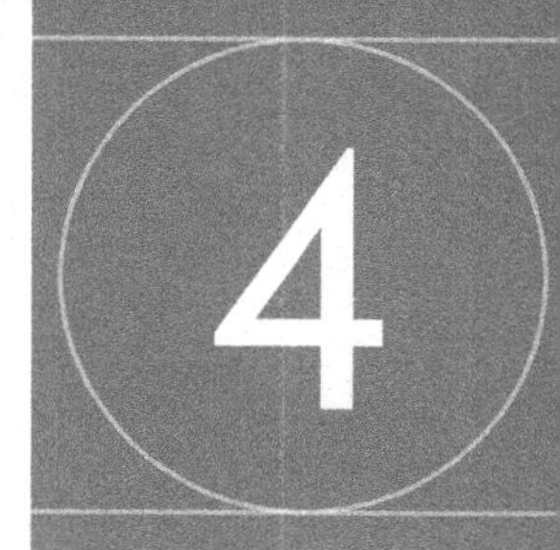

MECHANISM OF INJURY

Q The thoracic cavity extends from the first rib to which structure?

A Diaphragm

The thoracic cavity extends from the first rib to the diaphragm. The diaphragm level can vary anywhere from the fourth intercostal space (ICS) on exhalation to the lower costal margin (10th rib) on maximal inhalation.

▶ HINT

A penetrating trauma at the nipple level can result in either chest or abdominal trauma depending on whether the patient took a deep breath in or let a breath out.

Q A patient presents with a sternal fracture. What is the significance of the injury that the trauma nurse should be aware of?

A Force of impact

Fracture of the sternum requires a great force of impact and is associated with significant intrathoracic injuries, such as myocardial contusion and aortic dissection. The trauma nurse should be aware of the correlation between the sternal fracture and significant intrathoracic injuries, which may be life-threatening.

▶ HINT

Fractures of ribs 1 to 3, femur, and scapula all require a significant force of impact.

Q Which kind of mechanism causes an open pneumothorax: blunt or penetrating?

A Penetrating

An open pneumothorax is caused by penetrating trauma to the chest. It is also called a *sucking chest wound* and is caused by a large defect in the chest wall, causing equilibration of pressures between intrathoracic and atmospheric pressure. An open pneumothorax can also cause air to accumulate in the pleural space during inspiration, leading to profound hypoventilation and hypoxia.

▶ HINT

If the penetrating wound to the chest is greater than two thirds the diameter of the trachea, air will flow in and out of the wound (least resistance to airflow).

Q Which side (right or left) of the diaphragm is more likely to be injured following chest trauma?

A Left

The majority of diaphragm injuries from blunt trauma occur on the left side. The most common blunt injury is large posterior lateral tears on the left diaphragm. The right diaphragm may be more protected by the liver and requires a greater force of impact to injure, thus resulting in higher mortality. Lateral impact is the most common mechanism of injury to result in a diaphragm injury on the ipsilateral side.

HINT

Penetrating injuries to the diaphragm cause small tears and may have a delayed presentation of weeks to years later as the injury enlarges, and gradual herniation of stomach or bowel occurs.

Q What is the most common mechanism of injury that results in a pulmonary contusion?

A Compression–decompression

The mechanism of injury is commonly a compression–decompression impact on the thoracic cavity. This causes the lungs to be compressed between the anterior chest wall and the thoracic spine, increasing the pressure within the lungs. Contusions are a result of the increased pressure causing damage to the alveoli and capillaries, resulting in fluid crossing the alveolar-capillary membrane into the lungs.

HINT

Pulmonary contusions are commonly associated with chest wall injuries, including rib fractures.

Q A trauma patient is identified as having a sternal fracture. What cardiac injury is the most common after a significant blunt force impact to the chest?

A Cardiac contusion

Sternal fractures are commonly associated with cardiac contusions (cardiac injury) and pulmonary contusions (pulmonary injuries; Box 4.1).

Box 4.1 Associated injuries with sternal fractures

Chest wall bruises
Multiple rib fractures
Flail chest
Sternum fracture
Pulmonary contusion
Pericardial tamponade
Coronary artery laceration
Cardiac valve rupture

▶ HINT

Any injury that occurs as a result of a significant force of impact to the chest can be associated with myocardial contusion.

Q What is a common thoracic injury that occurs because of a sudden deceleration mechanism of injury?

A Thoracic aortic transection

The most common mechanism of injury for a thoracic aortic transection is a sudden deceleration mechanism of injury. The ligamentum arteriosum secures the aorta near the aortic arch, called the *level of the isthmus*. During a sudden deceleration, the aorta moves except at the point of the ligament, causing a transection at that level.

▶ HINT

The deceleration mechanism of injury can be horizontal (such as in a motor vehicle injury) or vertical (such as in a fall).

TRAUMATIC INJURIES

Q What is one of the most common injuries that occurs with a blunt trauma to the chest?

A Rib fracture

Rib fractures are probably the most common injury in blunt chest trauma. The fractures of ribs 1 through 3 are associated with significant intrathoracic injuries because of the force of impact required to fracture these ribs.

▶ HINT

Associated injuries with fracture of ribs 1 to 3 may include thoracic aortic transection, tracheobronchial, and vascular injuries.

Q What is an associated injury with the fractures of ribs 10 to 12 on the right side?

A Liver injury

A fractured rib can be displaced, causing injury to the underlying structures. On the right, ribs 10 to 12 cover the liver and on the left they cover the spleen. Fracturing of ribs 10 to 12 can cause injury to liver or spleen, depending on the side involved. Impacting ribs 4 to 12 can cause them to have a "bowing" effect, resulting in a midshaft fracture.

▶ HINT

Shoulder harness seat belts can cause fractures of ribs 10 to 12. The driver is at a greater risk for right-sided rib fractures and liver injury, whereas the passenger is at a greater risk for spleen injuries.

Q A patient presents in the ED with paradoxical chest wall movement following a motor vehicle collision (MVC). What would be the most likely injury the patient has sustained?

A Flail chest

A flail chest involves three or more fractures at two or more places resulting in a freely moving segment of the chest wall. Paradoxical movement of the chest wall is a hallmark sign in a flail chest (Box 4.2).

Box 4.2 Signs of flail chest

Dyspnea
Bruising of anterior chest wall
Crepitus
Position patient with fracture side down to splint chest wall
Paradoxical chest wall movement

▶ HINT

Sternal fractures may also cause a flail chest and paradoxical chest wall movement.

▶ HINT

Muscle spasms will splint the ribs, making a flail not always readily recognizable. Muscle relaxants will emphasize the presence of flail chest.

Q An injury to the internal mammary artery can result in what type of injury?

A Hemothorax

Hemothorax is caused by lung parenchymal lacerations, injuries to intercostal vessels, and injuries to the internal mammary artery. Both blunt and penetrating injuries to the chest can result in hemothorax.

▶ HINT

Hemothorax is a potential source of significant blood loss.

Q What is the most common site of injury in the trachea and bronchial area?

A Bifurcation of mainstem bronchus

Following blunt mechanism to the chest, the most common site of bronchial injury is at the bifurcation of the mainstem bronchus about an inch from the carina. If the injury does occur below the carina, the chest radiograph will show mediastinal air.

▶ HINT

Injury above the level of the carina can result in a delayed presentation, such as unresolved pneumothrorax, even after placement of thoracostomy tube.

Q What pulmonary injury is commonly associated with a flail chest?

A Pulmonary contusion

A blunt force significant enough to cause rib fractures and a flail chest can also cause the capillary vessels within the lungs to rupture, allowing blood to enter the interstitium and alveoli. Inflammation and edema develop in the lungs within a couple of hours after the injury. Lacerations to the lung tissue can also occur.

HINT

Pulmonary contusions may be small and localized with minimal symptoms, or large, involving one or both lungs and causing life-threatening symptoms.

Q Which cardiac chamber is most likely to be injured in a blunt mechanism of injury to the chest?

A Right ventricle

The right ventricle lies closest to the anterior chest wall and, because of its location, is more commonly injured following a blunt chest trauma. The atria are less commonly injured because they are smaller than the ventricles.

HINT

The complication of thrombus formation in the cardiac chambers is most common in the right ventricle because of the involvement of the right ventricle in blunt chest injuries.

ASSESSMENT/DIAGNOSIS

Q What diagnostic examination should be considered in patients with fractures of the first rib?

A Arteriogram

It may be difficult to visualize the first rib in a diagnostic chest x-ray and a fracture in this area may be missed. Arteriogram should be considered following fracture of ribs 1 through 3 because the force of impact and the vascular structures underlying those ribs can result in significant arterial injuries, including damage to the subclavian artery or vein.

HINT

Clavicle fracture is not usually serious, but a jagged edge of the clavicle bone may also injure the subclavian artery or vein.

Q What is the most definitive diagnosis for a bronchial injury?

A Bronchoscopy

An injury above the level of the carina may not demonstrate mediastinal air on chest radiograph. The most definitive diagnosis is with a bronchoscopy.

HINT

Bronchial injuries are commonly diagnosed by the presence of symptoms.

Q What is an obvious sign of a diaphragm injury with bowel herniation?

A Bowel sounds in chest

On assessment, bowel sounds heard in the chest, especially on the left side, indicate a significant diaphragm injury and bowel herniation into the thoracic chest. This is commonly associated with increased work of breathing and diminished breath sounds.

HINT

Diaphragmatic injuries are associated with hemothorax. Chest tubes should be placed cautiously to avoid injury to the herniated bowel.

Q What radiographic examination is most specific to diaphragm injury?

A CT or MRI

The most prominent feature found on a chest radiograph is elevation of hemidiaphragm and potentially a bowel pattern in the chest. Chest x-ray and ultrasonography may identify large diaphragmatic injuries but frequently miss smaller defects. CT or MRI are more sensitive in evaluating for injuries or to obtain better visualization of the anatomy of the thoracic structures.

HINT

Diagnostic laparoscopy is the most definitive diagnosis but is not indicated in all trunk trauma.

Q What is the finding on a chest x-ray that indicates the presence of a pulmonary contusion?

A Infiltrates

Infiltrates may be unilateral or bilateral and have the appearance of acute respiratory distress syndrome (ARDS). This is caused by inflammation and fluid in the lungs. Fluid can enter both the pulmonary parenchyma and alveoli, causing a "white out" of the lungs on chest x-ray.

HINT

Severe pulmonary contusions can progress into ARDS.

Q What is the most specific diagnostic study used to identify a thoracic aortic aneurysm?

A Arteriogram

A chest x-ray is a screening tool used on trauma patients and can identify a widened mediastinum (Box 4.3) but is not specific to a thoracic aortic aneurysm. An arteriogram is recommended to visualize the aorta. An invasive arteriogram is the most specific study for an aortic injury, but a CT arteriogram is less invasive and is used as a screening tool.

Box 4.3 Findings on chest x-ray for thoracic aortic injury

Widened mediastinum
Loss of aortic knob
Presence of left apical cap

HINT

The most common site for a traumatic aortic injury is the level of the isthmus.

Q A patient is admitted for 24-hour monitoring following an MVC resulting in a bent steering wheel. What injury may be suspected in this patient?

A Cardiac contusion

Cardiac arrhythmias, including life-threatening ventricular arrhythmias, may occur following cardiac contusion and requires cardiac monitoring for at least 24 hours.

HINT

Other workup of a patient with suspected cardiac contusion includes 12-lead EKG, cardiac enzymes, and an echocardiogram.

Q What diagnostic technique is commonly used to evaluate the chest for the presence of pericardial blood?

A Focused assessment sonography for trauma (FAST) technique

FAST is an ultrasound technique used to evaluate both abdominal and thoracic cavities. It is used to detect the presence of blood or fluid (effusion) in the pericardial space. The extended FAST (eFAST) may also be used to identify air and blood in the pleural space.

HINT

FAST has the advantage of being able to be performed rapidly in the ED for hemodynamically unstable trauma patients.

MEDICAL/SURGICAL INTERVENTIONS

Q Following the placement of a chest tube in a trauma patient, the nurse notes 1,500 mL of bloody output immediately on placement. What would the nurse expect the physician to do to manage this injury?

A Thoracotomy

A hemothorax with greater than 1,000 to 1,500 mL of blood on the initial insertion of a chest tube or greater than 200 mL/hr for 4 hours indicates the need for a thoracotomy. Accumulation of blood in the pleural space with a hemothorax can compromise ventilatory effort by compressing the lung tissue, resulting in hypoxemia as well as hemorrhagic shock caused by excessive loss of blood.

▶ HINT

Early surgical management for a large hemothorax is recommended to prevent complications of ongoing blood loss, empyema, and late fibrothorax.

Q What is the priority of care in patients with diaphragmatic injuries and herniated bowel?

A Airway and breathing

The herniation of bowel into the chest cavity increases the thoracic pressures and interferes with ventilation. The cornerstone of treatment of diaphragmatic injuries is intubation and ventilation to protect the airway.

▶ HINT

Placement of a nasogastric tube can assist with decompression of the bowel and limit herniation.

Q What type of mechanical ventilation may be considered in trauma patients with severe unilateral pulmonary contusion and severe hypoxemia?

A Independent lung ventilation (ILV)

ILV is considered in patients with significant unilateral pulmonary contusion and severe hypoxemia that cannot be corrected. Positive end-expiratory pressure (PEEP) is recommended in managing patients with pulmonary contusions, but in patients with unilateral lung involvement, the unaffected lung can become overdistended and the affected lung underventilated. This is called *maldistribution of ventilation*. ILV can provide PEEP into the affected lung without overdistending the unaffected lung.

▶ HINT

Pressure control modes of ventilation and high-frequency oscillatory ventilation (HFOV) may be used in patients with bilateral pulmonary contusions who have failed with conventional ventilation.

Q Following a paracentesis, the blood aspirated is placed in a container and agitated. If it does not form clots, this indicates the blood was aspirated from which space?

A Pericardial space

Blood aspirated from the pericardial space is defibrinated, so the blood does not clot. If the needle punctured the ventricle and aspirated blood is from the ventricular chamber, then the blood will clot.

▶ HINT

Blood from the pleural space is defibrinated and also does not clot.

Q A patient with cardiac contusion becomes hypotensive. What pharmacological intervention may be used to improve the patient's hemodynamic status?

A Dobutamine (Dobutrex)

Dobutamine is a positive inotropic agent that increases myocardial contractility. Patients with cardiac contusion frequently experience decreases in myocardial contractility and ejection fractions. Improving contractility will improve blood pressure and hemodynamics.

> **HINT**
>
> **Administering vasoconstrictive agents to increase blood pressures in patients with cardiac contusions may actually worsen their hemodynamics because of the increase in resistance (afterload) on the heart.**

Q A patient with a thoracic aortic injury presents to the ICU with a blood pressure of 194/98 mmHg and a heart rate of 106 beats per minute. The trauma nurse would expect that the physician would order which class of medication to lower the patient's blood pressure?

A Beta-blocker

A beta-blocker will block adrenergic activity and lower the blood pressure. This will lower the risk of further injury to the aorta and aortic rupture. Beta-blockers decrease the heart rate, also limiting injury to the aorta. Alpha-blockers, such as nipride, will lower the blood pressure but cause a reflex tachycardia that may worsen the aortic injury.

> **HINT**
>
> **Esmolol is a beta-blocker that is short acting and titratable. It is commonly used to manage the blood pressure in patients with traumatic aortic aneurysms.**

Q In a suspected tension pneumothorax, what intervention can be performed before a chest tube can be placed?

A Needle thoracentesis

If the patient is suspected of having a tension pneumothorax and is hemodynamically unstable, a needle thoracentesis can be performed to rapidly reverse the life-threatening symptoms. A 14-gauge (G) needle is placed in the second ICS, midclavicular on the affected side.

> **HINT**
>
> **The definitive treatment of tension pneumothorax is the placement of a chest tube to decompress the pneumothorax.**

Q What is a concern of intubating a patient with tracheobronchial injury?

A Further injury

The blind placement of an endotracheal tube on a patient with a tracheobronchial injury can cause further injury. A flexible bronchoscope can be useful in guiding the placement of the endotracheal tube, limiting the risk of further injury.

> **HINT**
>
> **Without a chest tube, positive pressure mechanical ventilation can worsen the pneumothorax without a chest tube by forcing air into the pleural space.**

NURSING INTERVENTIONS

Q What is the primary goal for managing a patient with rib fractures?

A Pain management

Management of rib fractures includes pain management, usually with oral analgesics. This can include opioids, nerve blocks, epidural, or intrapleural analgesia if pain is severe.

▶ HINT

In patients with flail chest, administration of analgesia will decrease pain and may relax the intercostal muscles, making paradoxical chest wall movement of flail more obvious.

Q During assessment of a trauma patient in the ED, the nurse notes diminished breath sounds on the left side with dullness to percussion. What is the most likely cause?

A Hemothorax

If diminished breath sounds on the affected side are found, this indicates a collapsed lung and is commonly found with a pneumothorax or hemothorax. The presence of dullness on percussion indicates the presence of fluid or blood such as a hemothorax. A pneumothorax will have hyperresonance with percussion over the affected side.

▶ HINT

Clinical presentation of hemothorax includes dullness to percussion, decreased breath sounds on affected side, and flat neck veins resulting from blood loss.

Q What type of dressing is recommended to manage an open-sucking chest wound before definitive treatment?

A Three-sided dressing

A three-sided dressing works as a flutter valve. It allows air to leave but not to reenter the pleural space. An occlusive dressing could result in a tension pneumothorax.

▶ HINT

A flutter valve may also be used to manage the open pneumothorax.

Q Following a blunt chest injury, a patient in the trauma ICU demonstrates subcutaneous air, cough, hemoptysis, and persistent subcutaneous emphysema. What is the most likely injury?

A Bronchial injury

Symptoms of a bronchial injury may be delayed by several days after injury. Bronchial injury is commonly recognized by the symptoms, especially an unresolving pneumothorax (Box 4.4).

Box 4.4 Symptoms of tracheobronchial injuries

Noisy breathing
Dyspnea
Airway obstruction
Hemoptysis
Cough
Hoarseness
Subcutaneous emphysema: neck, face, or suprasternal
Progressive mediastinal air
Persistent pneumothorax
Tension pneumothorax

HINT

Tracheobronchial injuries are more likely to be caused by a penetrating trauma and should cause a high suspicion.

Q A patient in the emergency room presents with a penetrating trauma of the left chest. If the patient continues to be unresponsive to fluids and remains hemodynamically unstable, then the trauma nurse should suspect which injury?

A Pericardial tamponade

Penetrating trauma is the most common mechanism of injury causing pericardial tamponade. A pericardial tamponade commonly presents with hemodynamic instability despite adequate fluid resuscitation. The development of tamponade produces a reduction in the filling of ventricles during diastole and a decrease in output during systole.

HINT

Cardiac tamponade is caused by bleeding into the pericardial sac as a result of a ruptured coronary artery, lacerated pericardium, or an injury to the myocardium in trauma patients.

Q What are the components of the Beck's triad which are associated with cardiac tamponade?

A Increased jugular venous distension (JVD), hypotension, and muffled heart sounds

The increased JVD is caused by impedance in filling the ventricle during diastole, hypotension is a result of a decrease in cardiac output, and muffled heart sounds occur because of the accumulation of blood in the pericardial sac. If the patient has other associated injuries with significant blood loss, the JVD may be absent (Box 4.5).

Box 4.5 Symptoms of pericardial tamponade

Increased jugular venous distension
Hypotension
Muffled or distant heart sounds
Pulsus paradoxus

(*continued*)

Box 4.5 Symptoms of pericardial tamponade (*continued*)

Pulsus alternans
Cyanosis
Dyspnea
Pulseless electrical activity
Tachycardia
Pericardial friction rub

HINT

Diminished amplitude of the QRS complex may also be associated with pericardial tamponade because of the fluid collection around the heart.

HINT

***Pulsus paradoxus* is the decrease in systolic blood pressure during inspiration, whereas *pulsus alternans* is an alternating weak and strong pulse.**

Q A trauma patient is admitted to the trauma ICU following a blunt trauma to the chest. The patient was intubated in the ED and is on a mechanical ventilator. One day posttrauma, the nurse notes an increase in peak inspiratory pressures (PIP). What would be the most likely cause?

A Pulmonary contusion

The combination of atelectasis, blood, fluid, and interstitial edema produces a decrease in pulmonary compliance and an increase in PIP. The findings of pulmonary contusions frequently occur within 24 to 48 hours after injury and are commonly associated with a blunt chest injury. The triad of physiological changes associated with pulmonary contusion is hypoxemia, intrapulmonary shunting, and reduced pulmonary compliance (Box 4.6).

Box 4.6 Symptoms of pulmonary contusion

Shortness of breath
Diffuse crackles
Tachypnea
Hypocarbia
Blood-tinged or bloody sputum
Wheezes
Increased work of breathing
Increased peak airway pressures
Infiltrates on chest x-ray
Tachycardia
Hypoxemia

HINT

ARDS may also present with an increase in PIP but will commonly occur 48 to 72 hours after a traumatic injury.

Q Following fluid resuscitation and patient stabilization, what is the most appropriate fluid management to prevent worsening of pulmonary contusions?

A Limit fluid intake

Trauma patients should not have excessive restrictions of fluid replacement during resuscitation. Fluid administration should obtain the goal of hemodynamic stabilization. After the trauma patient is stabilized hemodynamically, then restriction of fluids may limit pulmonary contusions and associated complications.

HINT

Restricting fluids initially in a hemodynamically unstable patient following a trauma can significantly decrease tissue perfusion and worsen outcomes.

Q A driver of a motor vehicle involved in a front-end collision suddenly develops short runs of ventricular tachycardia. What would be the most likely cause of the arrhythmias?

A Cardiac contusion

Complications of myocardial contusions include arrhythmias. These arrhythmias can range from supraventricular tachycardia (SVT) and atrial fibrillation (AF) to lethal ventricular arrhythmias. Atrioventricular (AV) blocks may also be associated with cardiac contusions (Box 4.7).

Box 4.7 Signs of cardiac contusion

Tachycardia
Decreased urine output
Hypotension
Chest pain
Increased jugular venous distention
Arrhythmias
ST segment changes (elevation)
T-wave changes

HINT

The most common arrhythmia with myocardial contusion is sinus tachycardia. Cardiac contusion can cause signs of decreased perfusion to tissues because of the decrease in ejection fraction and cardiac output.

Q A patient with multiple rib fractures on the right exhibits rapid shallow breathing and limited movement. What is the most appropriate intervention by the trauma nurse?

A Provide pain management

Patients with multiple rib fractures experience significant pain and breathing deeply increases the painful response. Managing the patient's pain can allow the patient to breath deeper and more effectively with less splinting. Splinting places the patient at an increased risk for atelectasis and pneumonia.

HINT

The use of multimodal pain management is recommended to manage pain to allow deeper breathing without the respiratory depression of opioids.

COMPLICATIONS

Q What is the life-threatening complication of a pneumothorax?

A Tension pneumothorax

In a tension pneumothorax, the air builds in the pleural space, becomes trapped, and the increased pressure causes the mediastinum to shift. The shifting of the mediastinal structures causes the compression of the aorta and inferior vena cava. This results in a life-threatening hemodynamic instability. Needle decompression, with 14- to 18-G angiocath at the second to third ICS midclavicular, is the emergency treatment until a chest tube can be placed.

HINT

The trauma nurse should palpate the trachea for deviation. The trachea will be deviated away from the side of the tension pneumothorax.

Q What is a long-term pulmonary complication of pulmonary contusions?

A Pulmonary fibrosis

Patients with pulmonary contusions are more likely to develop ARDS. Contused lungs from trauma commonly demonstrate fibrosis on chest x-ray within 1 to 6 years after injury. The vital capacity and air volumes are also significantly decreased because of the fibrosis.

HINT

Fibrosis occurs in ARDS, which has physiological effects that are very similar to those of pulmonary contusions following the injury or insult.

Q An echocardiogram may be used to evaluate a patient with a myocardial contusion several days after injury. What late complication of a cardiac contusion can be identified with an echocardiogram?

A Intracardiac thrombus

The decrease in contractility and ejection fraction, which occurs with contusion of the myocardium, can lead to blood stasis in the cardiac chambers and thrombus formation. The use of echocardiogram can identify the thrombus in the cardiac chambers. The identification of depression of myocardial contractility and cardiogenic shock can be identified early with echocardiogram and are complications of cardiac contusion.

▶ HINT

Transesophageal echocardiogram (TEE) is more sensitive than a transthoracic echocardiogram (TTE) approach in identifying intracardiac thrombus.

Q A trauma patient experiences pulseless electrical activity (PEA) during fluid resuscitation. What traumatic injury is most likely to have occurred?

A Pericardial tamponade

One of the causes of PEA is pericardial tamponade. This is the result of pericardial restriction of the heart, which limits filling of the cardiac chambers and the ability to mechanicaly contract. Electrical activity is not affected, so the patient has a discernable rhythm on the monitor, but no mechanical activity.

▶ HINT

Pericardial tamponade is considered to be a constrictive cardiomyopathy.

Q Which blunt cardiac injury has one of the highest mortalities?

A Cardiac rupture

Blunt forces to the chest increase the intrathoracic pressure resulting in the rupture of a cardiac chamber. This carries a high mortality. Transection of the ascending aorta is fatal in most cases.

▶ HINT

Emergency thoracotomy on a patient with blunt trauma cardiac arrest is rarely successful.

KNOWLEDGE CHECK: CHAPTER 4

1. The nurse receives a patient following a motor vehicle collision. The patient was an unrestrained driver, and the airbag did not deploy. The patient has a respiratory rate of 42 breaths per minute, obvious paradoxical movement of the chest wall, and presents in severe respiratory distress requiring intubation. The nurse is suspecting what type of injury?

   A. Three or more rib fractures on one side
   B. Fracture of the sternum
   C. Rib fractures involving ribs 4 to 6
   D. Clavicle fracture

2. Rib and sternal fractures are commonly associated with other severe injuries. Which of the following correctly matches the location of the injury to the associated complications?

   A. Left lower rib fractures and liver lacerations
   B. Right lower rib fractures and splenic rupture
   C. Sternal fracture with cardiac contusion
   D. Left lower rib fracture with great vessel injuries

3. A patient comes into the ED after involvement in a high-speed motor vehicle collision impacting a telephone pole. The patient is unresponsive on arrival with a blood pressure of 80/40 mmHg, absent pedal pulses, and bounding radial pulses. Chest x-ray reveals widened mediastinum. What is this patient's expected injury?

   A. Aortic injury at level of isthmus
   B. Pericardial tamponade
   C. Blunt cardiac injury
   D. Cardiac rupture

4. A patient presents to the ED with a machete lodged in the chest. The patient is hypotensive with pulsus paradoxus. The nurse is actively transfusing the patient with blood products and intravenous fluids are being administered. The patient suddenly becomes unconscious and cyanotic. Which intervention would be most appropriate in this situation?

   A. Pericardiocentesis
   B. Expedited transfer to the operating room
   C. Open thoracotomy
   D. Obtain an emergency arteriogram of the aorta

5. A patient with a pulmonary contusion has a decrease in pulmonary compliance and an increase in airway pressures. This is related to which of the following?

   A. Pulmonary interstitial edema
   B. Hypercarbia
   C. Air in the pleural space
   D. Blood clots in the lungs

(*See answers next page.*)

1. A) Three or more rib fractures on one side

Flail chest is defined as three or more fractures occurring in two or more places, resulting in a freely moving chest wall. Flail chest displays paradoxical movements, tachypnea, and frequently requires intubation with positive pressure ventilation. Fracture of the sternum is associated with myocardial contusions and intrathoracic injuries. Rib fractures 4 to 6 may cause a bowing effect in the chest, resulting in midshaft fracture. A clavicle fracture is not considered a serious injury and would not contribute to respiratory distress.

2. C) Sternal fracture with cardiac contusion

Sternal fractures are usually associated with heart or great vessel injury because of the location and force of impact. The angle of Louis is the most common fracture site of the sternum; it is adjacent to the second intercostal space (ICS). Left lower rib fractures may be associated with splenic injuries and rupture, not the right side. Right lower rib fractures may be associated with hepatic lacerations, not the left side.

3. A) Aortic injury at level of isthmus

Aortic injuries are usually the result of sudden deceleration mechanism of injury. The more common site of damage is the descending aorta at the level of the isthmus immediately below the arch. Pericardial tamponade will present with hypotension but will have distended neck veins and muffled heart sounds. Blunt cardiac injury may also have occurred due to the mechanism, but the symptoms are not descriptive of cardiac injury. Cardiac rupture is not as common and will typically result in death.

4. C) Open thoracotomy

The patient is exhibiting pericardial tamponade. An open thoracotomy in the ED is the most appropriate intervention for a hemodynamically unstable patient with a penetrating injury to the chest. Pericardiocentesis and surgical repair are acceptable treatments for a patient with pericardial tamponade, but an open thoracotomy would be more appropriate in this case because of the patient's declining status. An arteriogram of the aorta is not indicated in this situation. A cardiac injury should be suspected over an aortic transection based on mechanism of injury.

5. A) Pulmonary interstitial edema

Pulmonary contusions can be life-threatening because of hypoxemia, intrapulmonary shunting, and reduced lung compliance. Inflammation and edema occur after lung injury. The combination of atelectasis, interstitial edema, and the presence of blood and fluid produce a decrease in pulmonary compliance and an increase in airway pressure. Hypercarbia does not increase airway pressure. Pneumothorax and pulmonary embolism can cause an increase in airway pressures but are not always associated with pulmonary contusions.

6. A patient who suffered a femur fracture is 2 days postoperative and begins to report chest pain on inspiration. The nurse finds an oxygen saturation of 92% on 2 L via nasal cannula, a respiratory rate of 27 breaths per minute, and a heart rate of 112 beats per minute. Which of the following imaging studies is the most definitive diagnosis of a pulmonary embolism (PE)?

   A. Computed tomography angiogram (CTA) of chest
   B. Pulmonary angiogram
   C. Chest x-ray (CXR)
   D. Ventilation perfusion scan

7. Which of the following ventilation techniques is the most appropriate in the treatment of patients with pulmonary contusions to improve oxygenation?

   A. Increase positive end-expiratory pressure (PEEP).
   B. Maintain low plateau pressures.
   C. Decrease respiratory rate.
   D. Increase FiO_2 to 100%.

8. A patient comes in with a cardiac contusion and multiple rib fractures following a motor vehicle collision. The trauma nurse performs a 12-lead EKG and troponin levels. What other diagnostic procedures would be appropriate for this patient in the acute period?

   A. Transthoracic echocardiogram (TTE)
   B. Radionuclide angiography
   C. Transesophageal echocardiogram (TEE)
   D. Bronchoscopy

9. A patient admitted with a traumatic aortic aneurysm is most likely to have which one of the following performed during the surgical repair of the aorta to prevent complications?

   A. Autotransfusion from the chest tube
   B. Clamped aorta without distal canalization
   C. Partial left heart bypass
   D. Aortic bypass with autologous graft

10. What are the possible complications caused by the cross-clamping of the aorta to repair an aortic transection?

   A. Right lung pneumonia
   B. Myocardial infarction
   C. Graft infection
   D. Atelectasis

(*See answers next page.*)

6. B) Pulmonary angiogram

The diagnosis of PE is confirmed by a pulmonary angiogram, which is considered the most definitive diagnosis. A ventilation perfusion scan can recognize a high-probability ventilation/perfusion (V/Q) defect suspicious of a PE. A CTA scan can demonstrate one or more filling defects or obstructions in the pulmonary artery or pulmonary artery branches. CXR changes may be found but are nonspecific for a PE.

7. A) Increase positive end-expiratory pressure (PEEP).

PEEP is favorable to improve oxygenation because it allows pressure to remain in the alveoli at end expiration, recruits collapsed alveoli, and improves oxygenation. Lowering respiratory rates would not be beneficial to the pulmonary contusion patient. If tidal volumes are decreased or the patient is placed on pressure-controlled ventilation, the respiratory rate should actually be increased to maintain normal minute ventilation. Lower plateau pressures limit the trauma to the lungs but do not necessarily improve oxygenation. Increasing FiO_2 can improve oxygenation but 100% is not recommended unless all other attempts to improve oxygenation have failed.

8. A) Transthoracic echocardiogram (TTE)

TTE is indicated to assess cardiac function and determine ejection fraction. Cardiac contusions frequently result in decreased ventricular contractility and decreased ejection fractions. Radionuclide angiography and TEE may be used to evaluate cardiac function but are not typically used in the acute period and TEE is more invasive. Bronchoscopy is not indicated to evaluate cardiac injury.

9. C) Partial left heart bypass

During cross-clamping of the aorta to repair the aortic transection, the organs that are usually perfused distal to the site of the cross-clamp may become hypoperfused, resulting in multiple organ failure. Partial left heart bypass is commonly used to move blood around the cross-clamped area to perfuse organs distal to the cross-clamp. A clamped aorta without distal canalization can be performed, but the procedure has to be very quick to prevent hypoperfusion. Autologous grafts are not typically used and autotransfusion from chest tubes is not indicated in this surgical repair.

10. B) Myocardial infarction

Myocardial infarction can occur because of the increased resistance to the heart with the cross-clamped aorta. Organ dysfunction can also occur during this procedure because of the risk of hypoperfusion below the clamp. All the other answers are potential complications of the surgical repair of an aorta but are not specifically the result of the cross-clamping of the aorta.

Abdominal Trauma

5

MECHANISM OF INJURY

Q **The spleen is most commonly injured in which type of trauma: blunt or penetrating?**

A **Blunt**

Common organs injured by blunt mechanism are the solid organs such as spleen, liver, and pancreas. Entrapment of the abdominal wall against the vertebral column and compression of the abdomen increases the pressure within the abdominal cavity and causes solid organs to rupture. Hollow organs are able to collapse during the increased pressure.

HINT

Other mechanisms of injury in blunt trauma to the abdomen include changing of organ position and puncture of organs with bone fractures.

Q **During sudden deceleration in a blunt trauma, movement of abdominal organs most commonly causes tearing of which abdominal organ?**

A **Duodenum**

During energy transfer, shearing forces may cause tearing at the attachment points of ligaments. The duodenum is secured by the ligament of Treitz; therefore a sudden deceleration results in the tearing of the duodenum at the level of the ligament.

HINT

This is a similar mechanism to the tearing of the aorta during a sudden deceleration mechanism because of the arch secured by the ligamentum of arteriosum.

Q **Seat belts can increase injury to which body system?**

A **Abdomen**

Seat belts can change the patterns of blunt trauma by increasing abdominal injuries. They decrease the severity of injury and lower the number of traumatic brain injuries but can increase the abdominal trauma. Lap belts lie across the lower abdomen and can increase abdominal organ injuries. Other causes of abdominal trauma include handlebar injuries for patients on bicycles and motorcycles.

HINT

A bent steering wheel in a motor vehicle collision (MVC) is associated with more significant abdominal injuries to the driver.

Q Following an MVC, the driver wearing a shoulder harness during the collision is more likely to injure which abdominal organ?

A Liver

The harness seat belt is secured across the left shoulder to the right hip, with the belt lying across the area of the liver. On impact, the liver is compressed, resulting in an injury.

HINT

A passenger with a shoulder harness is more likely to damage the spleen.

Q Which mechanism, gunshot or stab wound, is more likely to result in an abdominal organ injury requiring surgical management?

A Gunshot wound

Gunshot wounds are associated with a 96% to 98% chance of a significant intra-abdominal injury requiring surgery and have a higher mortality rate than stab wounds. Stab wounds are associated with a 30% to 40% chance of injury needing surgery and have a lower mortality than gunshot wounds. Gunshot wounds are associated with a greater kinetic energy and destruction of tissue than stab wounds, which may not enter the peritoneum.

HINT

Gunshot wounds to the abdomen are more likely to have an exploratory laparotomy with minimal diagnostic workup before the surgery.

TRAUMATIC INJURIES

Q Where is the pancreas located in the abdominal cavity: the intraperitoneal or retroperitoneal space?

A Retroperitoneal space

The abdominal cavity is divided into the peritoneal and retroperitoneal spaces. The peritoneal cavity contains the stomach, small intestine, liver, gallbladder, transverse colon, sigmoid colon, upper one third of rectum, part of the bladder, and uterus. The retroperitoneal space contains part of the duodenum, ascending colon, descending colon, kidneys, part of the bladder, pancreas, and major vessels.

HINT

Retroperitoneal organ injuries can be more difficult to diagnose than intraperitoneal injuries.

Q Penetrating trauma to the back, flank, or buttocks can result in injury to which body system?

A Abdomen

The flank and back are regions of the abdomen, and penetrating injuries in these regions can result in trauma to the abdomen. Penetrating injuries to the diaphragm are harder to recognize than blunt injuries and may require laparoscopy or surgical exploration.

HINT

A missed occult injury to the diaphragm may have a delayed presentation of shortness of breath due to herniated stomach or bowel into the thoracic cavity.

Q Which diaphragm, right or left, is more likely to be injured in a blunt abdominal trauma?

A Left

Rupture of the left diaphragm is more common than the right because the liver protects the diaphragm on the right. Following a diaphragm injury, the stomach or small bowel may herniate into the thoracic cavity. Auscultation of the chest may reveal bowel sounds if herniated.

HINT

The presence of asymmetrical chest wall movement may indicate an injury to the diaphragm, liver, or spleen.

Q A nasogastric (NG) tube is placed following penetrating abdominal trauma and bloody aspirate is obtained. What organ is most likely injured?

A Stomach

Stomach injuries are commonly caused by penetrating trauma. The most common sign of a stomach injury is bloody gastric aspirate. Other signs include rapid onset of epigastric pain, tenderness, and signs of peritonitis.

HINT

Free air in abdomen indicates rupture of hollow organ.

Q Which abdominal organ is most likely to be injured in both blunt and penetrating trauma?

A Liver

The most frequently injured organ is the liver because of its size and location. It is a solid organ and hence is more commonly injured in blunt abdominal trauma. The driver using a shoulder harness is likely to injure the liver in an MVC due to the location of the belt over the liver. The liver is also commonly damaged with penetrating injuries because of its size in the abdominal cavity.

HINT

The high mortality caused by liver injury is the result of hemorrhage (early) or peritonitis and sepsis (late).

Q Which portion of the esophagus is most commonly injured following penetrating trauma?

A Cervical region

The esophagus is not commonly injured in trauma. If injured, the most common mechanism of injury is penetrating trauma, which occurs more frequently in the cervical region of the esophagus. The abdominal portion is rarely injured.

▶ HINT

Injury results in fluid accumulation in the lungs and respiratory distress.

Q In grading severity of injury, a hematoma of the spleen is blood accumulation in which part of the spleen?

A Capsular portion of the spleen

A hematoma in the spleen is an accumulation of blood in the capsular portion of the spleen. If the capsule ruptures, it is then called a *laceration*.

▶ HINT

A splenic hematoma can be monitored for a bleeding complication and managed with observation instead of surgical management.

ASSESSMENT/DIAGNOSIS

Q Which abdominal organ commonly presents with delayed onset of symptoms?

A Duodenum

Secretions in the stomach are acidic but are alkaline in the duodenum. Perforation of the stomach results in rapid, acute signs of peritonitis, whereas the spillage of alkaline fluid into the abdominal cavity is not an immediate irritant of the peritoneum. Duodenal ruptures may have referred pain to back, chest, shoulder, and testicles (retroperitoneal injury).

▶ HINT

Presentation may be delayed and is indicated by septic peritonitis (Box 5.1).

Box 5.1 Delayed presentation of duodenal injuries

Fever
Elevated white blood cell count
Jaundice
High intestinal blockage
Third-spacing fluid
Elevated bilirubin and amylase
Hypovolemia

Q Free air in the abdomen may indicate the presence of rupture to which type of abdominal organs?

A Hollow organs

Hollow organs are air filled and when ruptured will release "free air" in the abdomen. Solid organ rupture will not present with free air on radiographic x-rays.

HINT

Free air found on radiographic studies indicates the need for immediate surgery for significant organ injury.

Q Which diagnostic radiographic study is best able to identify the severity of organ injury?

A CT scan

Advantages of CT scan include the ability to grade the severity of injury, as well as to be able to view the retroperitoneal cavity and the intra-abdominal injuries. The ability to grade injuries allows for some patients to be observed following injury rather than undergo surgical management. The disadvantage is that there is a need to transport unstable patients to perform the CT scan.

HINT

An abdominal CT scan can identify the organ involved and the severity of organ injury thereby lowering the incidence of negative laparotomies.

Q What is bruising in the flank area due to bleeding in the retroperitoneal space called?

A Grey-Turner's sign

Grey-Turner's sign is ecchymosis (or bruising) in the flank area resulting from bleeding in the retroperitoneal space. Cullen's sign is ecchymosis around the umbilicus and indicates bleeding in the peritoneal cavity. The trauma nurse should inspect the patient's abdomen for bruising, abrasions, and lacerations, which may indicate intra-abdominal organ injury.

HINT

Grey-Turner's and Cullen's signs may not appear for several hours or days following the trauma.

Q While assessing the patient, the trauma nurse finds a "board-like" abdomen. What does this finding indicate?

A Peritonitis

A "board-like" abdomen is the result of involuntary spasm of abdominal muscles resulting from peritonitis. Muscle guarding is an increased voluntary contraction of the abdominal muscles in an effort to prevent pain.

HINT

Rebound tenderness is pain or abdominal activity following sudden withdrawal of stimulus such as fingers.

Q What is the advantage of a CT scan compared to a diagnostic peritoneal lavage (DPL)?

A Identification of retroperitoneal injuries

The advantage of a CT scan compared to DPL is the scan's ability to view the retroperitoneal cavity as well as intra-abdominal injuries. The other advantage is the CT scan's ability to identify the organ involved and grade the severity of injury. Disadvantages of CT scan include the expense and difficulty in scanning an unstable patient. CT scan is the diagnostic modality of choice in monitoring nonoperative solid visceral injuries.

▶ HINT

CT scan may miss injuries to the mesentery and small bowel, thus limiting the diagnostic effectiveness of CT scan for these injuries.

Q Which is the noninvasive and repeatable test that can be used to evaluate hemoperitoneum at the bedside following a blunt trauma?

A Abdominal ultrasound

Ultrasonography of the abdomen is preferred over abdominal CT scan in hemodynamically unstable trauma patients. It is a noninvasive, quick, inexpensive, and repeatable test that can be used to evaluate hemoperitoneum. Trained technicians are able to identify free fluid greater than 200 mL with an abdominal sonography.

▶ HINT

Ultrasonography is less reliable than CT scans for grading the severity of abdominal organ injuries and excluding hollow visceral injuries.

Q What is the ultrasonography technique used to rapidly evaluate the abdomen following a blunt trauma?

A Focused abdominal sonography for trauma (FAST) technique

FAST is a technique used to rapidly evaluate the abdomen for traumatic injuries. One of the advantages of using FAST in the ED is that the patient does not have to be transported to imaging to obtain a CT scan. Exploratory laparotomy is indicated in hemodynamically unstable patients with a positive FAST, indicating evidence of hemoperitoneum. It can estimate the amount of blood in the abdomen and identify candidates for observation, thus preventing unnecessary laparotomies. Extended focused abdominal sonography for trauma (EFAST) includes the cardiac window.

▶ HINT

A penetrating stab wound to the abdomen evaluated with the FAST technique can have false negatives.

Q Which abdominal organ is more difficult to evaluate for injury with a diagnostic laparoscopy?

A Bowel

A laparoscope can observe the diaphragm, liver, spleen, anterior stomach, uterus, ovaries, cecum, and sigmoid colon. It is more difficult for a complete examination of the bowel, flexures of colon, and retroperitoneum, and can miss injuries in these areas. Treatment of certain injuries can be performed during diagnostic laparoscopy such as ligating bleeders or closing lacerations.

HINT

Diagnostic laparoscopy may be indicated with penetrating injuries when there is a high likelihood that the injury is tangential to the abdomen.

Q A supraumbilical approach for a DPL is more accurate than below the umbilicus in a patient with what type of associated injury?

A Pelvic fracture

DPL is a procedure used to diagnose occult intra-abdominal bleeding in abdominal trauma. A below-the-umbilicus DPL performed on a patient with a pelvic fracture can result in a false positive due to bleeding caused by the pelvic fracture and an unnecessary exploratory laparotomy. The technique of performing the DPL above the umbilicus lowers this risk. Disadvantages of DPL include the inability to diagnose retroperitoneal injuries, inability to determine type or extent of injury, and potential of a missed ruptured hollow viscera if performed early after the injury.

HINT

Relative contraindications for DPL include advanced pregnancy, pelvic injuries, previous multiple abdominal surgeries, morbid obesity, advanced cirrhosis, and coagulopathy.

Q If an emergency DPL is performed in a patient with suspected abdominal trauma, what red blood cell (RBC) level would indicate a positive lavage?

A Greater than 100,000 mm^3

An RBC count greater than 100,000 mm^3 is considered positive with a DPL and is an indication for exploratory laparotomy (especially if the patient is hemodynamically unstable). Other signs of positive DPL frequently include white blood cell (WBC) levels greater than 500 mm^3, or elevated amylase, alkaline phosphate, or bilirubin in the lavage fluid.

HINT

If a DPL is performed, an elevated WBC has no diagnostic value in the early postinjury period (less than 4 hours).

Q What would be the best intervention in a hemodynamically stable patient with a grade II liver laceration?

A Observation

A hemodynamically stable grade II liver laceration can be observed without an exploratory laparotomy in most situations without other significant abdominal organ injuries. Observation of patients with abdominal organ injuries should include hemodynamic monitoring, frequent physical assessment, and serial labs (especially hemoglobin [Hgb] and hematocrit [Hct]).

> **HINT**
>
> **Unnecessary laparotomy can increase complications, length of stay, and mortality following stab wounds and blunt abdominal trauma.**

MEDICAL/SURGICAL INTERVENTIONS

Q What would be the most appropriate intervention for a patient with blunt abdominal trauma presenting with obvious signs of peritonitis?

A Exploratory laparotomy

Obvious signs of peritonitis are an indication for an exploratory laparotomy following a blunt abdominal trauma. Other indications for exploratory laparotomies indicate unexplained shock, impalement, evisceration of bowel or omentum, significant bleeding from NG tube, ongoing hemodynamic instability, or free air on x-ray.

> **HINT**
>
> **Signs of peritonitis should be recognized following an abdominal injury and include abdominal tenderness, board-like abdomen, elevated WBC count, fever, and other signs of sepsis.**

Q What is the first priority in an exploratory laparotomy following an abdominal trauma with hemodynamic instability?

A Locate the source and control hemorrhage

The first priority in exploratory laparotomy following abdominal trauma is to locate the source of bleeding and control hemorrhage. The second priority is to locate colonic injury to control fecal contamination, then identify injuries to abdominal organs and structures, followed by repair to the damaged tissues and organs. The third and fourth priority identifies injuries to abdominal organs and structures, and repair of damage to tissues and organs.

> **HINT**
>
> **The combination of bowel and liver injury significantly increases risk of posttraumatic infections.**

Q A penetrating trauma to the stomach results in devitalized tissue. What is the best surgical intervention for this patient?

A Debridement of devitalized tissue

Treatment of stomach injury includes debridement of devitalized tissue and closure with sutures or a partial gastrectomy if the injury is extensive.

HINT

Following stomach repair, an NG tube may be present for 3 to 5 days with specific instructions not to reposition the NG tube. Repositioning an NG tube after gastric repair can cause damage to the anastomosis or sutures.

Q What is the primary surgical management of small bowel injuries?

A Debridement and resection

The key to successful surgical repair of the small bowel is debridement. All devitalized tissue and marginally injured bowel should be resected. Most small bowel injuries can be closed after simple debridement, resection, and suturing.

HINT

All but 50 cm of the entire small bowel can be resected without compromise (total length is 260 cm).

Q During an exploratory laparotomy, the liver is noted to be profusely bleeding. What is the most commonly used technique to control bleeding called?

A Damage control

If intra-abdominal hemorrhage is severe, the trauma surgeon performs damage control by packing the liver bed, using fibrin glue (sealant made from concentrated fibrinogen and thrombin), and/or selective hepatic artery or portal vein ligation temporary closure, and planned reoperation to control coagulopathic bleeding. This is frequently referred to as *damage control surgery*.

HINT

After the damage control surgery, the trauma nurse assesses for uncontrolled hemorrhage, monitors coagulation studies, and administers agents to reverse the coagulopathy.

Q What is a common practice for treating a grade I liver laceration following a blunt abdominal trauma?

A Observation

Simple injuries (grade I to II) may be observed. A nonoperative course is taken for these minor hepatic injuries with no evidence of bleeding. If surgically managed, surgery usually includes sutures or application of topical agents to control bleeding or electrocautery.

HINT

This involves observation in the ICU or step-down unit (SDU) with frequent vital signs, complete blood count (CBC) and prothrombin time (PT)/partial thromboplastin time (PTT) monitoring.

Q What is a commonly used fecal diversion following a colon injury?

A Double-barrel transverse colostomy

Double-barrel transverse colostomy involves the complete division of the bowel, and each part is brought to the surface. One opening puts out stool and one puts out just mucus. Loop colostomies are easily constructed and taken down but may not completely divert fecal material from the distal segment of the colon. A colostomy is made either at the site of the colon injury or proximal to the site to protect distal repair.

▶ HINT

In a right colon injury, colostomies are avoided because of the difficulty of the procedure. Right colon injuries are typically treated with primary repair or hemicolectomy.

Q A grade V rupture of the spleen typically requires what type of intervention?

A Splenectomy

A splenectomy is the recommended procedure for a grade IV to V splenic injury. These injuries involve vascular injuries that produce major devascularization or completely shatter the spleen.

▶ HINT

Surgical repair of the spleen is called a *splenorrhaphy*.

Q What is a nonoperative interventional treatment of a splenic or liver injury used to control bleeding?

A Embolization

Embolization of splenic and hepatic arteries in patients with contrast extravasation and ongoing blood loss can be used to control the hemorrhage. This is a nonoperative management of abdominal bleeding from the liver or spleen.

▶ HINT

Grades IV and V liver or splenic injuries may require surgery because of the increased severity of injury.

NURSING INTERVENTIONS

Q Percussion over the right upper quadrant (RUQ) following an acute liver injury produces what type of sound?

A Dullness

Signs of traumatic liver injuries include tenderness over right lower ribs or RUQ, dullness to percussion, signs of peritoneal irritation, and increased abdominal girth.

Q Following a stomach injury and partial gastrectomy, the patient has an NG tube. What is a common order regarding the care of the NG tube?

A Do not reposition

The NG tube is placed intraoperatively. Repositioning the NG tube can cause injury to the anastomosis or sutures.

HINT

Following stomach repair postop an NG tube may be present for 3 to 5 days with an order not to reposition.

Q A Kehr's sign indicates the presence of which abdominal organ injury?

A Spleen

Symptoms of traumatic splenic injury include profound bleeding, positive Kehr's sign, Saegesser's sign, and Ballance's sign (Table 5.1).

Table 5.1 Signs of splenic injury

Saegesser's sign	Pain in the neck area because of irritation of the phrenic nerve
Kehr's sign	Pain radiates to the left scapula
Ballance's sign	Dullness over left flank

HINT

Pain associated with splenic injuries includes generalized abdominal pain with localized pain in the left upper quadrant (LUQ).

Q A patient presents in the trauma ICU with abdominal pain that worsens with movement and rebound tenderness. What is the most likely cause of the pain?

A Peritonitis

The symptoms of peritonitis include diffuse abdominal pain, rebound tenderness to board-like abdomen, which worsens with movement. Peritonitis frequently results from hollow organ rupture or spillage of bowel contents into the peritoneal cavity.

HINT

The Markel test is used to assess for peritonitis. Strike the patient's heel with a fist. If this elicits abdominal pain, it is a sign of peritonitis.

Q Which abdominal organ injury may lack peritoneal signs?

A Duodenum

Duodenal injuries frequently lack signs of peritonitis soon after trauma. This is because of the neutral to alkaline pH in the duodenum. The injury may produce abdominal pain and vomiting. After several days, the patient may develop leukocytosis and fever along with abdominal pain, indicating the presence of septic peritonitis.

HINT

A board-like abdomen indicates the presence of peritonitis.

COMPLICATIONS

Q Soon after blunt abdominal trauma and an exploratory laparotomy, the patient develops respiratory distress and bilateral fluffy infiltrates. What is the most likely complication?

A Abdominal compartment syndrome (ACS)

Intra-abdominal pressure (IAP) is a compartment pressure that can be monitored and measured. It is defined as a steady-state pressure concealed within the abdominal cavity. When the pressure increases in the abdominal cavity to the extent of causing organ dysfunction or failure, it is now known as *ACS*. ACS causes decreased tidal volume and increased ventilatory pressures leading to respiratory distress and bilateral fluffy infiltrates (Table 5.2).

Table 5.2 Three factors of abdominal compartment syndrome

Factors	Indications
Abdominal organ volume	Grossly swollen bowel (occupies several times the original space) Excessive crystalloid resuscitation
Presence of space-occupying substances (blood, ascites, tumor, free air)	Bleeding, leakage of abdominal contents, bowel edema Blood or blood clots
Abdominal wall compliance	Acute respiratory failure, abdominal surgery, major trauma/burns, prone positioning, central obesity

HINT

Closing an abdominal cavity after surgery can result in ACS with multiple complications, including acute respiratory distress, acute renal failure, dehiscence and evisceration of bowel, sepsis, and multiple organ failure (MOF).

Q What pressures can be monitored to assess for the presence of ACS?

A Bladder pressures

ACS monitoring is performed by the measurement of bladder pressure, which can be obtained through a Foley catheter. A normal IAP is approximately 5 to 7 mmHg, whereas the normal range in critically ill patients is from 5 to 15 mmHg of pressure. It is not uncommon to find a pressure of 15 to 20 mmHg in abdominal trauma patients or those with sepsis. ACS is defined as an IAP greater than 20 mmHg with organ involvement (Table 5.3).

Table 5.3 Grading intra-abdominal pressure

Grade	IAP
I	12 to 15 mmHg
II	16 to 20 mmHg
III	21 to 25 mmHg
IV	Greater than 25 mmHg

IAP, intra-abdominal pressure.

▶ **HINT**

IAP in morbidly obese patients often ranges from 9 to 14 mmHg.

Q What is the potential neurological complication of ACS?

A Increased ICP

There is a direct relationship between elevated IAP and ICP. The increased pressure is referred to the thoracic cavity from the abdominal region, increasing the thoracic pressure. This decreases the jugular venous drainage and increases the pressure within the cranium. This is very important in trauma patients with traumatic brain injuries.

▶ **HINT**

Refractory intracranial hypertension has been treated successfully using abdominal decompression or neuromuscular blocking agents (relaxes abdominal muscles thus lowering pressures).

Q What is the surgical management of ACS?

A Decompression

An excessively high IAP or progressive or refractory ACS typically requires a decompressive laparotomy. Many trauma surgeons leave the abdomen open following major laparotomies to prevent ACS.

▶ **HINT**

Surgical decompression of the abdomen frequently causes hypotension because the sudden perfusion of the mesenteric vascular bed.

Q Following a decompressive abdominal surgery, what type of wound coverage is recommended?

A Negative pressure dressing

Negative pressure systems control the abdominal contents, manage third-space fluids, and facilitate wound closure. Vacuum-assisted fascial closure (VAFC) systems provide constant tension on the abdominal wound edges, facilitating the ability to successfully perform a late fascial closure.

▶ **HINT**

The goal of temporary closure is to create a tension-free closure of the abdomen without elevating IAP.

Q What is a potential late complication of abdominal trauma involving the small intestines?

A Intestinal adhesions or obstruction

Internal scarring following abdominal surgery can result in intra-abdominal adhesions leading to obstruction (Box 5.2).

Box 5.2 Late complications of abdominal trauma

Peptic ulcers
Intestinal obstruction (adhesions or strictures)
Hernia (midline or ostomy sites)
Fistulas
Chronic abscesses
Cholelithiasis and cholecystitis

HINT

Duodenal fistulas cause acidosis secondary to loss of bicarbonate from pancreatic juices.

Q What is the major potential complication following a splenectomy that requires preventive management?

A Pneumococcal infections

A concern is an overwhelming postsplenectomy sepsis (OPSS), which can occur because of the loss of some immune responses. A large percentage of the OPSS occurs within 1-year postsplenectomy but can occur several years later. Pneumococcal infections are associated with high mortality following a splenectomy.

HINT

Before discharge, the vaccination Pneumovax needs to be given to a patient following a splenectomy.

Q What metabolic abnormality occurs with a draining fistula following stomach injury?

A Metabolic alkalosis

Fistulas that form after gastric injury repair cause metabolic alkalosis because of the loss of hydrogen chloride (HCL) and potassium (K+). The loss of gastric acids increases the pH.

HINT

Duodenal fistulas can cause metabolic acidosis secondary to loss of bicarbonate from pancreatic juices. Jejunal fistula produces low volumes of neutral pH fluid with little change in acid or base balance.

Q Which combination of abdominal organ injury has been found to increase mortality?

A Injury to both liver and colon

The combined intra-abdominal injuries of liver and colon have the highest mortality risk because of increased septic peritonitis. Intra-abdominal abscess formation occurs because of foreign-body fragments, necrotic tissue, blood, or bile remaining at site of injury. The combination of spillage of stool and blood clots leads to abdominal infections.

HINT

Postoperative fluid collections or abscesses can be drained by CT-guided placement of a catheter.

Q Which electrolyte abnormality commonly occurs following pancreatic injury?

A Hypocalcemia

Calcium is sequestered into the pancreas following an injury. Hypocalcemia presents with tetany, prolonged QT interval, and muscle cramping. Close monitoring of ionized calcium and treatment with calcium are important in the care of pancreatic trauma patients.

HINT

The life-threatening complication of hypocalcemia is torsades de pointes.

KNOWLEDGE CHECK: CHAPTER 5

1. Referring to the anatomy of the abdomen, what contains the stomach, small intestine, liver, gallbladder, transverse colon, sigmoid colon, upper third of rectum, part of the bladder, and the uterus?

   A. Peritoneal cavity
   B. Retroperitoneal space
   C. Splenic flexure
   D. Pleural space

2. Which of the following is a mechanism of injury to organs in blunt abdominal trauma?

   A. Entrapment between vertebral column and impacting forces
   B. Sudden decrease in uniform pressure
   C. Concussive injury
   D. Coup–contrecoup

3. A patient comes to the ED following a motorcycle collision. The patient was wearing a helmet and thrown from the bike about 10 ft. The patient just returned from receiving a CT scan of the head, neck, back, and abdomen. The results revealed a 2-cm liver laceration. The patient asks the nurse whether surgery is needed. What is the best response?

   A. "The liver laceration is 2 cm, it is categorized as a grade III, and most likely needs a surgical intervention."
   B. "The liver laceration is 2 cm, it is categorized as a grade I, and surgery is usually not warranted."
   C. "The liver laceration is 2 cm, it is categorized as a grade IV, and immediate surgery is needed."
   D. "The liver laceration is 2 cm, it is categorized as a grade II, and usually does not require surgery."

4. The nurse is assessing a patient with a blunt abdominal trauma injury. The patient has hypoactive bowel sounds, and abdominal pain. Blood pressure is 121/82 mmHg, heart rate is 99 beats per minute (bpm), respiratory rate is 20 breaths per minute with an oxygen saturation of 98% on 4 L via nasal cannula. What diagnostic study is the best choice with this clinical presentation?

   A. CT of the abdomen
   B. CT with intravenous contrast of the abdomen
   C. Diagnostic peritoneal lavage (DPL)
   D. CT with oral contrast of the abdomen

(See answers next page.)

1. A) Peritoneal cavity

The abdominal cavity is actually divided into the peritoneal cavity and the retroperitoneal space. These organs are present in the peritoneal cavity of the abdomen. The retroperitoneal space contains the duodenum, ascending colon, descending colon, kidneys, part of the bladder, pancreas, and major vessels. The pleural space is the thin, fluid-filled space between the visceral and parietal areas of each lung and does not contain any of these organs. The splenic flexor is not a compartment of the abdomen that contains organs.

2. A) Entrapment between vertebral column and impacting forces

Blunt abdominal trauma causes entrapment of organs between the vertebral column and the impacting forces. Solid organs commonly involved are the spleen, liver, and pancreas. The hollow organs, such as the stomach, tend to collapse with the increased pressure on the abdominal cavity. Blunt abdominal trauma causes a sudden increase (not decrease) in uniform pressure in abdominal cavity. Concussive injuries are usually a result of penetrating injury such as a gunshot wound or blast injury. Coup–contrecoup injuries are associated with brain injury, not abdominal trauma.

3. D) "The liver laceration is 2 cm, it is categorized as a grade II, and usually does not require surgery."

Liver injuries are scaled from grades I to VI. Lacerations that are 1 to 3 cm in length are categorized as grade II. Grades I to III are often successfully managed nonoperatively and through close observation. Lacerations less than 1 cm are categorized as a grade I, lacerations greater than 3 cm and deep into the parenchyma are categorized as a grade III. Grades IV to VI typically result in surgical management of the liver.

4. A) CT of the abdomen

CT is the most appropriate diagnostic study for the hemodynamically stable patient. CT of the abdomen with intravenous contrast aids in the diagnosis of active abdominal bleeding if the patient's presentation displays suspected abdominal bleeding. A plain CT of the abdomen would not show the vascular structures. Oral contrast CT scans reveal no significant benefit in the initial diagnosis and delay the treatment. DPL is a method used to detect intra-abdominal bleeding and is best utilized in the hemodynamically unstable patient.

5. The patient is currently in the ICU after being admitted yesterday with an abdominal injury. The original CT scan revealed abdominal bleeding. There is a repeat CT scan ordered for this morning. The patient was questioning why the test is being ordered so soon after the original scan. Which of the following rationales is the most accurate?

   A. A repeat CT scan evaluates ongoing bleeding.
   B. A repeat CT scan evaluates for a pseudoaneurysm.
   C. A repeat CT scan evaluates abdominal distention.
   D. A repeat CT scan evaluates stabilization of the injury.

6. A patient has suffered an abdominal gunshot wound. The abdomen is open and there is evisceration of abdominal contents. The nurse has secured an airway and cannulated two veins to infuse crystalloid solutions. How should the nurse address the abdominal wounds?

   A. Attempt to place abdominal contents back into the cavity.
   B. Place a sterile, moist dressing over the site.
   C. Irrigate the site and leave open.
   D. Place Vaseline gauze and cover with sterile dressing.

7. The focused assessment sonography for trauma (FAST) is a rapid, bedside examination that is most helpful when examining patients with hemodynamic instability. This is utilized to examine patients for which of the following?

   A. Small bowel obstruction
   B. Kidney contusion
   C. Colon laceration
   D. Intraperitoneal hemorrhage

8. A patient presented to the hospital with a blunt injury to the abdomen. The patient was admitted to the unit for close observation. Two days later, the patient spikes a fever of 102°F, has an elevated bilirubin level and a board-like abdomen, and is jaundiced. The nurse is highly suspicious of

   A. Liver failure
   B. Gallstones
   C. Sepsis
   D. Peritonitis

(*See answers next page.*)

5. D) A repeat CT scan evaluates stabilization of the injury.
Repeat or serial CT scans are usually ordered in patients with abdominal bleeding in order to evaluate the progression or stabilization of the bleeding, and to ensure a pseudoaneurysm does not develop. If a patient has abdominal distention, a CT scan may be warranted to evaluate the cause of the distention, but that is not a reason for serial or repeated CT scans in a patient with abdominal bleeding.

6. B) Place sterile, moist dressing over the site.
The nurse should never attempt to push abdominal contents back into the abdominal cavity; this increases the risk of infection. The care of the wound should be to place a sterile dressing over both the site and the intestines. Leaving it open to air causes drying and increases the risk of infection from exposure. Vaseline gauze is not recommended for the treatment of eviscerated intestines.

7. D) Intraperitoneal hemorrhage
FAST is indicated in trauma patients with suspected abdominal trauma. It allows evaluation of the chest, abdomen, and pelvis. It is used to identify intraperitoneal hemorrhage and is able to detect the presence of perisplenic fluid, perihepatic and hepatorenal space fluid, pericardial tamponade, and fluid that may be present in the pelvis. It is not used to evaluate the small bowel or colon for injuries. It is not able to identify a contusion.

8. D) Peritonitis
A delayed presentation of peritonitis is common with a duodenal tear because it spills alkaline fluid into the abdomen. The alkaline fluid causes less of an immediate irritation and delayed presentation of symptoms. Although patients in liver failure have an increased bilirubin level and jaundice, this typically does not occur within 2 days of the trauma. Gallstones are unlikely with this presentation of a trauma patient. The patient is febrile and has sepsis, but the source is more likely to be from peritonitis.

9. The American Association for the Surgery of Trauma (AAST) has developed a grading system for splenic injuries in order to guide proper treatment and interventions. What grade of splenic injury would involve a laceration of vessels producing devascularization to more than 25% of the spleen?

   A. Grade I
   B. Grade II
   C. Grade III
   D. Grade IV
   E. Grade V

10. Nonoperative management is the current standard of practice for patients who are hemodynamically stable with low-grade splenic injuries. Which of the following interventions would be considered the most important with this type of splenic injury?

   A. Bed rest
   B. Limited oral intake
   C. Serial hemoglobin (Hgb) and hematocrit (Hct) levels
   D. Repeat CT scan within 24 hours

(*See answers next page.*)

9. D) Grade IV

This would describe a grade IV splenic laceration. Grade I splenic injury includes a capsular tear less than 1 cm of parenchymal depth. Grade II is a 1- to 3-cm parenchymal injury without vessel involvement. Grade III is greater than 3-cm parenchymal depth or involvement of trabecular vessels. Grade V is a completely shattered spleen with devascularization. Grades I to III are less severe and are frequently managed with observation, not surgery.

10. C) Serial hemoglobin (Hgb) and hematocrit (Hct) levels

Serial Hgb and Hct lab work would identify bleeding, indicating need for follow-up radiographs or surgery. Current evidence reveals that routine follow-up CT scans can be omitted in stable patients with blunt splenic trauma because they do not change the course of management. Bed rest is typically indicated but monitoring for hemorrhage is most important. Limited oral intake would not be indicative in this situation.

Genitourinary Trauma

6

MECHANISM OF TRAUMA

Q What is the most common mechanism of injury for urethral injury?

A Straddle injury

Blunt mechanism usually results in posterior urethral injury. An example is a straddle injury, which occurs when the bulbous urethra is compressed against the symphysis pubis. Common causes are motorcycle collision, horseback-riding injuries, and bicycle injuries. Penetrating mechanism is secondary and includes gunshot wounds, stab wounds, self-instrumentation, and perineal impalement after falls.

HINT

Urethral damage is less common in women because the urethra is short, mobile, and protected by the symphysis pubis. There is a greater chance of injury in males because the urethra is longer and fixed by a ligament.

Q Are ureteral injuries more commonly a result of blunt or penetrating trauma?

A Penetrating

The most common cause for ureteral injury is penetrating trauma. A blunt mechanism of injury rarely causes ureter injuries. A severe deceleration mechanism may cause an avulsion of the ureter from the ureteropelvic junction.

HINT

Colon and bowel injuries commonly occur concomitant with ureter injuries.

Q What is the most common blunt mechanism of injury that causes bladder rupture?

A Seat belt injury

Seat belt injury in motor vehicle collisions (MVC) is the most common cause of a ruptured bladder and is frequently due to a full bladder. Compression of a full bladder by the lap belt during a sudden deceleration impact causes the dome of the bladder to rupture into the intraperitoneal space.

HINT

History of prior bladder surgery, irradiation, or malignancy may weaken the bladder and make the bladder more prone to rupture.

Q What injury may be associated with posterior urethral injuries?

A Pelvic fracture

Posterior urethral injuries may accompany pelvic fractures. Presence of a known pelvic fracture and blood at the meatus would be a significant red flag for the presence of urethral injury.

HINT

Remember, blood present at the meatus indicates that the trauma nurse should not attempt to insert an indwelling bladder catheter.

Q What type of genitourinary injury can occur with intercourse?

A Penile fracture

Penile fracture can occur with forceful bending of the erect penis during intercourse. Amputations of the penis or testicle can occur because of self-mutilation, assaults, and industrial trauma.

HINT

Blunt trauma to the scrotum can result in rupture of the testicles.

TRAUMATIC INJURIES

Q What traumatic injury is most commonly associated with extraperitoneal bladder rupture (EBR)?

A Pelvic fracture

The majority of EBR ruptures occur with pelvic fractures. A cystography is recommended in patients with pelvic fractures because of high association of bladder injuries.

HINT

Acetabular fractures are not commonly associated with bladder injuries.

Q Which kidney is most commonly injured in a trauma?

A Right kidney

The right kidney is the most frequently injured because of its lower position and less protection from the posterior rib cage. Increased injuries to the kidneys occur with a deceleration mechanism, back and flank trauma, or rib fractures.

HINT

Kidneys are well protected from trauma by the vertebral column, are surrounded by perirenal fat pads, capped by the adrenal glands, and protected anteriorly by abdominal viscera.

Q What is the most commonly injured structure within the renal system?

A Kidney

The kidney is the most commonly injured organ within the renal system. Blunt mechanisms of injury account for the majority of these injuries.

▶ HINT

Kidney damage can cause significant blood loss and a life-threatening injury. Avulsion of the renal artery and complete loss of blood flow to the kidney is called a *pedicle injury*.

Q Following a straddle injury, if the Buck's fascia remains intact, the ecchymosis is confined to which structure?

A Penis

The urethra is divided into the anterior and posterior compartments. The anterior urethra is composed of the bulbar and penile urethra. The narrowest portion of the urethra is the meatus. The posterior urethra is composed of prostatic and membranous urethra, and neurovascular erectile mechanism, which runs posterolateral and adjacent to the posterior urethra. If Buck's fascia is intact, the ecchymosis of urethral disruption is confined to the penis or perineum.

▶ HINT

Symptoms of urethral injury depend on whether the anterior or posterior urethra is injured in the trauma.

ASSESSMENT/DIAGNOSIS

Q What is a common finding that would require urological imaging to be performed?

A Hematuria

Gross hematuria requires a series of urological imaging to diagnose an injury to the renal system. Microscopic hematuria in the presence of hemodynamic instability should also be an indication for an evaluation. Gross hematuria is a cardinal sign of kidney and bladder injuries.

▶ HINT

Hematuria is not always present in all urological injuries but is an indication for a urological radiographic series.

Q What is the gold standard diagnostic study used to identify renal injury?

A CT scan

A CT scan is the gold standard for evaluating the renal system following blunt trauma. A CT scan can be used to identify injury to the kidneys and grade the severity of the injury (Table 6.1). A CT arteriogram and venogram may also be used to identify vascular injuries to the renal artery or renal vein. An MRI is equivalent to a CT in identifying and grading the severity of the renal injury. An MRI is more capable of differentiating an intrarenal hematoma from a perirenal hematoma.

Table 6.1 Renal injury scale

Grade I	Contusion	Microscopic or gross hematuria with normal urologic studies
Grade I	Hematoma	Subcapsular, nonexpanding without parenchymal laceration
Grade II	Hematoma	Nonexpanding perirenal hematoma confined to renal retroperitoneum
Grade II	Laceration	<1 cm parenchymal depth of renal cortex without extravasation
Grade III	Laceration	>1 cm parenchymal depth of renal cortex without collecting system rupture or urinary extravasation
Grade IV	Laceration	Parenchymal laceration extending through the renal cortex, medulla, and collecting system
Grade IV	Vascular	Main renal artery or vein injury with contained hemorrhage
Grade V	Laceration	Complete shattered kidney
Grade V	Vascular	Avulsion of renal hilum that devascularizes the kidney

HINT

Ultrasound has not been found to be accurate in identifying injuries of the renal system.

Q What diagnostic study is most frequently used to evaluate ureteral injuries?

A Intravenous pyelogram (IVP)

IVP is a diagnostic study used to view the kidneys, ureters, and bladder. Contrast dye is administered intravenously. Obtain consecutive x-rays to evaluate renal function; identify extravasation of dye from the kidneys, ureters, or bladder; and determine devitalized segments of the kidney or abnormal ureteral deviation. An IVP has a high false-negative rate in penetrating injuries and is not reliable for diagnosis in that population.

HINT

No single diagnostic test can be used to evaluate the renal system and an IVP may be combined with cystogram and CT scan.

Q What diagnostic study should be performed before cystogram if the patient presents with blood at the meatus?

A Retrograde urethrogram

A retrograde urethrogram is used to evaluate the urethra and diagnose urethral rupture by presence of extravasation of dye (Box 6.1). It may be performed before a cystogram to ensure the urethra is intact without injury before inserting a catheter into the bladder to perform the cystography.

Box 6.1 Indications for retrograde urethrogram

Straddle injury
Significant deceleration mechanism
Blood at meatus
High-riding prostate
Perineal butterfly hematoma
Scrotal or perineal crepitus
Inability to pass indwelling catheter

HINT

Although blood at the meatus and a high-riding prostate are commonly associated with urethral injury, the absence of such findings does not rule out the presence of urethral injury.

Q What is the diagnostic study that is best used to identify a bladder rupture?

A Cystogram

CT of the abdomen is inadequate to identify a bladder rupture. A cystogram is the most accurate diagnostic study and can be used to differentiate intraperitoneal bladder rupture (IBR) from an EBR. The normal bladder is shaped like a teardrop. It may appear distorted by the presence of a pelvic hematoma. Cystography is the most sensitive test for a submucosal tear of the bladder wall.

HINT

CT cystography is another option used to evaluate the integrity of the bladder and is about equal to a conventional cystography.

Q What is the diagnostic study of choice to identify urethral injuries?

A Retrograde urethrogram

A retrograde urethrogram is used to identify the presence of both anterior and posterior urethral injury. The presence of extravasation of dye indicates an injury.

HINT

It is also important to use the retrograde urethrogram to determine whether the injury is partial or complete.

MEDICAL/SURGICAL INTERVENTIONS

Q What is an indication for surgical management of kidney injury?

A Pedicle injury

A pedicle injury is the avulsion of the renal artery from the aorta, resulting in complete loss of blood flow to the kidney. The kidney is mobile in the retroperitoneum, and the main renal artery connected to the aorta undergoes excessive stretch, causing arterial injury. The injury may be an avulsion or rupture of the intimal layer, forming a thrombus, causing arterial occlusion and renal ischemia.

▶ HINT

Indications for surgical management also include ongoing hemorrhage, penetrating mechanism, and a pulsatile or expanding renal hematoma.

Q What is the nonoperative management of hematuria in a stable patient?

A Bed rest

For patients presenting with gross hematuria who are hemodynamically stable, bed rest may be ordered for 24 to 72 hours, or until hematuria is clearedin patients presenting with gross hematuria but are hemodynamically stable.

▶ HINT

Nonoperative management of renal trauma may include angiography and embolization to control bleeding.

Q What is the purpose of a stent being placed in the ureter following surgical repair?

A To maintain patency

A stent is placed in ureters to maintain alignment, ensure patency during healing, ensure tension-free anastomosis, and prevent urinary extravasation. Surgical management of ureteral injuries typically involves debridement and anastomosis of the ureters with the goal of watertight closures. If large segments of the ureters are damaged, a transureteroureterostomy can be performed, in which one ureter is anastomosed to the other.

▶ HINT

Extravasation of urine can cause the development of a uroma.

Q What is the most common nonoperative management of an EBR?

A Suprapubic catheter

A suprapubic catheter is placed to drain urine and allow the bladder to heal. The catheter is usually left in place for 7 to 10 days and then the bladder is reevaluated by cystogram for continued extravasation. If extravasation persists, the catheter may remain in place for another 7 to 10 days. The majority of bladder ruptures can be managed with catheter placement and drainage alone. IBR may require surgical repair, intraperitoneal irrigation, and catheter placement.

▶ HINT

An indication for surgical management EBR includes avulsion of the bladder, neck, or concomitant injury to vagina or rectum.

Q A complete injury of the anterior or posterior urethra typically requires what type of management?

A Placement of suprapubic catheter

Complete disruption of the anterior or posterior urethra is an indication for a suprapubic catheter to be placed for urinary diversion. The patient may undergo an observational period while the associated pelvic fracture and hematoma stabilize. Definitive management may include surgical repair or reconstructive procedure.

HINT

An incomplete injury may be managed with a urethral-placed catheter by a urologist.

NURSING INTERVENTIONS

Q What clinical finding would be a contraindication for the placement of an indwelling bladder catheter?

A Blood at the meatus

If blood is present at the meatus, under no circumstances should a Foley catheter be placed. Other contraindications to insertion of a bladder catheter include scrotal hematoma, perineal hematoma, or high-riding prostate.

HINT

If resistance is met with insertion of a bladder catheter, stop the insertion. If the bladder catheter is inserted without a urine return, do not inflate the balloon.

Q A patient presenting with hematuria and flank pain following an MVC may have experienced injury to which urological structure?

A Kidneys

A common presentation of kidney trauma is hematuria and flank pain. Hematuria is an important sign for injury to several of the urological structures, but, in combination with flank pain, it is more likely indicative of an injury to the kidneys.

HINT

Ureter injuries will not have hematuria in 20% to 45% of the cases.

Q The presence of vaginal bleeding following a straddle injury in a female may indicate what type of injury?

A Urethral injury

Although women are less likely to experience urethral injuries, the presence of vaginal bleeding, external genitalia, or significant incontinence in the presence of pelvic fractures should be a high suspicion of a urethral injury.

▶ HINT

Men are more likely to experience urethral injuries because they have longer urethras.

Q What type of bladder injury may present with an inability to void and acute abdominal signs?

A IBR

A complete rupture of the dome of the bladder results in extravasation of urine into the peritoneal cavity. The common presenting signs include an inability to void and acute abdominal signs such as abdominal pain or tenderness, fever, and peritoneal irritation. IBR is also associated with shock symptoms of hypotension and tachycardia (Table 6.2).

Table 6.2 Symptoms of intraperitoneal and extraperitoneal bladder rupture

Intraperitoneal Bladder Rupture	Extraperitoneal Bladder Rupture
Suprapubic tenderness	Pain with urination
Peritoneal irritation	Suprapubic tenderness
Ileus	Reddened suprapubic area
Inability to void	Necrosis of tissue suprapubic area
Hypotension	
Fever	
Abdominal pain	
Abdominal tenderness	

▶ HINT

EBR usually occurs at the lateral end or base of the bladder and is associated with pelvic fractures.

Q What is the triad of symptoms found in urethral injuries?

A Blood at meatus, inability to void, and distended palpable bladder

The classic triad of symptoms includes blood at meatus, inability to void, and distended palpable bladder (Table 6.3).

Table 6.3 Symptoms of anterior and posterior urethral injuries

Anterior Urethral Injury	Posterior Urethral Injuries
Perineal pain	Inability to void
Blood at meatus	Blood at meatus
Penile and perineal edema	Distended bladder
Distended bladder	Butterfly perineal bruising
Inability to void (occasionally be able to void)	High-riding prostate with rectal exam
Scrotum swelling	
Ecchymosis of scrotum	
Necrosis of scrotal tissue (late sign)	

HINT

The diagnostic test used to evaluate for presence of urethral injury is a retrograde urethrogram.

COMPLICATIONS

Q What is a complication of a delayed presentation of a ureter injury?

A Peritonitis

Delayed presentation appears as peritonitis. These symptoms include onset of fever, development of an ileus, abdominal mass, and hematuria, as well as an increase in serum creatinine levels (Box 6.2).

Box 6.2 Complications of ureteral injuries

Infection
Ureteral strictures
Urinary ascites
Uroma
Fistula formation with bowel

HINT

Delayed presentation injuries may be managed initially with endoscopic or interventional procedures followed by delayed surgical management.

Q What is the most common complication of urethral injury managed with a suprapubic catheter alone?

A Stricture formation

The placement of a suprapubic catheter alone without a urethral-placed bladder catheter has a high incidence of stricture formation in the urethra. This is typically managed with urethroplasty (Box 6.3).

Box 6.3 Complications of urethral injuries

Impotence
Strictures
Incontinence
Obstruction

KNOWLEDGE CHECK: CHAPTER 6

1. A patient arrives to the ED following a motor vehicle collision (MVC). The patient was restrained, and the airbag deployed. What injuries should the nurse suspect when a lap belt is utilized?

   A. Injuries to the colon and the bladder
   B. Injuries to the bladder and the pancreas
   C. Injuries to the stomach and the colon
   D. Injuries to the small intestine and the stomach

2. A patient has sustained a straddle injury after a horseback-riding accident. The patient is complaining of suprapubic pain and is unable to urinate. The nurse suspects a bladder injury and knows that treatment modalities differ according to the type of bladder injury. Which of the following diagnostic procedures would be most appropriate to diagnose a bladder injury?

   A. Pelvic x-ray
   B. CT cystography
   C. Bladder ultrasound
   D. Kidney, ureter, and bladder (KUB) x-ray

3. A patient came into the ED after a bicycle injury. The patient hit a curb, flew off the bike, and landed on their back. The patient complains of lower back pain and abdominal tenderness. Considering the method of injury, what would be the most probable injury sustained?

   A. Kidney rupture
   B. Acute tubular necrosis
   C. Hemorrhagic injury to the kidney
   D. Vascular damage to the renal artery

4. A patient was sitting on a glass table that broke, causing a penetrating injury to the pelvis. The basic metabolic panel results came back with blood urea nitrogen (BUN) = 26, creatinine level = 2.1 mg/dL, glucose = 99 mg/dL. A pyelogram is obtained, and results are pending. In the meantime, the patient becomes febrile and develops hematuria and a firm abdomen. The nurse suspects:

   A. Peritonitis
   B. Ureteral injury
   C. Kidney injury
   D. Sepsis

5. A 32-year-old male patient had a bicycle accident, landed on the crossbar, and sustained a straddle injury. He is experiencing an inability to void, blood at the meatus, and butterfly bruising to the scrotal area. These symptoms are expected with what type of injury?

   A. Medial urethral injury
   B. Anterior urethral injury
   C. Posterior urethral injury
   D. Injury at Buck's fascia

(See answers next page.)

1. A) Injuries to the colon and the bladder

The mechanism of injury is usually a crush injury of air-filled organs, such as the colon, and fluid-filled organs, such as the bladder. These are the most commonly injured organs from the use of a seat belt. The stomach is located higher in the abdominal cavity and injury is less likely to be caused by a seat belt injury. The pancreas is retroperitoneal and is less likely to be injured with a lap belt. The small intestines can be involved with sudden deceleration but is not typically involved with lap belt mechanism.

2. B) CT cystography

The classifications of bladder injuries include partial-thickness wall contusions, extraperitoneal rupture, and intraperitoneal rupture. The classification is made based on a retrograde cystography or CT cystography. A pelvic x-ray is used to recognize pelvis fractures but cannot identify bladder injuries. Bladder ultrasound and a KUB x-ray will not identify bladder injuries.

3. D) Vascular damage to the renal artery

Deceleration forces usually result in vascular damage to the renal artery. As there is minimal collateral circulation to the kidney, any type of ischemic injury could lead to tubular necrosis but would not be the immediate injury for this patient. Bleeding injuries would be more likely if there has been a deep penetrating injury to the site. Rupture of the kidney presents in a hemorrhagic shock state.

4. B) Ureteral injury

The presentation of the patient can be mistaken for peritonitis, but the correct answer is ureteral injury. The clue would be the hematuria, elevated creatinine, and taking into account the mechanism of injury. Ureteral injures are only present with hematuria about 40% of the time but are most common with penetrating-injury trauma patients. Kidney injury is possible but unlikely because there is no complaint of flank pain, and the mechanism of injury would not match. Renal injuries are usually caused by deceleration, not penetration. Sepsis is inconclusive because of the incomplete workup, lack of white blood cell (WBC) count, and lactic acid level.

5. C) Posterior urethral injury

Straddle injuries occur when the bulbous urethra is compressed against the symphysis pubis, and usually result in a posterior urethral injury. Posterior injuries present with blood at the meatus, inability to void, bladder distention, butterfly bruising, and a high prostate with rectal examination for male patients. Anterior urethral injuries present with perianal pain, blood at the meatus, perianal edema, scrotal swelling in male patients, cellulitis, and ecchymosis. Buck's fascia surrounds the anterior urethra, corporal bodies, and penile skin. A medial urethral injury is not medically recognized.

Obstetrical Trauma

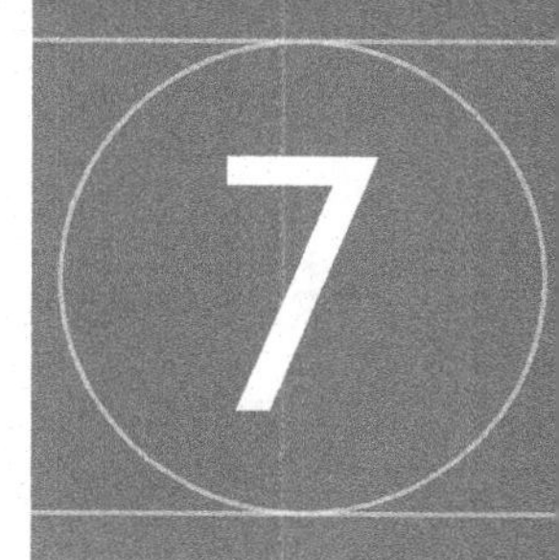

MECHANISM OF INJURY

Q What is the most common mechanism of injury for obstetrical trauma?

A Motor vehicle collision (MVC)

A frequent mechanism for trauma in pregnant patients is an MVC. As a driver of the vehicle, during impact, the steering wheel can cause damage to the gravid abdomen. Third trimester holds the greatest risk because of the enlarged abdomen being closer to the dash and steering wheel.

▶ HINT

Other mechanisms of injury in pregnant trauma patients include falls, domestic violence, and gunshot wounds.

Q Gait disturbances of a pregnant patients can lead to what type of traumatic injury?

A Falls

Falls may be common because of gait disturbances and altered balance. The relaxation of the pelvic girdle ligaments causes changes in balance. An increase in fatigue and risk of presyncopal and syncopal episodes in pregnant patients also contribute to falls.

▶ HINT

The enlarged uterus contributes to the imbalance and, as the pregnancy progresses through the trimesters, fall risks increase.

Q What is a significant risk of fetal death when a pregnant patients is in a house fire?

A Carbon monoxide poisoning

Burns and smoke inhalation during pregnancy can cause carbon monoxide poisoning, which can be fatal to the fetus. Carbon monoxide poisoning is most commonly associated with house fires. Battering and spousal abuse during pregnancy are other mechanisms of injury and the pregnancy may be the precipitating factor in some domestic violence cases.

▶ HINT

Fetal survival is directly related to gestational age.

TRAUMATIC INJURIES

Q What is a common genitourinary traumatic injury during the third trimester of pregnancy?

A Bladder rupture

The bladder is more elevated and compressed by the uterus in pregnant patients, therefore it is more likely to rupture with blunt force trauma. There is also an increase in glomerular filtration rate (GFR) and urinary frequency (Box 7.1).

Box 7.1 Genitourinary electrolyte abnormalities

Increased glomerular filtration rate
Glycosuria
Hypocalcemia
Hypophosphatemia
Hypomagnesemia
Decreased serum creatinine levels

HINT

Calcium, phosphate, and magnesium levels may decrease during pregnancy and require monitoring following a trauma.

Q What is the most common maternal injury that results in fetal death?

A Pelvic fracture

Maternal pelvic fractures carry the highest risk for fetal death. The fetal death may be caused by several different mechanisms of injury, including direct fetal injury, placental abruption, and maternal shock.

HINT

Pregnant patients are at an increased risk for hemorrhage following pelvic fractures due to vascular dilation in the pelvic region.

Q What organ is frequently injured in blunt trauma to the abdomen during the third trimester?

A Uterus

During the third trimester, the uterus is located in the abdomen. Abdominal trauma will likely damage the uterus due to the size and location during the third trimester.

ASSESSMENT/DIAGNOSIS

Q What information would be important when obtaining a history of a pregnant trauma patient?

A Gestational age of the fetus

When obtaining a medical history in a pregnant patients following a trauma, the following information should be included: gestational age, status of pregnancy, parity, maternal Rh factor, and delivery history. The trauma nurse should determine whether the patient has had a previous cesarean section (C-section), which may direct the delivery, if necessary.

▶ HINT

The trauma nurse should also question the pregnant trauma patient regarding history of any previous abortions or premature deliveries.

Q What is a common respiratory physiological change that results in hypocarbia?

A Chronic hyperventilation

Pregnant patients commonly have $PaCO_2$ levels of 25 to 30 mmHg with chronically compensated respiratory alkalosis because of chronic hyperventilation. This must be taken into account when interpreting the arterial blood gas (ABG). Normal respiratory changes with pregnancy include a chronic state of hyperventilation, increased tidal volumes by as much as 40%, and increases in vital capacity by 100 mL to 200 mL (Box 7.2).

Box 7.2 Normal respiratory changes in pregnancy

Tachypnea
Hypocarbia
Increased tidal volume
Increased vital capacity
Elevated diaphragm
Elevated PaO_2
Decreased functional residual capacity

▶ HINT

Normal physiological changes that occur during pregnancy can affect the assessment, interventions, and outcomes during a trauma.

Q What changes occur with the circulating blood volume in pregnant patients?

A Increased blood volume

Normal cardiovascular change with pregnancy includes hypervolemia. The blood volume increases by the 10th week, with an increase of as much as 50% by the 34th week of pregnancy. Acute blood loss can lead to a decrease in perfusion to the uterus and fetus (Box 7.3).

Box 7.3 Cardiovascular changes in pregnant patients

Hypervolemia
Tachycardia
Left-axis deviation
T-wave flattening or T-wave inversion
Elevated ST segments
Q-waves
S3 gallop

HINT

The normal hypervolemic state during pregnancy can mask a 30% gradual blood loss or 10% to 15% acute blood loss. Signs of hypovolemia (tachycardia and hypotension) may be delayed in a pregnant trauma patient.

HINT

Heart rate can increase by 15 to 20 beats per minute (bpm) by the second trimester of pregnancy; therefore, if the heart rate in a pregnant trauma patient reaches 70 bpm, this is considered to be bradycardia.

Q What is the assessment technique used to evaluate the fetus in a trauma patient?

A Fetal heart tones (FHTs)

Following a trauma, the pregnant patients should have FHT assessed to identify fetal distress. FHTs are audible with Doppler by weeks 10 to 12. A normal FHT is 120 to 160 bpm, and rates more than 160 bpm or less than 120 bpm are signs of distress. FHT is the fifth vital sign in pregnancy. FHT should be continuously monitored if fetus greater than 23 weeks' gestation. If under 23 weeks' gestation, a brief assessment of fetal viability is adequate. Continuous cardiotocographic monitoring is recommended following a trauma or the presence of meconium.

HINT

Fetal tachycardia progressing to bradycardia suggests fetal anoxia.

Q What is the purpose of palpating the abdomen of the pregnant trauma patient when assessing the fetus?

A To assess fundal height

The uterus is palpable between weeks 12 and 14 and is located at the top of the umbilicus between weeks 18 and 22. A palpated fundal height is used to determine gestational age in weeks of the fetus. Fundal height is measured by determining the distance from the symphysis pubis to the top of the uterus.

▶ HINT

Fundal height that is higher than the expected gestational age may indicate an abruptio placentae or uterine rupture.

Q What is the diagnostic study used to identify an abruptio placentae?

A Ultrasound

Abdominal ultrasound is used to assist with the diagnosis of an abruptio placentae. It is not 100% sensitive, but in combination with vaginal bleeding, it can be used to assist with the diagnosis (Box 7.4).

Box 7.4 Role of ultrasound in pregnant trauma patients

Determination of gestational age
Determination of fetal cardiac rate and rhythm
Localization of placenta to determine presence of abruptio placentae
Assessment of amniotic fluid volume
Fetal well-being
Determine fetal injury
Identifying fetal demise

▶ HINT

Dark red vaginal bleeding is a cardinal sign of an abruptio placentae.

Q What is a sign of imminent delivery in a pregnant patient?

A Crowning

Crowning occurs when the fetus's head is visible upon vaginal assessment during contraction. If the delivery is imminent, emergency medical services (EMS) will deliver before transport. The visual assessment of the vagina should be done if the contractions are less than 5 minutes apart or the patient is experiencing the urge to push.

▶ HINT

Nonobstetric staff should not perform a digital exam to gauge cervical dilation.

MEDICAL/SURGICAL INTERVENTIONS

Q Following a fatal MVC, when should a C-section be performed?

A During cardiopulmonary resuscitation (CPR)

Perimortem C-section is determined by the gestational age and duration of maternal arrest. A viable fetus is above 23 to 28 weeks' gestational age and it should be performed within 4 to 5 minutes of the cardiac arrest. The C-section should be performed while CPR is in progress.

Q What is different about placing a chest tube on a pregnant trauma patient?

A The tube is placed 1 to 2 intercostal spaces (ICSs) higher

The uterus becomes an abdominal organ in the third trimester, which elevates the diaphragm. This requires a chest tube to be placed at 1 to 2 ICSs higher than normal placement.

Q What is the primary issue with administering vasoactive medications to a pregnant patient?

A Placental hypoperfusion

The uretoplacental vasculature is highly sensitive to vasopressors and will lead to decreased placental perfusion and fetal demise.

HINT

Pregnant trauma patients should receive fluid resuscitation primarily to increase the blood pressure (BP) and avoid vasopressors if possible.

Q Which is the priority of care when managing a pregnant trauma patient, mother or fetus?

A Mother

Maternal well-being is the priority of care over interventions for the fetus. Interventions to save the mother will often improve the survivability of the fetus.

Q What is the rapid intervention required for abruptio placentae to improve fetal survivability?

A C-section

Prompt recognition and immediate C-section will improve survivability of the fetus following abruptio placentae. C-section is recommended in maternal instability or fetal compromise. Abruption may follow after even a minor trauma and should be monitored for closely. If the patient is stable, a vaginal delivery may be attempted.

HINT

In situations of fetal demise, vaginal delivery is the preferred method of delivery.

NURSING INTERVENTIONS

Q In what position should the trauma nurse place the pregnant trauma patient while lying on the stretcher?

A Tilted to the left side

If a pregnant patients in the third trimester is lying supine, the enlarged uterus compresses the vena cava and aorta, impeding venous return and cardiac output. The pregnant trauma patient should be tilted to her left side while maintaining spine precautions.

▶ HINT

Placing a pregnant patient supine can result in hypotension.

Q When obtaining x-rays on a pregnant trauma patient, what should the nurse do?

A Place a lead apron over patient's abdomen

When obtaining radiographic studies on a pregnant trauma patient, shield the uterus with a lead apron. This decreases the radiation exposure of the fetus.

▶ HINT

The use of MRI is preferred to CT when evaluating a pregnant trauma patient because of the exposure of radiation with CT scans.

Q In what position would the trauma nurse place the pregnant patient with a prolapsed cord?

A Trendelenburg's position with knee–chest position

If a cord prolapse is present following a trauma, relieve cord compression by placing the patient in Trendelenburg's position with knee–chest position, if the mother's injuries allow.

▶ HINT

In a fetus with a prolapsed cord, insert a gloved hand into the vagina and cradle the cord in the palm of the hand with the fingertips elevating the fetus.

Q When delivery is imminent, in a fetus presenting in normal head-down position, what body part is most likely to become obstructed?

A Shoulder

Shoulder dystocia occurs when the shoulders obstruct preventing the delivery. Once the shoulders are delivered, the rest of the body will quickly follow (Box 7.5).

Box 7.5 Potential complications of imminent delivery

- Breech position
- Shoulder dystocia
- Excessive bleeding pre- and postdelivery
- Prolapsed cord

▶ HINT

Never pull the infant out. This can damage sinal nerves.

Q What method is used to clear the airway of a newborn infant?

A Suction the infant's mouth

Suctioning the infant's mouth and sometimes nose will assist with clearing the airway immediately after birth. After birth, keep the infant at the vagina to prevent under or over transfusion. Clamp the cord in two places about 6 to 8 inches from the abdomen and cut the cord in between the clamps.

▶ HINT

Do not milk the cord.

COMPLICATIONS

Q Because of the relaxation of the gastroesophageal sphincter during advanced pregnancy, what is a potential complication of pregnant patients?

A Aspiration

Pregnant patients experience relaxation of the gastroesophageal sphincter, delayed gastric emptying, and ileus, which can all contribute to vomiting and aspiration. Abdominal palpation assessing for tenderness is not reliable in the pregnant patient as abdominal guarding, tenderness, and rigidity are normal findings.

▶ HINT

Assume that the pregnant patient has a full stomach and is at risk for vomiting and aspiration. Placement of a nasogastric (NG) tube is recommended.

Q Immobilization of a pregnant trauma patient places the patient at a high risk for what complication?

A Thromboembolic event

Fibrinogen and factors VI, VIII, and IX increase during pregnancy, whereas circulating plasminogen levels decrease. This increases the risk of thromboembolism with immobilization. Coagulation studies do not typically change during pregnancy.

▶ HINT

Anemia can occur during pregnancy because erythrocyte production may not be maintained during pregnancy.

Q A pregnant trauma patient is complaining of a headache and is noted to be hypertensive. What is the most likely complication of the pregnancy?

A Preeclampsia

Obstetric complications, such as eclampsia or preeclampsia, may present as changes in vision, headache, hypertension, edema, proteinuria, and seizure activity. Preeclampsia involves gestational hypertension, which is defined as a systolic BP greater than 140 mmHg or diastolic BP greater than 90 mmHg. The difference between preeclampsia and eclampsia is the presence of seizures in the latter (Box 7.6).

Box 7.6 Symptoms of preeclampsia

Hypertension
Headache
Edema of hands, face, and sacrum
Visual changes
Nausea
Abdominal pain
Proteinuria
Albuminuria
Elevated creatinine and BUN
Decrease urine output

BUN, blood urea nitrogen.

▶ HINT

The most severe form of eclampsia is called the *HELLP syndrome*: *H*emolysis, *E*levated *L*iver enzymes, *L*ow *P*latelets.

▶ HINT

A complication of preeclampsia is acute kidney injury.

Q The mother reports no fetal movement after a traumatic injury. What would that indicate?

A Fetal demise

No fetal movement following a trauma indicates fetal demise. FHT and ultrasound can be used to determine presence of fetal heart activity and determine viability of the fetus.

▶ HINT

Premature labor may indicate fetal injury or demise.

Q Differentiation of amniotic fluid and urine can be determined by testing the fluid for what?

A pH

Following a trauma and suspected premature rupture of membranes (PROM), differentiation of amniotic fluid from urine may be determined by checking the pH of the fluid. Amniotic fluid has a pH of 7.0 to 7.5, whereas urine is more acidic and has a pH of 4.8 to 6.0. The physician may check the fluid for ferning appearance under a microscope.

▶ HINT

Evidence of fluid pooling in the vagina, or leaking from the cervical os when the patient coughs, or when fundal pressure is applied, will help determine PROM.

Q A pregnant trauma patient is admitted for PROM. After 2 days, the patient exhibits an elevated white blood cell (WBC) count and fever. What is the most likely cause?

A Amniotitis

Amniotitis is an infection of the amniotic membranes following PROM. Signs of amniotitis include elevated WBC, maternal tachycardia, tender uterus, temperatures higher than 101°F or 38°C, and fetal tachycardia.

▶ HINT

Elevated WBC and fever indicate infection; the hint in the previous question is the reference to PROM.

Q What would be a sign of premature labor following a trauma?

A Bloody show with ruptured membranes

The trauma nurse needs to recognize signs of labor that include a bloody show, ruptured membrane, and increased frequency of contractions. Following a trauma, the fetus is assessed for viability and injuries before the premature labor is stopped. If the fetus is found to be viable, labor can be inhibited with medications such as tocolytics (ritodrine hydrochloride, magnesium sulfate).

▶ HINT

When timing frequency of contractions during labor, they are timed from beginning of one to the beginning of the next.

Q What is a predominant sign of an abruptio placentae in a pregnant trauma patient?

A Vaginal bleeding

Abruptio placentae occurs when the placenta separates or pulls away from the uterine wall, causing disruption of maternal–fetal circulation. An abruptio placentae most commonly occurs within 2 to 6 hours after the initial trauma and almost all occur within 24 hours. Early recognitionof an abruptio placentae and treatment will increase the chance of survival for the fetus (Box 7.7).

Box 7.7 Signs of abruptio placentae

Vaginal bleeding
Premature labor
Abdominal pains
Expanding fundal height
Maternal shock
Fetal distress
Uterine rigidity

HINT

If the tissue covers the os following the abrupto placentae, there may not be vaginal bleeding.

Q What complication has a high maternal mortality and almost universal fetal mortality?

A Uterine rupture

Uterine rupture is rare but is associated with a high risk of maternal death and almost universal fetal death. Uterine ruptures involve the fundus portion of the uterus. The severity can vary (Box 7.8).

Box 7.8 Signs of uterine rupture

Maternal shock
Abdominal distension
Irregular uterine contour
Palpable fetal parts
Abnormal FHTs/fetal distress
Abdominal rigidity

FHTs, fetal heart tones.

Q What laboratory finding is the most specific to disseminated intravascular coagulation (DIC)?

A Elevated D-dimer

DIC is a potential complication with pregnant trauma patients. It presents with abnormal bleeding, bruising, petechiae, and organ dysfunction. The laboratory findings include an elevated prothrombin time/partial thromboplastin time (PT/PTT), decreased fibrinogen, decreased platelets, and increased D-dimer. There are many coagulopathies that will elevate the coagulation times and decrease the platelets, but DIC is the only coagulopathy that will elevate the D-dimer. The D-dimer measures the by-product of a clot.

▶ HINT

DIC is the only coagulopathy that causes the body to clot first and bleed second.

Q Direct fetal injury can occur with maternal blunt abdominal trauma. What parts of the fetus are more likely injured?

A Skull and brain

Direct fetal injury is rare. It can occur with blunt maternal abdominal trauma and most often involves the fetus' skull and brain. Deceleration injuries can be the mechanism of injury. Penetrating injuries to the abdomen can cause direct fetal injury because in late gestation, the uterus is in the abdominal cavity. In this situation, the fetus is more likely to die than the mother.

▶ HINT

If pelvic fracture occurs when the fetus's head is engaged in the pelvic canal, it can crush the skull of the fetus.

Q An antigen–antibody reaction can occur if the mother is Rh negative or positive?

A Negative

Antigen–antibody reaction can occur if the mother is Rh negative. When the fetus is Rh positive and the mother is Rh negative, the mother is at risk for an antigen–antibody reaction from the mixing of fetal–maternal blood, causing a thrombolytic reaction. Kleihauer–Betke (KB) assay blood test can detect fetal blood cells in maternal circulation and can quantify the amount. Even minor trauma can causes sensitization of maternal–fetal hemorrhage.

▶ HINT

Anti-D immunoglobulin G (IgG) needs to be given within 72 hours of trauma if the mother is Rh negative.

KNOWLEDGE CHECK: CHAPTER 7

1. Which of the following is the physiological reason a pregnant patients is commonly involved in falls?

   A. They have more syncopal episodes.
   B. The pelvic girdle ligaments relax and develop a wide-stance gait.
   C. They experience bradycardic episodes.
   D. They experience transient ischemic attacks (TIA).

2. What mechanism of injury typically has the lowest mortality rate in the pregnant patient subjected to trauma?

   A. Gunshot wound
   B. Stab wound
   C. Motor vehicle collision
   D. Fall

3. A 28-week pregnant patient comes in after being involved in a severe motor vehicle collision (MVC). The patient has shallow breathing, blood pressure of 89/48 mmHg, a heart rate of 52 beats per minute (bpm), and is currently being intubated. The patient loses a palpable pulse, and cardiopulmonary resuscitation (CPR) efforts are being initiated. Which of the following is a priority of care at this time?

   A. Assessment of fetal heart tones (FHT)
   B. Vaginal examination and an assessment for vaginal bleeding
   C. Emergency cesarean section (C-section) within 5 minutes of cardiac arrest
   D. Ultrasound for gestational age

4. When a pregnant patient presents with a blood pressure of 90/72 mmHg, what should be the first nursing intervention to address the situation?

   A. Repeat the blood pressure measurement.
   B. Place the patient in reverse Trendelenburg position.
   C. Assess the patient for symptomatic hypotension.
   D. Place the patient on her left lateral side.

5. A 22-year-old pregnant patient in their third trimester has arrived at the ED in respiratory distress. The patient was eating pistachios and got a shell lodged in their trachea. The shell was successfully retrieved and the patient is currently complaining of a sore throat and cough. An arterial blood gas (ABG) is collected and the results are pH = 7.36, PaO_2 = 104 mmHg, SaO_2 = 95%, $PaCO_2$ = 30. Which of the following is the most correct interpretation of this ABG?

   A. Mild compensating respiratory acidosis
   B. Normal
   C. Compensated metabolic acidosis
   D. Respiratory alkalosis

(*See answers next page.*)

1. B) The pelvic girdle ligaments relax and develop a wide-stance gait.
Pregnant patients are at an increased risk for falls because they experience increased fatigue, relaxation of the pelvic girdle ligaments, altered balance, and gait disturbances. These cause balance issues, and an enlarged uterus with a growing belly shifts the body's center of gravity forward, making it even harder to stay upright. Syncopal episodes, bradycardia, and TIA are not common reasons for falling and may be a complication.

2. D) Fall
Falls are the second leading cause of injury during pregnancy. Motor vehicle collision is the number one cause of death in pregnant patients. Penetrating injuries cause trauma to the pregnant patient, with gunshot wounds having a higher mortality rate than stab wounds.

3. C) Emergency cesarean section (C-section) within 5 minutes of cardiac arrest
Emergency C-section needs to be initiated within 5 minutes to improve survival of both the mother and fetus, and resuscitation measures need to be continued throughout the C-section. FHT, ultrasound, and vaginal examinations are important assessments of the fetus but the delay would affect outcomes of both the fetus and mother.

4. D) Place the patient on her left lateral side.
Positioning the patient on the left lateral side increases circulation because it keeps the uterus off the vena cava, and allows for improved blood return and cardiac output, as well as flow to the fetus, uterus, and kidneys. The nurse may repeat the blood pressure, but it would be more effective if the nurse positioned the patient, and then repeated the blood pressure. Placing the patient in reverse Trendelenburg position increases the blood pressure in nonpregnant patients but placing on the left side promotes increased venous return in a pregnant patient. Even if the patient is not symptomatic of hypotension, left-side positioning increases needed circulation and perfusion.

5. B) Normal
These are normal ABG readings for a pregnant patient. Normal parameters for pregnant patients are pH of 7.35 to 7.45, PaO_2 of 101 mmHg to 104 mmHg, SaO_2 greater than 95%, $PaCO_2$ of 25 mmHg to 35 mmHg.

PART III

Clinical Practice: Extremity and Wound

Musculoskeletal Trauma

8

MECHANISM OF INJURY

Q What type of vertebral fractures can occur when people jump from a significant height and land on their feet?

A Compression fractures

Compression fractures of the lumbar spine frequently occur when people fall or jump on their feet from significant heights. A common triad of fractures occurs with these types of falls that include calcaneus, thoracolumbar, and bilateral wrist fractures. The triad is caused by the person landing on their feet (calcaneus fracture), the force causing compression fractures in the thoracolumbar spine, and the person falling forward on their wrists (bilateral wrist fractures).

▶ HINT

A direct impact on the top of the head can also cause compression fractures of the cervical spine and is called *axial loading*.

Q A motor vehicle/pedestrian collision causes a typical pattern of injury. What is this called?

A Waddell's triad

Motor vehicle/pedestrian injury commonly presents with a pattern of injury called *Waddell's triad*. The three injuries include bilateral femur fractures, blunt chest injury, and traumatic brain injury. This is classic with children who turn to face the approaching vehicle. The impact of the vehicle bumper occurs at the level of the femur (bilateral femur fractures), the child is thrown onto the hood of the vehicle (chest trauma), and then continues to fall off the car, landing on the head (traumatic brain injury).

▶ HINT

Adult motor vehicle/pedestrian collisions may have a slightly different pattern of injury as adults will commonly turn to avoid being hit by the vehicle.

Q Where is the most common point of impact on the dash in a seat-belted front-seat passenger during head-on collision?

A Bilateral knees

A front-seat passenger in a motor vehicle collision (MVC) may sustain injury to bilateral knees from the impact of the dashboard, and hip fractures or posterior dislocations may be caused by the posterior directional force.

▶ HINT

If the passenger is not restrained with a shoulder harness, then the face is typically the point of impact is typically the face hitting the dashboard.

Q A history of frequent fractures or various stages of healing fractures may indicate what in pediatric patients?

A Child abuse

History of multiple fractures and ED visits, or various stages of healing fractures, in children may be a sign of child abuse and should be further investigated. At ages 2 years and younger, ribs are very bendable and less likely to fracture, therefore rib fractures in children younger than 2 years indicate a significant force and should create a high suspicion of child abuse. Spiral fractures are a result of a "twisting" mechanism and are uncommon unintentional injuries in young children. A simple fall does not cause spiral fracture in children. A corner fracture or bucket handle fracture in a child is also especially predictive of child abuse as these occur with intentional injury.

▶ HINT

A *corner fracture* is a piece of bone avulsed from the fragile growth plate caused by a shearing mechanism, whereas a *bucket fracture* is similar but involves a larger piece of avulsed bone.

Q What is a common fracture that occurs in an older adult person following a fall?

A Femoral neck fracture

Fractures of the femoral neck are common in older adult patients. With osteoporosis, the older adult patient's bones may actually fracture during ambulation causing the fall versus the fracture being the result of the fall itself.

▶ HINT

The comorbidities of osteoporosis and osteoarthritis in older adult patients increase their risk of fractures.

Q What type of amputation involves a cut with well-defined edges?

A Guillotine

An amputation caused by a cut or guillotine type of mechanism has well-defined edges and is easier to reimplant. Crush injuries causing an amputation result in soft-tissue damage and are less likely to be able to be reimplanted. A forceful stretching and tearing away of the tissue causing an amputation is called an *avulsion injury*.

▶ HINT

A clean guillotine amputation has the most success of reimplantation.

TRAUMATIC INJURIES

Q What type of fracture results in a great amount of nerve and vascular injury?

A Displaced fracture

Bone disruption or displacement following an injury can result in injury to surrounding tissue, nerves, and blood supply. Trauma to the surrounding structures and bone can be caused by both blunt and penetrating injuries.

HINT

Musculoskeletal trauma includes injuries to bone, joints, muscle, ligaments, nerves, and blood vessels.

Q What type of injury may have occurred when there is a laceration over the site of the fracture?

A Open fracture

An open fracture occurs when the skin integrity over or near the fracture is open; this is typically a complete fracture. The bone may or may not be protruding from the wound. An incomplete fracture occurs when the bone integrity is not completely disrupted. Open fractures are graded in severity (Table 8.1).

Table 8.1 Grade of open fracture

Grade	Description
Grade I	Minimal soft-tissue damage
Grade II	Wounds >2 cm with a crush injury
Grade III	Associated with extensive tissue damage

HINT

The trauma nurse should consider any lacerations or open wounds in the vicinity of the fracture an open fracture.

HINT

Grade III open fractures have a large amount of wound contamination and are associated frequently with nonviable tissue.

Q What is the name of the fracture when the bone bends and the fracture is an incomplete fracture?

A Greenstick fracture

A greenstick fracture occurs when the bone bends and the fracture is incomplete. A comminuted fracture refers to the splintering of bone into multiple pieces following a blunt injury. In a displacement fracture there is a lack of alignment of the ends of the bones; an impaction injury occurs when the bones are wedged into each other.

> **HINT**
>
> **Greenstick fractures are more likely found in pediatric trauma patients than adults.**

Q What is the systemic response to a fat emboli called?

A Fat embolism syndrome

Fat embolism is the presence of fat particles within the microcirculation. Fat embolism syndrome is the systemic response and manifestation of fat embolism. Large numbers of patients with long-bone fractures have fat globules present in the blood, but only a few have symptoms of fat embolism.

> **HINT**
>
> **Symptoms of fat embolism syndrome are similar to a pulmonary embolism and can be indistinguishable from acute respiratory distress syndrome.**

ASSESSMENT/DIAGNOSIS

Q What would a low ankle–brachial index (ABI) indicate following a lower limb traumatic injury?

A Decrease perfusion

ABI measures the systolic blood pressure (SBP) in the ankles and is divided by the SBP in the brachial area. An ABI of 1 is normal, whereas an ABI of less than 0.9 indicates occlusive disease, and an ABI of less than 0.45 indicates significant decrease in blood flow.

Q When assessing an extremity following a fracture, the nurse notes the patient has paresthesia. What type of injury is associated with the fracture?

A Nerve injury

Both motor and sensory abnormalities should be assessed following an extremity injury. The neurovascular examination of an extremity includes the five Ps: pain, pallor, pulseless, paresthesia, and paralysis. Of the five Ps, pain, paresthesia, and paralysis correlate to nerve injury, whereas pallor and pulselessness are used to assess arterial supply distal to the site of injury.

> **HINT**
>
> **A nerve that is lacerated or that has sustained significant injury may cause a loss of sensation to the affected extremity distal to the site of injury.**

Q An abnormal externally rotated leg may indicate what type of fracture?

A Pelvic fracture

Pelvic fractures can be a result of external rotation, lateral compression, abduction, and shearing forces. The trauma nurse should have a high suspicion for a pelvic fracture if the trauma patient has an abnormal rotation of a leg, especially an externally rotated leg.

▶ HINT

If a patient has sustained a pelvic fracture, the trauma nurse should assess for associated injuries such as blood at the meatus (renal trauma) and hemodynamic instability (hemorrhage in the pelvic region).

Q When performing an extremity assessment on a trauma patient, to what should the trauma nurse compare the affected extremity?

A The unaffected extremity

The trauma nurse should compare the affected extremity to the unaffected when performing assessment of the color, pulse, length of limb, sensory abnormalities, and function. When assessing the trauma patient, note whether the patient has full range of motion in all extremities unless contraindicated.

▶ HINT

Palpate pulses proximal and distal and compare the pulses to the opposite side for strength and quality.

Q What is the bedside assessment that can be performed to assess for the stability of a pelvis?

A Press the iliac crests together

To assess for pelvic fractures and pelvic stability, the trauma nurse may press the iliac crests toward the midline noting any instability or increased pain. An unstable pelvic fracture exists when there is a fracture in more than one place of the pelvic ring, resulting in displacements on the ring.

▶ HINT

Never "rock" a pelvis if an injury is suspected. This may cause further damage to the internal structures.

Q What initial diagnostic studyis used to identify fractures?

A Radiographs

Radiographs are used to identify fractures following extremity trauma. Recommended radiographs of an extremity should be of at least two views because a fracture may not be seen with just a single view. Common views obtained to identify a fracture are anterior–posterior and lateral views. An arteriogram should be obtained if there is a suspected injury to the vasculature with an extremity injury. A duplex Doppler ultrasonography may be used as an alternative to an angiogram and can be performed in the ED.

▶ HINT

Crepitus noted during palpation of an extremity indicates the possibility of an underlying fracture and a radiograph should be obtained.

Q What monitoring should be used in patients with suspected pulmonary embolism?

A Oxygen saturation

The use of continuous oxygen saturation monitoring is recommended to identify periods of transient hypoxia following a long-bone fracture because of fat embolism. Clinical symptoms of fat embolism include hypoxia, tachycardia, tachypnea, dyspnea, fever, and chest pain.

▶ HINT

Hypoxia as a result of a fat embolism is refractory to high levels of FiO_2 (fraction of inspired oxygen) and decreases lung compliance as a result of intrapulmonary shunting.

Q What is the clinical symptom of a fat embolism that can be used to distinguish fat embolism from a pulmonary embolism?

A Petechiae

The appearance of petechiae on the upper trunk, axilla, chest, conjunctiva, and mucous membranes is a hallmark sign of a fat embolism and is present in about 50% of the cases. There is no specific test to diagnose fat embolism.

▶ HINT

This petechial rash usually resolves within 24 hours of the fat embolism syndrome.

Q What is considered to be the hallmark of compartment syndrome?

A Pain that cannot be controlled with pain medications

Pain that goes beyond pain medications is a hallmark sign of compartment syndrome, whereas pain on passive movement is an early sign of compartment syndrome. Pain on passive movement is assessed by moving the distal portion of the extremity and determining the presence of pain (e.g., calf injury can be assessed by the examiner moving the foot up and down).

▶ HINT

Compartment syndrome can produce pain beyond pain medications, paresthesia, and paralysis (or weakness of the involved extremity) early in the presentation.

Q What finding on assessment of an extremity at risk for compartment syndrome would indicate irreversible tissue injury?

A Loss of a pulse

Pulses and capillary refill remain intact in the presence of compartment syndrome because it involves the collapse of arterioles and veins, not the major arteries. In compartment syndrome, once a pulse is lost, it is too late to salvage the extremity because of irreversible tissue damage.

▶ HINT

A presentation of compartment syndrome may include a decrease in the sensation of the affected extremity because of the damage of the nerves within the fascial compartment; this is an earlier sign than a loss of a pulse.

Q What is considered a normal compartmental pressure in an extremity?

A 10 mmHg

Compartment pressures in the extremeties can be measured in patients suspected of experiencing compartment syndrome. A normal compartment pressure is 10 mmHg. A compartmental pressure greater than 30 mmHg requires a surgical open fasciotomy to relieve the pressure.

HINT

The physical examination may be primarily used to recognize compartment syndrome.

Q Compartment syndrome in the forearm and wrist can be assessed by asking the patient to perform what movement?

A Flexion and extension of fingers

The volar compartment contains flexors and pronator muscles of the forearm and wrist, median and ulnar nerves, and ulnar and radial arteries. Compartment syndrome occurring in the volar compartment presents with weakness in flexors of finger and thumb. The trauma nurse can assess the volar compartment by having the patient extend and flex a thumb and finger or perform finger abduction or adduction movements.

HINT

The patient typically maintains fingers in a flexed position and experiences pain on extension.

MEDICAL/SURGICAL INTERVENTIONS

Q When would an extremity trauma become a higher priority of care in a multisystem trauma patient?

A With potential loss of limb

Injury to an extremity is not considered a high priority in managing a multiple trauma patient unless it involves a potential loss of limb or hemodynamic instability. Vascular injuries are of a higher priority because of lack of perfusion to the extremity and potential loss of limb.

HINT

A loss of pulse distal to the extremity injury indicates vascular involvement and may require surgical management to restore perfusion to the limb.

Q When immobilizing a limb following a traumatic injury, how much of the extremity should be immobilized?

A The joint above and below injury

Proper immobilization includes immobilization of the joint above and below the injury. An extremity that has an obvious deformity, crepitus, edema, or vascular compromise should be immobilized. Immobilization devices should be checked frequently and monitored for swelling, with padded splints placed to prevent further injury. Air splints may be used to decrease edema.

HINT

Any rigid material can be used as a splint and, in lower extremities, one limb can be splinted against the other. Splinting of a pelvic fracture may be performed with a folded sheet that is clamped or knotted in the front.

Q The trauma nurse knows not to reposition which type of fracture when immobilizing an extremity with a splint?

A Open fracture

In an open fracture with protruding bone or a comminuted fracture, do not reposition the extremity to immobilize the fracture. Excessive manipulation of a fractured extremity can cause further injury to surrounding structures and increase bleeding into tissues.

HINT

If the nurse suspects any neurovascular compromise from an external splint, the splint should be removed, adjusted, and reapplied.

Q What is the primary goal of placement of external fixators on a pelvic fracture?

A Limit blood loss

An external fixator is frequently used to stabilize pelvic fractures and limit blood loss. External fixation is accomplished with percutaneous pins connected to a rigid frame. Therapeutic embolization in interventional radiology is also used to control hemorrhage associated with pelvic fractures.

HINT

Damage-control procedures may be required to prevent hemorrhage and death.

Q What type of medication is frequently ordered following vascular repair?

A Antithrombotics

Following surgical vascular repair in patients with extremity trauma, anticoagulation or antiplatelet therapy may be initiated to prevent formation of clots and graft occlusion. Vasopressors should be used cautiously because of the significant vasoconstriction in the peripheral circulation, causing loss of perfusion to the affected limb.

HINT

Frequent neurovascular checks should be performed following vascular injury and surgical repair.

Q What is the best intervention to decrease the incidence of fat emboli?

A Fixation of fracture

Long-bone fracture is associated with higher incidence of fat emboli. The best intervention to prevent fat embolism is to fixate the fracture. Early stabilization and fixation of the long-bone fracture has been shown to decrease the incidence of fat embolism. Immediate stabilization of long-bone fracture is not always possible in multisystem trauma patients with life-threatening injuries but should be performed as soon as possible to prevent fat embolism.

▶ HINT

Manipulation of an extremity with a long-bone fracture can increase the risk of fat embolism.

Q Following a traumatic amputation, what is the best initial method used to prevent further blood loss from the remaining stump?

A Direct pressure

The initial management of a traumatic amputation is to control the blood loss. This should be attempted first by applying direct pressure to the wound. If this does not control the blood loss, then apply a tourniquet as close to the stump as possible to minimize the amount of tissue ischemia caused by the tourniquet.

▶ HINT

Most amputated parts experience vasoconstriction, which limits the blood loss.

Q What specific care of the amputated part increases the time from amputation to reimplantation?

A Placing the part on ice

Appropriate care of the amputated body part is to remove the dirt and debris from the part, then wrap it in gauze dressing moistened with saline. The amputated part should then be wrapped in a towel, enclosed in a sealed bag, and placed on ice. Cooling the extremity increases the time to reimplantation. Cooling the amputated part decreases the metabolic rate and inhibits bacterial growth.

▶ HINT

The amputated part should not be directly exposed to the ice or submerged in ice to prevent frostbite and further tissue damage.

Q In the ED, what is the best cleansing solution to use on the amputated part?

A Aqueous penicillin

Initial emergency care of the amputated part is to wash it with isotonic solution then wrap it in sterile gauze moistened with a solution of aqueous penicillin (1,000,000 U in 50 mL Ringer's lactate). Do not use antiseptics, hydrogen peroxide, iodine, or other solutions on the amputated part.

▶ HINT

The use of betadine on the amputated part can cause the extremity to be unable to be reimplanted and should be avoided.

Q What systemic complication of a trauma can limit the ability to reimplant and salvage an amputated extremity?

A Hypotension

The extent of the skeletal and soft-tissue damage, and the duration of the limb ischemia are clinical variables used to predict whether the limb is salvageable. Severe hypotension worsens the chances of being able to reimplant an extremity because of ischemic injuries.

HINT

The probability of successful reimplantation in older adult victims is not as good as in younger patients.

Q A loss of bone in a lower extremity amputation limits reimplantation because of what complication?

A Limb length discrepancy

A large loss of bone in lower extremity amputations results in limb length discrepancy and poor ambulation. In these cases, reimplantation should be avoided and a prosthesis used for ambulation. Preservation attempts of amputated parts fail because of the presence of severe inflammation or infection, significant soft-tissue necrosis, and severe functional deficit.

HINT

Lower extremity reimplantation requires preservation of protective sensation for successful usage and ambulation.

Q What body parts can tolerate a greater warm ischemia time?

A Fingers

Ischemic time begins at the time of injury, and muscle fibers are very sensitive to lack of oxygen and demonstrate damage after 30 minutes of ischemia. Digits contain tendinous tissue and ligaments, which can tolerate a longer ischemic time than the more proximal limbs, which have a greater muscle mass. Digits can tolerate an increase in warm ischemic time to 24 hours and cold ischemic time to 48 hours.

HINT

Candidates for reimplantation include amputation of scalp, hand, foot, nose, or penis (Table 8.2).

Table 8.2 Reimplantation: Indications and contraindications

Indications for Reimplantation	Contraindications for Reimplantation
Proximal to distal interphalangeal of the digit	Severe crush or avulsion injuries
Younger age	Multiple levels of amputations
Occupational value of digit	Lower extremity with limb length discrepancy
Bilateral hands	
Multiple digits	
Thumb	

▶ HINT

Lower extremity reimplantation is less likely to be successful because of limb length discrepancies or loss of sensation in the sole of the foot.

Q What pharmacological therapy is frequently utilized to prevent a decrease in perfusion to the reimplanted extremity?

A Antiplatelet medication

Aspirin or other antiplatelet medications are commonly administered following reimplantation to prevent platelet aggregation and loss of perfusion to the reimplanted part. Antiplatelet drugs improve arterial flow to the reimplanted extremity, lowering the incidence of procedures to revascularize the extremity.

▶ HINT

Instruct the patient to avoid smoking postoperatively because of its vasoconstrictive effects, which cause hypoperfusion.

Q What is the primary surgical intervention for a compartment syndrome?

A Fasciotomy

A fasciotomy is the opening of the fascial compartment to decrease the pressure on surrounding structures (muscle, nerve, and vessels).

▶ HINT

Each extremity has more than one compartment and the extremity may require more than one fasciotomy (Table 8.3).

Table 8.3 Extremity compartments

Extremity	Number of Compartments
Thigh	2
Calves and feet	4
Upper extremity	3
Forearms	2
Hand	4

NURSING INTERVENTIONS

Q What is the initial intervention for a trauma nurse to use to control bleeding from a wound?

A Direct pressure

A priority of care with musculoskeletal injuries is to control bleeding. It is recommended that direct pressure on an actively bleeding wound should be utilized first to control the blood loss. Tourniquet use may be recommended to prevent severe hemorrhage following a mangled extremity injury and, once placed, should be left on until surgical management is available.

HINT

Improper or prolonged placement of a tourniquet can cause nerve paralysis and extremity ischemia.

Q What is the recommended method to control severe blood loss following a traumatic extremity injury?

A Tourniquet

Applying direct pressure to a wound to control bleeding is the recommended first intervention to establish hemostasis. But severe bleeding that continues despite direct pressure may require a tourniquet to control blood loss and hemorrhagic shock. Bleeding may also be controlled with cautery and suturing.

HINT

Scalp injuries typically require sutures to control blood loss.

Q What do muscle spasms following a traumatic fracture cause in the patient?

A Pain

Pain management is a big concern for the trauma nurse caring for patients with traumatic fractures. Pain is caused by the bony fracture, tissue injury, tissue ischemia, and nerve injury. Muscle spasms can contribute to the pain and may be managed with muscle relaxants. Regional anesthesia with nerve blocks may be used to control pain following a fracture associated with a large amount of pain.

HINT

Pain management is a big concern for the trauma nurse caring for patients with traumatic fractures throughout their hospitalization.

Q Following a traumatic amputation how should the extremity be positioned?

A Elevated

Elevating the stump or the remaining portion of the extremity limits edema and swelling.

HINT

In compartment syndrome, the extremity should be positioned level to the heart.

Q Once an extremity part is reimplanted, what should the nurse assess for on the reimplanted part?

A Perfusion

Assessment of perfusion for the reimplanted extremity includes frequent neurovascular checks, Doppler tones, pulse oximetry, and surface temperature probes. A decrease in oxygen saturation or temperature of a reimplanted extremity indicates tissue hypoperfusion.

▶ HINT

A decrease of 2.5°C may indicate a decrease in perfusion to the limb.

Q Following reimplantation of a hand, the nurse notes the fingers are cool to the touch, nail beds are pale, and there is a delay in capillary refill. What is the most likely complication?

A Arterial congestion

Arterial congestion is a potential complication following reimplantation of a body part. The reimplanted part appears mottled and pale, has a sluggish capillary refill, is cool to the touch, and the tissue turgor may appear "prune like" in arterial congestion. This indicates hypoperfusion and may require revascularization of the extremity.

▶ HINT

If the trauma nurse suspects arterial congestion in a reimplanted part, the extremity should be lowered to below the heart level, dressings loosened or removed, and the physician informed.

Q During assessment of a reimplanted traumatically amputated extremity, the nurse notes the extremity appears to have a bluish discoloration, but a brisk capillary refill remains. What is the most likely complication?

A Venous congestion

Venous congestion of a reimplanted body part appears as cyanotic, is cool to the touch, with a brisk capillary refill, and tense skin turgor. The management of venous congestions is to elevate the affected extremity while maintaining alignment, and to change or remove tight dressings. Medical leeches are frequently used if the reimplanted body part develops venous congestion.

▶ HINT

Leech therapy is not indicated if the complication is impaired arterial flow. Leeches are used to assist with reestablishing venous outflow.

Q What commonly used laboratory finding is used to assess for muscle injury following a crush mechanism of injury?

A Creatine kinase (CK)

CK levels elevate in patients with crush injuries because of the release of CK from the muscle when injured. Potassium levels can also rise following crush injuries because of the release of intracellular components. Disruption of the muscle cell membrane, which releases myoglobin and other components (serum glutamic-oxaloacetic transaminase [SGOT], lactate dehydrogenase [LDH], CK, glucose, potassium) into the bloodstream.

▶ HINT

Rhabdomyolysis is caused by the filtering of the myoglobin in the kidneys, causing acute kidney injury.

Q Which electrolyte abnormality is most commonly associated with crush injury and acute renal failure caused by rhabdomyolysis?

A Hyperkalemia

Potassium elevates following crush injuries because of the release of intracellular components following cellular injury. Potassium is primarily found intracellularly and is released with traumatic crush injuries. Hyperkalemia is most commonly found early and typically peaks within 12 to 36 hours after a crush injury. The hyperkalemia can be managed with kayexalate, insulin, and dextrose; bicarbonate infusion; or a beta agonist. Calcium gluconate can be administered as a cardioprotectant in hyperkalemic cases.

▶ HINT

Hyperkalemia may be identified early by the presence of peaked T waves on the EKG.

Q What is a sign commonly used to determine compartment syndrome in a patient unable to communicate abnormal sensation or pain in the affected extremity?

A Tautness of skin

A patient unable to communicate pain or abnormal sensation in the affected extremity can contribute to a missed compartment syndrome. Patients unable to verbalize pain following an extremity injury require frequent assessment of the affected extremity for firmness, tautness of skin, and the presence of skin blisters.

▶ HINT

The complication of an untreated compartment syndrome can be more severe than a fasciotomy.

Q In what position should the nurse place the patient's extremity if compartment syndrome is suspected?

A Neutral position

An extremity suspected of having compartment syndrome should be maintained in a neutral position. Elevating the extremity may further compromise perfusion to the extremity. Allowing it to be lower than the level of the heart will increase edema and worsen compartment syndrome.

▶ HINT

Remove any constricting dressings or casts from the extremity suspected of developing compartment syndrome.

COMPLICATIONS

Q What is a life-threatening complication of pelvic fractures?

A Hemorrhage

The pelvis contains a large vascular blood supply, including a large venous plexus, therefore injuries to the pelvis can result in significant blood loss and hemorrhagic shock. Posterior fractures of the pelvis have a greater incidence of hemorrhagic complication than injuries to the anterior portion of the pelvis. A femur fracture may lose up to 1,500 mL of blood following an injury, and a loss of about 700 to 750 mL can be attributed to tibial or humeral fractures.

HINT

Assess for significant blood loss that may be associated with extremity trauma and bone fractures.

Q What type of pelvic fracture has the greatest risk of complications and mortality?

A Open pelvic fracture

Complications associated with an open pelvic fracture include injury to the perineum, rectum, and genitourinary structure (especially the bladder).

Q What is a complication of a hip dislocation?

A Avascular necrosis

A complication of a hip dislocation is avascular necrosis of the femoral head. Dislocation of the knee may cause damage to the peroneal nerve, and to the popliteal artery and vein. Posterior knee dislocation is associated with a higher incidence of vascular injury.

HINT

Early surgical repair of hip dislocations may lower the incidence of avascular necrosis.

Q What type of fracture most commonly develops the complication of an infection?

A Open fracture

Infections following fractures occur with the greatest incidence in open fractures. Infections may involve the wounds or bone. Complication of an infection leads to delayed wound healing, osteomyelitis, and even sepsis.

HINT

Close observation by the trauma nurse for signs of sepsis is recommended following an open fracture and extremity wounds.

Q What body system is most frequently involved with fat embolism syndrome?

A Lungs

Fat particles in the circulation cause damage to the capillaries and may involve eyes, skin, and heart, but the lungs are most commonly affected. An elevated intramedullary pressure following trauma causes fat to be released through open venous sinusoids and obstructs flow in the pulmonary capillaries. There is also a systemic response beyond the pulmonary capillaries, which may be a result of the release of free fatty acids, causing a release of inflammatory mediators.

HINT

Fat embolism syndrome presents with signs of dyspnea and hypoxia.

Q What is a complication of a crush syndrome following trauma to an extremity?

A Rhabdomyolysis

Crush syndrome is a condition in which prolonged muscle compression leads to muscle necrosis and the release of myoglobin. Rhabdomyolysis is a form of acute kidney injury in which there is a large amount of injured muscle releasing myoglobin in the blood (myoglobinemia) and is filtered through the kidneys (myoglobinuria).

▶ HINT

Rhabdomyolysis causes reddish to brownish urine, frequently described as "cola" or "tea" colored.

Q An elevated pressure in the osteofascial compartment results in injury to which component of the bundle first?

A Muscle

An osteofascial compartment is a sheath of fascia that binds the muscle and the neurovascular bundles. Compartment syndrome is an elevated pressure within the osteofascial compartment that results in ischemic injury to muscle, nerve, and vascular structures. It occurs most commonly because of a compression or crush-type injury but can also occur from an external source such as wraps, casts, or air splints.

▶ HINT

The onset of compartment syndrome is usually 6 to 8 hours after injury.

Q What is considered a severe complication of an untreated compartment syndrome?

A Amputation

A severe complication of an untreated compartment syndrome is an amputation caused by severe muscle damage and necrosis (Table 8.4).

Table 8.4 Comparison of complications: Compartment syndrome and fasciotomy

Complications of Compartment Syndrome	Complications of Fasciotomy
Crush syndrome	Bleeding
Foot drop	Damaged neurovascular structures
Gross muscle necrosis	Infection
Amputation	Inadequate decompression

▶ HINT

Performing a fasciotomy on an extremity with internal fixation can result in decreased stabilization of the fracture.

▶ HINT

Crush syndrome as a result of a compartment syndrome causes myoglobinuria, hyperkalemia, metabolic acidosis, and acute kidney injury.

KNOWLEDGE CHECK: CHAPTER 8

1. There are different types of pelvic fracture stabilization devices that can be utilized to manage unstable pelvic fractures. Which of the following stabilization methods is the best at controlling hemorrhage?

   A. Wrap the pelvis in a folded sheet clamped at the front
   B. Air splint device
   C. Pneumatic antishock garment
   D. External fixator

2. An obvious open femur fracture should be addressed promptly once airway, breathing, and circulation are stable. Which of the following is the priority of care for the open fracture?

   A. Reducing the fracture
   B. Assessing for signs of infections and osteomyelitis
   C. Immediate surgery
   D. Application of a sterile dressing

3. The nurse receives a patient with an obvious open fracture to the arm. The extremity has glass and debris in the wound. Every time the nurse attempts to irrigate the wound, the patient screams in pain. What should the nurse do first to address this situation?

   A. Notify the physician of the patient's noncompliance.
   B. Notify the physician for the need for analgesic orders.
   C. Inform the patient of the importance of removing the debris and attempt to irrigate the wound again.
   D. Cover the wound with a sterile dressing and administer the ordered antibiotics.

4. A 78-year-old woman fell and attempted to brace her fall by reaching out her arm. She is complaining of right shoulder pain. What vascular structure is most likely to be damaged with shoulder injuries?

   A. Axillary artery
   B. Brachial artery
   C. Brachial plexus
   D. Radial artery

5. A 15-year-old patient was attempting to jump off a roof into a pool when they missed the pool and landed on the pavement. The patient has a calcaneus fracture and bilateral wrist fractures. What other injuries should the nurse suspect with this mechanism of injury?

   A. Vertebral fractures
   B. Sacral fractures
   C. Pelvic fractures
   D. Femur fractures

(*See answers next page.*)

1. D) External fixator

Considerable blood loss requires immediate stabilization by external fixation. Stabilization of pelvic fractures is commonly performed by wrapping the pelvis in a folded sheet knotted or clamped at the front; this is not as effective a method for controlling hemorrhage, however. An air splint is filled with air and used to temporarily immobilize an injured extremity, not a pelvic fracture. Pneumatic antishock garments have been used short term to stabilize the pelvis but external fixation is more definitive.

2. D) Application of a sterile dressing

Motor and sensory assessment, stabilization of the extremity, immobilization of the extremity, and application of a sterile dressing to the open wound all take priority in an open femur fracture injury. Infection and osteomyelitis are complications of an open femur fracture but are not an early finding, and do not need to be assessed with the initial presentation of an open fracture. Open fracture should not be reduced in the immediate period due to further trauma to tissues and surrounding structures. Immediate surgery may not be the priority depending on the patient's other injuries.

3. B) Notify the physician for the need for analgesic orders.

The nurse should notify the physician of the need for pain management so that proper irrigation and cleansing can be performed with the patient as comfortable as possible. The initial wound care includes removal of gross contaminates from the wound and covering exposed bone or tissue with a sterile saline dressing. The patient should be informed of the importance of cleaning the debris and the significance of treatment and infection prevention; however, pain is the fifth vital sign and should be addressed. A significant complication of fractures is infection; therefore antibiotics are indicated, but the wound still requires appropriate cleansing.

4. A) Axillary artery

If there is vascular or nerve involvement associated with a humeral fracture, it usually is caused by the axillary nerve or axillary artery. Rarely, the brachial artery, brachial plexus, or radial artery are involved with a shoulder injury. Identification of an anterior or posterior bulge may suggest a dislocation. Tenderness and swelling often are diffuse, making it difficult to detect clear point tenderness.

5. A) Vertebral fractures

Considering the mechanism of injury, thoracolumbar vertebral compression fractures should be suspected. The upward force of the impact when the patient jumped compresses the vertebral bodies resulting in burst fractures. Sacral, pelvic, and femur fractures are all possibilities, but vertebral fracture should have the highest suspicion.

6. A 24-year-old patient was involved in a motor vehicle collision (MVC). They were restrained and the airbag deployed. The patient's right patella came in contact with the dashboard and caused a patellar fracture. Knowing that the impact of the injury was forceful enough to injure the patella, what other injuries may be associated?

   A. Posterior hip dislocation
   B. Dorsalis pedis artery injury
   C. Compartment syndrome
   D. Femur fracture on the opposite leg

7. A patient came to the ED with an open femur fracture. The bleeding has been controlled and the patient is hemodynamically stable. The nurse goes to splint the site. What splint would be recommended for this injury?

   A. Rigid splint
   B. Traction splint
   C. Soft splint
   D. Contraction splint

8. A physician places orders for a patient with an open fracture. Which of the following is the most appropriate order for an open fracture?

   A. Irrigate with hydrogen peroxide.
   B. Change dressing frequently.
   C. Apply occlusive petroleum dressing.
   D. Irrigate the site with normal saline and apply sterile dressing.

9. Which of the following injuries can lose about 1,000 mL to 1,500 mL of blood?

   A. Vertebral fracture
   B. Femur fracture
   C. Hip dislocation
   D. Tibial fracture

10. This type of fracture has distal and proximal fracture sites wedged into each other:

   A. Displaced fracture
   B. Complete fracture
   C. Greenstick fracture
   D. Impacted fracture

(*See answers next page.*)

6. A) Posterior hip dislocation

The impact of the injury to the patella may also cause an associated posterior hip fracture or dislocation, popliteal artery injury (not dorsalis pedis artery), and a femur fracture in the affected leg. Compartment syndrome is a complication typically of a crush injury, not a patellar fracture.

7. B) Traction splint

A traction splint would be most appropriate for tibial and femur fractures. Rigid splints are made of plastic, metal, or cardboard and are used for extremities such as an injured forearm. Soft splints are devices like air splints and slings used to treat an injured arm, wrist, or hand. Contraction splint is not a recognized splint type.

8. D) Irrigate the site with normal saline and apply sterile dressing.

Open fractures should be irrigated with normal saline and a sterile dry dressing applied to the site. Frequent dressing changes are contraindicated because they increase the risk of bacterial contamination with each wound exposure. Applying a petroleum dressing or irrigating with hydrogen peroxide is not indicated and may cause harm.

9. B) Femur fracture

Femur fractures can result in a collection of 1,000 mL to 1,500 mL of blood in the thigh. Femur fractures present with pain, shortening of the affected leg, external or internal rotation, edema or deformity of the thigh, and possible neurovascular compromise. Tibial fractures lose up to approximately 750 mL of blood. Hip dislocation and vertebral fractures cause minimal blood loss.

10. D) Impacted fracture

An impacted fracture has distal and proximal fracture sites wedged into each other. A displaced fracture has proximal and distal fracture edges out of alignment, a greenstick fracture occurs when the bone buckles or bends, and a complete fracture is when there is total interruption in bony continuity.

Surface and Burn Trauma

9

MECHANISM OF INJURY

Q What is the most common mechanism of injury for a burn in children between the ages of 2 and 4 years of age?

A Scald injuries

The age group of 2 to 4 year olds (toddlers) is most commonly associated with scald injuries, whereas in adults, injury is usually most commonly caused by a flammable liquid.

HINT

Hot water from faucets, showers, and bathtubs is the leading source of scald burns in children.

Q Which type of fire causes the majority of fire-related deaths?

A Structural fires

Structural fires are responsible for the majority of burn-related deaths but only account for 5% of the hospital admissions. Cigarette smoking and alcohol consumption are common factors in fatal structural fires.

HINT

In older adult people, a significant number of burns are related to nightwear (i.e., robes, gowns).

Q What complication of fire-related injuries is a common cause of fatality?

A Smoke inhalation

Most fire-related deaths have smoke inhalation as a major contributor to fatality.

HINT

Inhalation of toxic substances (carbon monoxide, hydrogen cyanide, and other gases) in a structural fire is one of the leading causes of death.

Q What is the usual cause of a thermal burn?

A Flame

Thermal burns are usually a result of events generating heat, flames, or both.

HINT

An explosion increases the risk of the patient sustaining other trauma, especially penetrating injuries, in addition to flame or heat burns.

Q What might a burn with well-demarcated lines and no splash patterns on a child indicate?

A Child abuse

Always assess whether the pattern of the burn is suspicious for abuse. A scald injury on a child with well-demarcated lines and no splash injuries may indicate child abuse.

HINT

Children who pull pans of hot liquid on themselves commonly present with a burn pattern in the shape of Africa, with a large area of burn on top and a small area on the bottom.

Q What is a common source of electrical burn injuries?

A Lightning strikes

Electrical burns can be a result of lightning strikes or direct contact with an electrical current. The trauma nurse should determine the voltage, type of current, location of the electrical source's contact, length of contact, and whether the patient sustained any loss of consciousness following a direct contact to the electrical source.

HINT

Electrical current has a contact site, which is the point of entry, and an exit site at a distal location.

Q Which causes a more serious chemical burn, acid or alkaline chemicals?

A Alkaline

Caustic chemical agents, including acids, alkalines, and petroleum-based products, may produce chemical burns when in direct contact with skin or mucous membranes (direct ingestion). Alkaline chemical burns are usually more serious than acid burns because they penetrate the tissue more deeply. Alkaline chemicals are present in many household cleaning products and in wet cement.

HINT

The extent of the tissue damage and injury from chemical burns may continue to progress after the initial exposure.

Q A contaminated wound should be allowed to heal by what type of closure?

A Tertiary

Contaminated wounds should be cleaned, debrided, and left open to close by tertiary healing. Closing a contaminated wound with primary closure increases the risk of infection. The advantage of a primary closure is less scarring but it is used for clean cuts and lacerations. Primary intention closure can be accomplished by closure of the wound initially with sutures, staples, tape, or glue.

▶ HINT

Wounds that have minimal tissue loss and are cleaned can usually be closed by primary repair.

TRAUMATIC INJURIES

Q What two components determine the extent of a burn injury?

A Extent and depth

Classification of burn severity is based on the extent and depth of the injury. The extent of injury depends on the intensity and strength of the causative agent, the duration of exposure, and the conductance of the tissue involved. An example is a ring that can continue to burn a finger because of the heat of the metal, which can produce severe tissue injury.

▶ HINT

Other contributing factors for determining the severity of injury in burn patients is preexisting illness and associated injuries.

Q The zone of coagulation in a burn wound indicates what type of injury?

A Irreversible injury

Zone of coagulation is the area of irreversible cell death and involves the most severe area of the burn with the most intimate contact with the heat source (Table 9.1). This tissue is considered to be irreversibly injured and consists of necrotic tissue.

Table 9.1 Zones of burn–wound injury

Zone of Hyperemia	Zone of Stasis	Zone of Coagulation
Involves peripheral and superficial area of the burn wound	Injury is less superficial	Involves the most severe area of the burn with the most intimate contact with the heat source
The zone appears erythematous, indicating a first-degree burn	Caused by vascular damage and the inflammatory response	Irreversible cell death
	Edema forms in the next 24 to 48 hours	The tissue is necrotic
	Reversible area of injury if treated in a timely manner	

▶ HINT

After 3 to 4 days, loss of tissue viability in the zone of stasis causes the burn wound to become larger and deeper.

Q What is the phase of burn management that begins with hemodynamic instability and fluid shifts?

A Resuscitative phase

The resuscitative phase begins with an initial hemodynamic response and lasts until capillary integrity is restored and the plasma volume is replaced. The capillary leak allows for the loss of fluids, electrolytes (especially sodium), and plasma proteins into the tissues. The shift of fluids into the interstitial space causes intravascular volume loss and hypovolemia.

▶ HINT

Fluid is also lost through the wound, contributing to the hypovolemia.

Q What is the clinical sign that signifies the onset of the acute phase of burns?

A Diuresis

Diuresis is the onset of the acute phase of burn injury. This onset of diuresis is caused by the fluid shifting from the interstitial space back into the vascular space. The initial fluid loss into tissue occurs immediately from the burn wounds.

▶ HINT

In partial-thickness wounds, the greatest fluid loss occurs on the day of injury although in full-thickness injuries the greatest fluid losses peak by day 4 postburn.

Q Which of the layers of skin contain sweat glands and hair follicles?

A Dermis layer

The dermis layer, which is the second layer of skin, contains the sebaceous glands, sweat glands, vessels, nerves, and hair follicles. The dermis is not able to regenerate if completely damaged. Fat, muscle, and subcutaneous tissue are below the dermis layer and the outermost layer, the epidermis, is avascular.

▶ HINT

Injury to the dermis layer of skin may result in the loss of hair and inability to sweat in the previously damaged area.

Q What is a burn wound that affects the epidermis only called?

A Partial-thickness burn

A partial-thickness burn injury is superficial and involves the epidermis layer only. This used to be called a *first-degree burn* (Table 9.2).

Table 9.2 Burn depth

Term	Layers Involved
Partial thickness (first degree)	Epidermis
Superficial partial thickness (second degree)	Epidermis and upper part of dermal layer
Deep partial thickness (second degree)	Epidermis and most dermis
Full thickness (third degree)	Epidermis, dermis, and underlying subcutaneous tissue
Full thickness (fourth degree)	Involves muscle and bone

HINT

Epidermis and dermis layers are affected in second-degree burns.

Q What is the typical extent of injury for electrical burns?

A Deep muscle

Electrical burns involve both cutaneous and deep muscle damage, commonly resulting in an amputation. The contact wound may not appear severe but can have extensive subfascial tissue damage (Box 9.1). The path of the electricity may follow along bone (bone does not conduct well), and transverse through internal organs and structures (nerves, tendons, blood vessels) to exit the skin in a location distal to the initial contact. The exit wound may have more extensive tissue injury and muscle necrosis.

Box 9.1 Determinants of severity of electrical injuries

- Voltage
- Duration of contact to electrical source
- Resistance of the tissue
- Surface area of contact

HINT

The external damage may not reflect the actual damage to the tissues. The average-size burn wound associated with electrical injury is approximately 5% of the total body surface area (TBSA).

HINT

Tissue damage is determined by the current density; the smaller the area that comes in contact with the electricity, the greater the tissue damage.

Q Besides the type of chemical, what is another variant that may determine the extent of injury with a chemical burn?

A Duration of contact

The amount of damage sustained to the skin and tissue depends on the chemical agent, the duration of contact with the skin or tissue, and the concentration of the chemical. Chemicals break down cell walls and destroy intracellular proteins, resulting in cellular death. The longer the chemical remains in contact with the tissue, the greater the damage to the tissue.

HINT

Management of chemical burns is by copious irrigation for extended periods of time to wash the chemical away and decrease contact time.

Q What type of injury causes a partial-thickness injury as a result of rubbing the skin across a hard surface?

A Abrasion

An abrasion is an injury caused by the friction of skin rubbing against a hard surface and typically is a partial- or full-thickness injury. A puncture is an open wound that is deeper than it is wide. An avulsion is typically a full-thickness injury caused by a ripping or tearing mechanism of injury. The wound edges do not approximate and are typically jagged, which requires debridement.

HINT

When the skin is traumatically torn or pulled away from the soft tissue it is called a *degloving injury*.

ASSESSMENT/DIAGNOSIS

Q What are the cardiovascular signs of burn shock?

A Tachycardia and narrowed pulse pressure

Burn shock results in hypovolemia and hypoperfusion. This triggers the autonomic nervous system and the release of catecholamines. The cardiovascular effects then include tachycardia and vasoconstriction. The hypotension that occurs is a result of the decrease in circulating blood volume.

HINT

The initial sign of narrowed pulse pressure is a result of the hypotension and vasoconstriction, which occurs before onset of hypotension.

Q What is the sign frequently used to indicate correction of hypovolemia?

A Increased urine output

Signs of hypovolemia include decreased blood pressure, oliguria, and peripheral edema. These are characteristics of a burn shock. A sign frequently used at the bedside indicating adequate resuscitation of a hypovolemia is an increase in urine output or reversal of burn shock.

▶ HINT

Urine output reflects renal perfusion.

Q A patient's burn wounds are described as mottled, red, and "weeping." What is the most likely depth of burn?

A Superficial partial thickness

Superficial partial-thickness (second-degree) burns appear mottled, red to pale ivory, and are moist (weeping serous fluid; Table 9.3). Blisters form and are very painful because of exposed nerve endings.

Table 9.3 Burn–wound classification

Depth of Wound	Appearance of Wound
Partial thickness	Local pain, erythema without blisters (bullae), dry, skin blanches
Superficial partial thickness	Mottled, red to pale ivory, moist, forms blisters and is very painful
Deep partial thickness	Mottled; large areas of waxy, white discoloration; decreased moisture; skin does not blanch or prolonged blanching exists
Full thickness	White, cherry red, brown, or black and dry, hard and leathery; may or may not have blisters and thrombosed veins

▶ HINT

Burn wounds will have different degrees of depth within the wound.

Q In the rule of palms for an adult patient, the patient's palm represents how much of the patient's body surface area?

A About 1%

The patient's palm represents about 1% of the patient's body surface area and may be used to determine the surface area burned. This is called the *rule of palms*.

▶ HINT

The rule of palms is a quick and easy way to estimate the amount of body surface area burned but is not the most accurate method.

Q What chart is considered a more accurate assessment of the amount of body surface area burned?

A Lund and Browder chart

The Lund and Browder chart may be used to estimate the amount of body surface area burned and is a more accurate assessment because it takes into account the changes in body surface area related to the growth of the individual. The size of the burn is a predictor of survival, with the greater body surface area burns having the highest predicted mortality.

HINT

The presence of irregular or scattered burns can be estimated by using the palm of the patient's hand and can supplement the Lund and Browder chart in determining the size of the burn wound.

Q A child's head counts for how much body surface area when doing the rule of nines to determine the extent of burns?

A About 18%

The rule of nines is used to estimate the extent of burn wounds. The rule of nines divides the TBSA into sections of 9% or multiples of nine, except for the perineum, which is equal to 1%. An adult's head counts for 9% of the TBSA, whereas a child's head is 18% (Table 9.4).

Table 9.4 Rule of nines

Adult	Pediatric
Head: 9%	Head: 18%
Upper extremity: 9%	Upper extremity: 9%
Perineum: 1%	
Lower extremity: 18%	Lower extremity: 14%
Front: 18%	Front: 18%
Back: 18%	Back: 18%

HINT

The rule of nines is an estimation of the body surface area involved and may be used in adults and children older than 10 years.

Q What diagnostic test would the trauma nurse expect the physician to order for a burn patient with an altered level of consciousness (LOC)?

A A CT scan of the head

A change or altered level consciousness requires a CT scan to assess for an associated brain injury. Burn trauma should not cause an altered LOC. Presence of altered LOC may indicate a traumatic brain injury.

HINT

Associated traumatic injuries must be identified and managed in the same manner as in any patient without a burn.

Q What is an observational assessment finding that would provide the trauma nurse with a high suspicion of inhalation injury?

A Singed nasal, facial, and eyebrow hairs

In the initial assessment, the nurse assesses for soot; carbonaceous sputum; and singed nasal, facial, and eyebrow hairs. These findings indicate the patient is at a high risk for inhalation injury.

▶ HINT

Early intubation in burn patients with the signs of inhalation injury may prevent a loss of airway when swelling occurs. Hoarseness, stridor, and audible breathing are indicative of partial obstruction and indicate potential for complete obstruction of the airway.

Q What is the gold standard for diagnosing and evaluating the severity of inhalation injuries?

A Bronchoscopy

The gold standard diagnosis of inhalation injury includes bronchoscopy to identify carbonaceous debris in the tracheal and bronchial area as well as mucosal ulcerations.

▶ HINT

On the examination, a gold-standard question is looking for the most specific or diagnostic answer, not necessarily what is performed the most frequently.

Q What is a diagnostic test used to determine the presence of carbon monoxide poisoning following a house fire?

A Serum test

Serum levels of carbon monoxide can be measured to assess for exposure and toxicity. Toxic levels of carboxyhemoglobin are 25% to 35% and a lethal level is greater than 60%.

▶ HINT

In carbon monoxide poisoning, the pulse oximetry demonstrates a significant discrepancy from an arterial blood gas.

Q What is a clinical sign of carbon monoxide poisoning and cyanide toxicity?

A Altered LOC

Exposure to a large amount of carbon monoxide can cause an altered mental status and should be suspected in burn patients with a decrease in LOC. Delayed sequelae of elevated carbon monoxide levels include headaches, irritability, personality changes, loss of memory, confusion, and gross motor deficits that present within days to several weeks.

▶ HINT

Remember, a burn injury should not cause an altered LOC. Any neurological abnormalities should clue the trauma nurse to the presence of a traumatic brain injury or toxicities.

MEDICAL/SURGICAL INTERVENTIONS

Q What is a priority of care in a burn patient in the initial phase of resuscitation and fluid shifts?

A Obtaining an airway

Fluid shifts that occur with burn-injured patients cause significant peripheral edema, including in the region of the upper airway. Airway swelling can occur rapidly during the initial shock phase following burn injuries and an airway should be obtained before the airway swells.

▶ HINT

Patients with large burns, burns of the face and neck, or obvious inhalation injury should be intubated before the fluid resuscitation to prevent the loss of an airway.

Q What is used to determine the amount of fluid resuscitation to administer to a burn patient within the first 24 hours?

A Size of the burn

The amount of fluid resuscitation is determined by the size of the burn, so estimation of surface area burned is very important to guide initial care for partial- and full-thickness burns. The extent of the burn wound is the percentage of TBSA burned.

▶ HINT

Superficial (first-degree) burns do not have open wounds through which plasma is lost so they do not require fluid resuscitation.

Q What prehospital care should be done for the burn wound?

A Cover with a sterile sheet

Covering burns that are greater than 10% of the TBSA with a dry, clean sheet can protect the wounds from contamination. At the scene, the prehospital personnel should not spend time at the scene to clean the burn wounds but transport immediately to hospital.

▶ HINT

Do not apply any topical antimicrobial creams or ointments in the emergency stage before wound assessment can be performed in the hospital.

Q What is a potential complication of cooling a burn wound in the field?

A Hypothermia

Cooling burn wounds should occur within the first 20 minutes to be most effective. It is recommended to cool the burn wound with running cool water (not cold) for at least 5 minutes and should not be continued for greater than 20 to 30 minutes after the initial burn. If the patient begins to shiver, stop the cooling process. Cooling burn wounds in patients with large body surface area wounds can cause hypothermia and may not be recommended. Attempt to keep the patient warm even if cooling the burn wound (Box 9.2).

Box 9.2 Prehospital care of burns

Remove all jewelry to stop the burning.

Cool with running water.

Cover with sterile or clean cloth.

Do not use ice on burn wounds.

Do not use butter or other home remedies on burn wounds.

▶ HINT

Direct application of ice should not be used to cool burn wounds because of the potential of causing frostbite.

Q With a burn wound larger than 15% of body surface area, what is a priority of care for the patient's stabilization?

A Fluid resuscitation

Patients with burn wounds will third-space large volumes of fluid, resulting in hypovolemia. The fluid resuscitation is based on the percentage of body surface burned. The management of the fluid resuscitation in a burn patient requires the knowledge of the time of injury, careful estimation of burn size and depth, accurate patient weight, and a Foley catheter. Formulas are used to calculate the amount of fluids required in the first 24 hours following a burn trauma.

Q What type of fluid should be added to the resuscitation of a pediatric burn patient?

A Dextrose

Infants and young children should receive intravenous fluid with 5% dextrose at a maintenance rate in addition to the fluid resuscitation with lactated Ringer's solution or normal saline. Children have more limited glycogen storage than adults and frequently experience hypoglycemia in the early postburn stage.

▶ HINT

Monitor pediatric patients' blood glucose levels frequently during the early stages of their burn management.

Q What is the most commonly used intravenous fluid for burn resuscitation in an adult patient?

A Lactated Ringer's solution

Lactated Ringer's is commonly used to resuscitate an adult burn patient during the resuscitation phase. Other isotonic solutions, such as normal and hypertonic saline, and colloids may also be used during resuscitation. The most commonly used formula to calculate fluid resuscitation needs in adult burn patients is the modified Parkland formula, but there are many different acceptable formulas that can be used to determine the volume required during resuscitation (Box 9.3).

Box 9.3 Modified parkland formula

Volume of lactated Ringer's solution = 2 mL × body weight (in kg) × % of TBSA burned (partial or full thickness only)

TBSA, total body surface area.

HINT

The fluid resuscitation of a burn patient occurs over 24 hours, with one half of the calculated amount being administered within the first 8 hours and the remaining half infused over the following 16 hours.

HINT

Children with burn injuries may require an increase in fluids during resuscitation compared with an adult with the same burn. The child requires more precise calculation and assessment of hemodynamics because of the limited reserve (Box 9.4).

Box 9.4 Pediatric fluid calculation

Volume of lactated Ringer's = 3 mL × body weight (in kg) × % of TBSA burned (partial or full thickness only)

TBSA, total body surface area.

Q What is an indication for performing a chest wall escharotomy?

A Elevating peak inspiratory pressures

If the patient is on a mechanical ventilator, restriction of chest wall motion and elevating peak airway pressures are indications for a chest wall escharotomy. Extremity escharotomy can also be performed with extremity circumferential burns. The incision of the escharotomy extends the entire length of the burn wound, down through the eschar and superficial fascia to a depth sufficient to allow the cut edges of the eschar to separate. The escharotomy site should be covered with topical antimicrobial agents.

HINT

The most common type of burn requiring a fasciotomy is high-voltage electrical injury, or those patients with significant soft tissue, long-bone, or vascular injury.

Q What is the initial intervention for a patient experiencing carbon monoxide poisoning?

A Administer 100% oxygen

Elevated carboxyhemoglobin or cyanide levels should be initially managed by placing the burn patient on 100% oxygen at the bedside. The administration of 100% oxygen in patients with elevated oxyhemoglobin levels can lower the half-life of carbon monoxide from 2.5 hours to 40 minutes.

HINT

Accumulation of carbon monoxide is commonly found in patients burned in structural fires, so the question probably provides a hint in the scenario of a house fire.

Q What is the initial intervention for most chemical contamination?

A Irrigation

The decontamination procedure is important to limit the amount of tissue injury that occurs following contact with a caustic chemical. The typical management of chemical burns is irrigation with water or normal saline until pain subsides. Alkaline chemical burns require more extensive and longer irrigation with water than acid burns. Dry or powdered chemicals should be brushed off the skin initially with a dry towel before water is applied. Substances containing lime can become corrosive to skin when water is added so the powdered substance must be brushed off before water irrigation is used (Table 9.5).

Table 9.5 Neutralization of chemicals

Chemical	Neutralization in Addition Irrigation
Hydrofluoric acid	Calcium chloride gel
Tar and asphalt	Petroleum-based gels
Phenols	50% polyethylene glycol

HINT

The trauma nurse should attempt to identify the causative agent and contact a regional poison center to identify the characteristics of the substance and neutralization methods specific to the agent.

Q What can be applied to tar or asphalt on skin to decrease heat and burning?

A Petroleum products

Tar or asphalt on skin will continue to contain heat and burn. The tarred area needs to be cooled initially using petroleum products such as mineral oil or neomycin sulfate.

HINT

Cooling hot tar-covered skin with water will not stop the burning process.

Q What is a priority for patients potentially contaminated with radiation?

A Minimize contamination of others

Patients presenting to the ED with the potential exposure to radiation should be placed in an area away from other patients to prevent contamination. Healthcare clinicians should protect themselves from exposure to the patient's clothing and skin. Appropriate protective gear should be worn when providing care to radiation-exposed patients.

▶ HINT

The patient exposed to radiation should not be undressed because of the potential of aerosolizing the contaminant; therefore, clothing should be saturated with water before being removed.

Q What is the wound care recommended for nonviable skin and tissue?

A Debridement

Nonviable tissue is debrided to decrease the risk of infection and facilitate new tissue growth. Sharp debridement is commonly performed by the physician and nurses perform a gentler debridement while cleansing burn wounds. Large blisters may be broken and gently debrided, but small blisters may be left intact.

▶ HINT

Gentle cleansing of the burn wound with tepid water and mild soap is used to remove debris, loose skin, and bacteria and cleanse the wound.

Q Where is Sulfamylon cream usually applied for burn–wound care?

A Cartilage

Sulfamylon is frequently used on ears and noses that are burned. It should not be used on burns on the body because of its potential to cause metabolic acidosis. Silvadene is a cream used more often on burns that cover a large body surface area. It is a broad-spectrum antibiotic that is painless.

▶ HINT

Silvadene is not effective against deep burn–wound infections.

NURSING INTERVENTIONS

Q What is an important component of the initial current history the trauma nurse should obtain from the patient or emergency medical personnel?

A Mechanism of injury

It is important to determine the details of the injury in a burn patient. The cause of the burn, determining whether it occurred in a closed space, the time of injury, and whether any associated injuries or related trauma occurred are the important answers for the trauma nurse to determine.

▶ HINT

The time of injury (as well as extent of burns) is used to determine adequacy of fluid resuscitation at the time of entry into the trauma hospital.

Q A child is admitted to the trauma hospital with burns on their lower extremities. The scald burn wound is well demarcated. What should the trauma nurse suspect regarding this injury?

A Child abuse

Scald wounds on a child that are well demarcated indicate that the child was forcefully held in the hot water. If a child falls into hot water accidentally, they will splash around and the scald burn wounds will be irregular.

▶ HINT

Consider that the burn may be child abuse when treating a burned child, especially if the child is younger than the age of 2 years.

Q While administering fluids during the initial resuscitation phase of a burn injury, what should the trauma nurse assess to assist with assuring adequate fluid resuscitation?

A Urine output

Urine output is frequently used to assess for adequate resuscitation following a burn injury. This is particularly important in electrical burns because the actual amount of body surface area involved is not visible and the typical formulas underestimate the fluid requirement. The goal for the urine output in an adult burn patient is a minimum of 30 to 50 mL/hr and 1 to 2 mL/kg/hr for children under 30 kg.

▶ HINT

On the test, a rate of 0.5 to 1 mL/kg/hr may be used as a minimum urine output in an adult patient.

Q To maintain homeostasis, what is a nursing intervention that the trauma nurse should perform for a burn patient?

A Keep the patient warm

Burn patients will lose their body heat from the loss of skin. Hypothermia can affect other body systems, including potentiation of a coagulopathy. Maintaining a warm hospital room and resuscitating with warm fluid will assist with the warming of the burn patient. Patients with burns covering more than 50% of their total body surface require room temperatures higher than 86°F (30°C; Box 9.5).

Box 9.5 Nursing interventions in the ED

Observe cardiac monitor for life-threatening arrhythmias.
Administer warm fluids to avoid hypothermia.
Place a gastric tube for gastric distension.
Insert an indwelling bladder catheter to assess urine output.
Remove all jewelry, especially jewelry that is circumferential such as rings and bracelets.
Obtain peripheral access with large-gauge intravenous catheters.
Avoid placing the intravenous catheter into the burn wound, if possible.

HINT

One liter of room temperature fluid administered rapidly can lower the patient's body temperature by 1 degree.

HINT

Common life-threatening arrhythmias following burn injuries include atrial fibrillation, ventricular fibrillation, and asystole.

Q What type of assessment should be performed by the trauma nurse with circumferential extremity burns?

A Palpation of pulses

Assessment of a patient with burns to the extremities includes frequent palpation of pulses (radial, ulnar, posterior tibial, dorsalis pedis). The absence of flow or progressive diminishing of the pulse requires further assessment with a Doppler ultrasound.

HINT

A Doppler ultrasound assessment of the distal palmar arch vessels in the upper limb and the posterior tibial artery in lower limbs are the most reliable locations to determine the need for an escharotomy.

Q What should be a priority of care throughout the burn patient's course of wound healing?

A Pain management

Pain management is very important in the care of a burn patient, even with large amounts of full-thickness wounds. Areas of the burn wound that are full thickness do not have sensory or pain perception but surrounding the full-thickness injury are components of the burn that are less deep that maintain sensation and are very painful. Burn wounds have a variety of injury thicknesses, so they are painful.

HINT

When burns are severe, opioids should be administered via an intravenous route initially for better absorption, bioavailability, and improved pain management.

Q What is the concern for the trauma team members when handling a patient with chemical contamination?

A Exposure to the chemical

When a patient with chemical skin contamination presents to the ED, the trauma nurse should determine whether the causative agent could pose a risk for healthcare clinicians and ensure appropriate protective gear and decontamination procedures are utilized. The trauma team should be protected from contamination when handling a patient with chemical exposure or burns by using gloves, gowns, masks, and goggles.

▶ HINT

An example of a potential exposure injury is phenol that gets absorbed through the skin, which can cause liver and kidney damage.

Q When the physician is to suture a laceration of an ear, should the trauma nurse gather lidocaine with or without epinephrine for use as a local anesthetic?

A Without epinephrine

Epinephrine as a local anesthetic can help with some blood loss because of its vasoconstrictive properties, but in some smaller areas of the body, it may negatively affect perfusion. The suturing of the ears, digits, penis, and end of the nose should be done with a local anesthetic without epinephrine to prevent ischemia to these areas.

Q What is the reason for suturing without prior shaving of hair?

A Risk of infection

Shaving hair can actually increase the risk of infection as a result of multiple skin cuts and is not routinely recommended. Any hair removal required for suturing or wound care should be done with scissors or clippers, and not a razor.

▶ HINT

Eyebrows should never be shaved when suturing the face.

COMPLICATIONS

Q What is a potential complication of the initial fluid resuscitation in a burn-injured patient?

A Volume overload

Volume overload can occur as a result of the massive fluid resuscitation during the initial phase of a burn injury. Even though extravascular fluid shifts occur during the initial phase, the volume resuscitation can lead to complications of heart failure, acute respiratory distress syndrome (ARDS), elevated intraabdominal pressure, and increased intracranial pressure in high-risk patients. The goal in fluid resuscitation with a burn patient is to provide enough to improve organ perfusion, but not too much to avoid volume overload complications. Therefore, assessment of hemodynamics is important.

▶ HINT

Adding hypertonic saline at some point during the fluid resuscitation can lower the total volume requirements and improve urine output by shifting fluid back into the vascular space.

Q What electrolyte abnormalities are found with massive resuscitation of normal saline solution in the initial burn injury?

A Hypernatremia and hyperchloremia

Normal saline solution has a higher sodium and chloride content than blood, so administering large volumes can elevate the sodium and chloride levels. Lactated Ringer's replaces the sodium loss that occurs with burn shock with a sodium concentration of 130 mEq/L but does not cause hypernatremia. If hypertonic saline is used during resuscitation, the trauma nurse needs to frequently assess sodium levels, which should not be greater than 160 mEq/L.

HINT

The hyperchloremia metabolic acidosis causes a nonanion gap metabolic acidosis.

Q What is the primary complication of the fluid shift in the initial phase of burn injury?

A Organ dysfunction

In burn shock, fluid shifts out of the vascular space, resulting in hypovolemia. The hypovolemia results in hypoperfusion and affects all organs of the body.

HINT

Organ dysfunction occurs in the resuscitative phase of burn shock because of hypoperfusion.

Q What contributes to the tissue oxygen deficit in burn patients?

A Increase in metabolism

The hypermetabolic state following a burn injury is associated with an increase in oxygen demand and oxygen consumption. The patient is hypovolemic (because of third-spacing) with a decrease in tissue perfusion, therefore, the delivery is decreased and the demand is increased, further worsening the tissue-oxygen deficit. The hypermetabolism occurs within 24 to 48 hours postburn.

HINT

Tachypnea, fever, and tachycardia are frequently present because of the hypermetabolic state of the severely burned patient.

Q A circumferential burn to the chest can cause interference with what physiological function?

A Ventilation

A chest circumferential burn can cause difficulty with ventilation and the trauma nurse should be assessing for shortness of breath and increased work of breathing. If the patient is on a mechanical ventilator, the peak inspiratory pressures increase. The patient with circumferential burns frequently require an escharotomy to improve ventilation.

HINT

Escharotomy of the chest may be required before transportation to a burn center to prevent ventilation complications during transport.

Q What is a pulmonary complication that is found in victims of fires in small spaces?

A Asphyxiation

Asphyxiation occurs when the blood has a decreased amount of oxygen and there is an increase in the amount of carbon dioxide or toxic substances. Victims of fires in small spaces, such as a car or a house, frequently experience hypoxemia and asphyxia because the combustion of the fire consumes oxygen, leaving less than 21% of oxygen to breathe.

HINT

Administer oxygen by a 100% nonrebreather mask at a flow rate of 12 to 15 L/min in the initial management of a patient with burns and carbon monoxide poisoning.

Q Following a burn injury in a house fire, the patient has a pulse oximetry reading of 100% saturated, but the arterial blood gas comes back with a saturation of 82%. What is the most likely cause of this discrepancy?

A Carbon monoxide poisoning

Carbon monoxide, when inhaled, binds the oxygen receptor sites on the hemoglobin. It has a greater affinity for hemoglobin than oxygen. The affinity of hemoglobin to carbon monoxide is 200 to 300 times greater than oxygen and prolonged binding of hemoglobin decreases the oxygen-carrying capacity of the hemoglobin. Pulse oximetry monitors are unable to differentiate hemoglobin bound with oxygen from that bound with carbon monoxide. The arterial blood gas (SaO_2) is more accurate and shows the low oxygen saturation that occurs with carbon monoxide poisoning.

HINT

When caring for a patient who has sustained burn injuries in closed-space fires, arterial blood gases should be monitored to identify oxygen saturation abnormalities.

Q The upper airway can be injured in burn patients. What is the primary cause of injury?

A Inhalation injury

Direct inhalation injury is usually limited to the upper airway with the inhalation of superheated air. Inhalation of smoke and other toxins can damage the upper airway. Some gases formed during the fire combustion, when inhaled, produce harmful acids and alkali leading to edema and ulcerations in the lower airway. Inhalation injuries occur most commonly in patients trapped in a closed, smoke-filled space and not all inhalation injuries have associated facial cutaneous burns.

HINT

Hot gases and steam can also directly injure the airways through direct thermal damage.

Q What is the complication of smoke inhalation?

A Respiratory failure

Smoke inhalation extending into the alveoli leads to alveolar edema, loss of surfactant, and collapse of the lung units. ARDS is a complication of this alveolar damage. Other pulmonary complications include pulmonary edema, decreased lung compliance, tracheobronchitis, and pneumonia.

▶ **HINT**

The debris and secretions can overcome the airway's ability to clear the smoke and soot particles contributing to the atelectasis and alveolar collapse.

Q Besides carbon monoxide poisoning, what is a common poisoning that occurs from inhalation of gases in a house fire?

A Cyanide poisoning

Cyanide poisoning is a result of inhalation of burning polyurethanes, silk, paper, and wool, and commonly is associated with house fires. Cyanide interferes with the ability to produce adenosine triphosphate (ATP) at the cellular level by binding cytochrome oxidase. The loss of ATP can eventually result in cellular death. The administration of inhaled amyl nitrate and intravenous sodium nitrate is used to treat cyanide poisoning in patients in house fires. The nitrates work by converting iron in the hemoglobin to methemoglobin. Methemoglobin attracts the cyanide molecules, unbinding the cyanide from the cytochrome oxidase, which is needed to produce ATP.

▶ **HINT**

The side effect of the nitrates is hypoxemia because methemoglobin interferes with the ability of hemoglobin to bind and carry oxygen.

Q What laboratory value should the trauma nurse monitor in a patient with suspected cyanide poisoning?

A pH

A complication of elevated cyanide levels is a persistent metabolic acidosis and should be monitored in the clinical setting (Table 9.6). The arterial blood gas should be obtained to frequently evaluate the arterial pH.

Table 9.6 Complications of smoke inhalation

Complication	Onset
Acute pulmonary insufficiency	Immediate to early
Pulmonary edema	Occurs 48–72 hours after injury
Bronchial pneumonia	Occurs 48–72 hours after injury

▶ **HINT**

Reminder, a patient with metabolic acidosis hyperventilates to lower the $PaCO_2$. Hyperventilation is a sign of cyanide toxicity.

▶ **HINT**

The examination may use questions about complications with a hint provided in the scenario that refers to the timing of onset of complications.

Q What is a common cardiac complication following electrical burn injuries?

A Cardiac arrhythmias

Cardiac arrhythmias may be common because of the effects of the electrical current on the heart's intrinsic pacemaker. Cardiac arrhythmias can occur following any type of electrical current injury or burn (Box 9.6).

Box 9.6 Complications of electrical burns

- Rhabdomyolysis
- Cardiac arrhythmias
- Cataracts
- Neurological injuries
- Devitalized muscle and amputations
- Bone fractures
- Wound infections
- Vascular disruption, hemorrhage, and thrombi
- Cervical and spine injuries

HINT

Cardiac abnormalities may be evident on admission to the ED within several hours of the electrical burn.

Q Following an electrical burn injury, the patient's urine is noted to be dark brown. What is the most likely cause?

A Rhabdomyolysis

Urine with myoglobin is a brownish red color, almost tea or cola colored. Extensive muscle damage from the electrical burn causes the release of myoglobin (protein pigment in muscle), which is then filtered and excreted in the urine (myoglobinuria). Myoglobinuria can cause acute renal failure, which is called *rhabdomyolysis*. If pigment (myoglobin or hemoglobin) is present, urine output of at least 100 to 150 mL/hr must be maintained.

HINT

Sodium bicarbonate and mannitol may be administered in patients with myoglobinuria to alkalinize the urine and flush the myoglobin through the renal system.

Q What is the term used to describe the complication of permanent marking of the skin following an abrasion?

A Tattooing

Dirt and debris can be ground into the skin with an abrasion. If the abrasion is not thoroughly cleaned, it may leave a permanent stain or dark discoloration called a *tattoo*.

HINT

Facial abrasions are most susceptible to tattooing.

Q Following the loss of a large surface area of tissue, what is a potential complication the trauma nurse should be aware of?

A Hypothermia

Abrasions that cover greater than 40% of the TBSA are susceptible to heat loss and hypothermia. The trauma nurse should ensure the patient is being warmed, especially when large losses of skin and tissue have occurred.

HINT

The trauma room temperature should be warm and intravenous fluids should be warmed prior to administration.

Q What animal bite has the highest wound infection rates?

A Cat bites

Cat bites tend to have a greater risk of infection than dog bites because the fangs of cats are smaller and longer, causing a deeper puncture. Deep-puncture wounds carry a greater risk of infection because they are deeper wounds that can trap bacteria. Dog bites tend to have more of a tearing effect and bleed more than cat bites, thus clearing some of the bacteria from the wound.

HINT

Puncture and lacerations of the hands carry a risk of wound infection and osteomyelitis because the bones are so close to the surface.

Q The management of contractures and correction of functional deficits occur during which phase of burn injury?

A Rehabilitative phase

The rehabilitative phase involves prevention of complications and treatment of contractures, job retraining, and correction of other functional deficits. Correct positioning of the patient's burned extremities prevents contractures in the acute period and prevents the need to correct a contracture.

HINT

Rehabilitation begins on admission.

Q To prevent contractures, what is the correct position of a hand with burns?

A Separated fingers

Patients with hand burns require a splint to keep the fingers separated and the wrist cocked-up to prevent contractures. Patients with burns to the neck area should have the neck maintained in a neutral position and avoid pillows being placed behind the head, which causes neck flexion and contractures.

▶ HINT

Splints should be assessed frequently for skin breakdown.

Q Burns to the face may result in difficulty performing what activity of daily living?

A Eating

Burns on the face and head may cause problems with the patient's ability to talk, eat, swallow, or drink. Burns of the hands can interfere with many other activities of daily living and with many careers. Patients with burns on their feet may have difficulties with ambulation and running. Perineal area burns can result in urinary- and bowel-elimination difficulties, cause a greater incidence of urinary tract infections, and may interfere with the patient's sexual activity.

▶ HINT

Burns on the arms require occupational therapy and burns on the feet and lower extremities need physical therapy.

Q What complication can occur if the patient exposes the new skin following a burn to sun?

A Altered pigmentation

If the new skin is allowed to tan, this may cause it to have a permanently blotched appearance. Patients should be told to wear sunscreen with high sun protection on burned areas to prevent further thermal damage and pigmentation changes.

▶ HINT

Newly healed skin may be sensitive to heat and areas of the healed burn can be numb; therefore, instruct the patient to test the water of a bath or shower before entering.

Q What are commonly used to prevent hypertrophic scarring on extremities during rehabilitation?

A Pressure garments

Pressure garments used on the extremities can help limit the amount of hypertrophic scarring, which can develop during the wound-healing stages. To decrease the amount of scarring, silicone gel sheets and elastomer molds may also be used to soften and flatten skin.

▶ HINT

Use of pressure garments may be recommended for 2 to 3 hours a day over the next 1 to 2 years.

KNOWLEDGE CHECK: CHAPTER 9

1. Which of the following is considered the number one cause of fatal fires?
   - A. Cigarettes
   - B. Cooking
   - C. Candles
   - D. Arson

2. Which of the following areas of the body is the most commonly involved burn area?
   - A. Lower extremities
   - B. Face
   - C. Neck
   - D. Upper extremities

3. There are three classification zones of burns based on the extent and depth of the injury. Which of the following zones is described as less superficial and is a result of vascular damage and inflammatory response resulting in compromised tissue perfusion?
   - A. Zone of hyperemia
   - B. Zone of stasis
   - C. Zone of coagulation
   - D. None of the above

4. Which of the following depths of burn wounds has thrombosed veins, muscle, and/or bone involvement?
   - A. Superficial burn
   - B. Partial-thickness burn
   - C. Full-thickness burn
   - D. None of the above

5. A patient came in with third-degree burns to the anterior torso sustained from a pot of boiling water. The patient is experiencing diuresis following the third-spacing and edematous tissue. What phase of burn shock is this patient presenting?
   - A. Resuscitative phase
   - B. Acute phase
   - C. Recovery phase
   - D. Rehabilitation phase

6. Following a partial-thickness burn, when would the greatest amount of fluid loss resulting in hypovolemia occur?
   - A. 4 days postburn
   - B. 3 days postburn
   - C. 2 days postburn
   - D. 1 day postburn

(See answers next page.)

1. A) Cigarettes

Cigarette-smoking accidents are the number one cause of fatal fires. This is typically because a person carelessly discards or abandons the smoking materials and ends up igniting trash, bedding, or upholstered furniture. Cooking equipment is the leading cause of home fires and of injuries in home fires. Candle fires are not very common, but one out of three fatal candle fires in the home occurred when the candles were used for light because of a power outage. Incidence of arson has decreased over the past 30 years but remains the leading cause of property damage in the United States.

2. D) Upper extremities

The upper extremity of the body is the most commonly burned area of the body, followed by the head-and-neck regions. This may be the result of using the arms in an attempt to shield the face or body or in cases of carrying flammable material/explosives. Lower extremities tend to be the least commonly burned body part.

3. B) Zone of stasis

This accurately describes the zone of stasis. If resuscitation is promptly initiated following a burn injury, it may restore blood flow to the zone of stasis, allowing tissue to survive. The zone of hyperemia involves the most peripheral and superficial areas of the burn; it is erythema of a first-degree burn. The zone of coagulation is the area that contains irreversible cell death and involves the most severe burn area, which had the most intimate contact with the heat source.

4. C) Full-thickness burn

Full-thickness burns are as also called *third-* and *fourth-degree burns*. These burns may have charring, dark brown, or white skin and will be hard to the touch. Pain is usually only present at the periphery of the burn. Superficial burns (first-degree) have red skin and pain at the site. Partial-thickness (second-degree) burns have blisters, intense pain, white or red skin, and are moist or mottled but do not involve muscle or bone.

5. B) Acute phase

The resuscitative phase begins with the hemodynamic response and lasts until capillary integrity is restored and the plasma volume is replaced. The acute phase starts with the onset of diuresis of edematous fluid mobilized from the interstitial space and continues until the closure of the burn wound. The last phase, the rehabilitation phase, includes prevention and correction of functional deficits, contracture releases, psychological support, and job retraining. The recovery phase is not a recognized phase of the three phases of burn shock.

6. D) 1 day postburn

The greatest amount of fluid loss for partial-thickness burns occurs on the first day of injury (within 24 hours). Full-thickness burns have the greatest fluid loss at 4 days postburn.

7. Which of the following is a systemic complication that is commonly associated with burns?

   A. Acute respiratory distress syndrome (ARDS)
   B. Traumatic brain injury (TBI)
   C. Peritonitis
   D. Adrenal insufficiency

8. A patient came into the ED after receiving second-degree burns to the right hand from a hot liquid spill. The patient has a dressing applied to the site by the paramedic team; blood pressure is 119/82 mmHg, heart rate is 98 beats per minute, respiratory rate is 20 breaths per minute, oxygen saturation is 97% on room air, and pain is scored 8/10 on a 1 to 10 pain scale. What should the nurse do next?

   A. Place the patient on a nonrebreather face mask.
   B. Administer ordered morphine sulfate.
   C. Infuse intravenous normal saline.
   D. Replace the dressing to the site.

9. A 22-year-old patient was found unconscious in a running car inside a garage. The patient was brought to the ED. What would be the first intervention for this patient?

   A. 100% FiO_2 via nonrebreather
   B. 50% FiO_2 via partial face mask
   C. 6 L oxygen via humidified nasal cannula
   D. 4 L oxygen via nasal cannula

10. Fluid resuscitation needs to be a priority in treating patients with greater than 20% total body surface area (TBSA) burns or greater than 10% in the pediatric or older adult populations. Using the Parkland formula for a 154-pound man with a 40% TBSA, what would be the amount of isotonic fluid that needs to be administered within 24 hours?

   A. 11,200 mL
   B. 2,800 mL
   C. 24,640 mL
   D. 6,160 mL

(See answers next page.)

7. A) Acute respiratory distress syndrome (ARDS)

ARDS is commonly associated with burn patients. The physiology of burns includes an increase in capillary permeability. This leads to fluid extravasating into the lungs, causing interstitial and intra-alveolar fluid. TBI can occur in any trauma but is not associated primarily with burns. Peritonitis and adrenal insufficiency are not commonly associated with burn injuries.

8. B) Administer ordered morphine sulfate.

The patient with a second-degree burn should be medicated for pain. This patient is hemodynamically stable with an uncompromised airway and adequate evidence of perfusion. A dressing is already applied and the intravenous fluids may be continued with the management of pain.

9. A) 100% FiO_2 via nonrebreather

A patient with carbon monoxide poisoning should be immediately placed on 100% FiO_2 (fraction of inspired oxygen). This will accelerate the clearance of the carbon monoxide and promote oxygenation, oxygen carrying by hemoglobin, and tissue perfusion. The other answers do provide oxygen but are not enough to sufficiently clear carbon monoxide.

10. A) 11,200 mL

The Parkland formula is: 4 × weight (kg) × body surface area. In this patient: 4 × 70 kg × 40 = 11,200 mL. Hint: The 154 pounds needs to be converted to kilograms by dividing 154 by 2.2.

PART IV

Clinical Practice: Special Considerations

Psychosocial Issues of Trauma

Q What is one of the main reasons patients and families may have a difficult response to a traumatic event?

A Because it is an unexpected event

A traumatic or sudden event results in patients and families being unprepared for the injury (Box 10.1). The unexpected injury disrupts the normal routine and is not expected.

Box 10.1 Common psychological responses of patients to trauma

Anxiety
Fear
Pain
Isolation
Grief
Embarrassment (lack of privacy)

HINT

Trauma is frequently seen as something that "happens to other people."

Q What happens to normal coping mechanisms during a crisis?

A They become ineffective

A crisis is a sudden unexpected threat or loss of the basic resources of life that occurs when people's normal coping mechanism become ineffective. Trauma patients and their families frequently experience crisis immediately following the trauma and during various periods throughout their hospitalization.

HINT

Normal coping mechanisms may not be sustained for long periods of time during a crisis because of mental exhaustion.

Q All the unfamiliar sounds, sights, and constant stimulation experienced in the hospital can lead to what sensory abnormality?

A Sensory overload

Sensory overload is a common experience that occurs following severe trauma. It involves abnormal sounds such as unfamiliar voices and alarms, unfamiliar lines and tubes, unpleasant and unusual smells, and constant stimulation.

HINT

The loss of day and night routines and the associated sleep deprivation experienced in a hospital contribute to the sensory overload (Box 10.2).

Box 10.2 Ways to prevent sleep deprivation

Dim lighting at night
Sleep masks for patients to limit light
Grouping nursing interventions

Q What is a premorbid condition that influences the response of the patient to the traumatic event?

A Preexisting mental illness and/or personality disorder

A preexisting emotional disorder, mental illness, or personality disorder influences the patient's perception and response to the traumatic event. The patient's past experiences with healthcare and hospitalizations, either negative or positive, may also influence the patient's response to the trauma.

HINT

Other influences of patient's reactions to a traumatic event include religious, spiritual, and philosophical beliefs as well as educational level and socioeconomic status.

Q During the resuscitative phase of a trauma, what is the most common concern or fear of the patient?

A Fear of death

The fear of death or disability is a common concern of the patient during the initial resuscitation in the prehospital and ED. Severe pain is commonly associated with death.

HINT

The patient may initially only focus on what was lost and not what is still intact. They may be unable to see any part of their life that is not affected by the injury.

Q During resuscitation of a patient following a severe traumatic injury, the patient may exhibit behaviors of agitation. This may be a fear of what?

A Loss of self-control

The trauma patient may exhibit avoidance behavior, agitation, and/or verbal and physical hostility. This is typically a result of their experience of a loss of self-control and fear of what is happening.

HINT

An intervention to assist the patient during this phase is to get the patient's attention and have the patient listen to your voice as you provide instructions or explanation.

Q What is a major concern for patients during the critical care stage?

A Pain

The patient's focus begins to shift from fear of dying to fear of altered function or appearance. One of the biggest concerns or fears during this stage is pain. Other issues include sleep deprivation, development of delirium, and anxiety. These can negatively affect outcomes.

HINT

Many trauma patients have no recall of their experience in the ICU.

Q Following a traumatic injury, during the recovery phase the patient displays periods of anger and guilt. What are these signs of?

A Grief

Grief may be experienced following a trauma as a result of the loss of a body part, function, or even a loss of control. Grief is commonly displayed in stages of anger, guilt, bargaining, and depression. Patients may experience all these stages or only some of them.

HINT

These are the same stages of grief following the loss of a loved one.

Q No matter how critical the situation, the family needs to maintain a sense of what?

A Hope

Hope can be for improvement of their loved one's status or for recovery (Box 10.3). Hope can also be for their loved one not to suffer at the end of life.

Box 10.3 Psychosocial needs of the patient

Need for information
Need for compassionate care
Maintenance of hope

HINT

Hope can be the only positive emotion the patient or family may experience.

Q Frequently, what is the initial response of family members when receiving bad news regarding loved ones?

A Shock and denial

Most people are unprepared for the impact of a sudden injury or loss and react with shock and denial. They may also exhibit anger at the person relaying the information about their loved ones. Family reactions are dependent on past coping mechanisms, experience with loss, and current situations (Box 10.4).

Box 10.4 Common reactions of family members

Anxiety
Shock
Fright
Denial
Hostility
Distrust
Guilt
Remorse
Bargaining
Depression
Denial
Hope

HINT

Family members also move through the stages of grief and may not be at the same stage as the patient.

Q Families commonly go through phases regarding interactions with their loved one and staff members in the hospital. What is the primary reaction in the vigilance phase?

A Wanting to be at the bedside 24/7

The typical initial response of family members following a traumatic injury to their loved one is to feel the need to be at the patient's bedside every minute of the day. This is commonly called *vigilance*. They express concerns about being gone because of their fear of something bad happening in their absence, fear that they may miss speaking to the physician, or that their loved one may "wake up" while they are gone.

HINT

Nurses need to take the initiative and call family frequently with updates of the patient's status, which establishes a trusting relationship.

Q The trauma ICU nurse has been receiving frequent calls from different family members regarding the status of the patient. What would be the best response by the nurse?

A To establish a contact person

This is a common issue with patients in the ICU. The constant calls from family and friends seeking updates can be distracting and interfere with nursing care of the patients. Setting up a contact person within the family to whom healthcare staff can provide information regarding the updated status of the patient alleviates some of the calls.

HINT

Phone calls to the contact person from other family members and friends can also overwhelm the contact person. Nurses need to recommend methods for handling the calls (Box 10.5).

Box 10.5 Suggestions for dissemination of information

Establish a website with updated information, status, and progress.
Establish a chain of calls to deliver information to a larger number of people.
Develop an updated outgoing message daily on the phone.
E-mail updates to the group.
Text updates to the group.

HINT

Encourage immediate family members to have down time. "Allow" them to screen their calls.

Q The husband of a trauma patient in the ICU is found standing by his spouse's bedside without talking to them. What would be an appropriate response by the nurse?

A Encourage the husband to talk to them.

Families frequently do not know what to say to the patient or to talk about at the bedside. The nurse should encourage family and friends to normalize their conversations, for example, talk about daily happenings at work and home. Avoid talking only about the illness, injury, or treatments. If the patient is unresponsive, then talk about their hobbies, likes, or favorite activities. This is a component of a coma stimulation program.

HINT

Encourage family members to keep a diary at home and then talk to the patient from the diary. A role of the nurse is to assist with finding things to talk about when with their loved ones.

Q A physician enters the room of a comatose patient and begins to talk to the family about the prognosis over the patient's bed. What would be the best response of the nurse?

A Ask them to step outside the patient's room.

Asking the physician and the family member to step away from the patient's bedside is the best response of the nurse. Avoiding talking over the patient's bed about the patient's medical condition is the best practice.

HINT

Comatose patients are believed to be able to hear.

Q During family conferences, what is a common problem encountered when medical healthcare clinicians are informing the family of the patient's diagnosis and treatments?

A Use of medical jargon

When speaking with patients and family members, healthcare clinicians should avoid the use of medical jargon. Healthcare clinicians are frequently perceived as "speaking a different language." Nurses frequently play the role of "interpreter" for the physicians.

HINT

Nurses should regularly attend family conferences to help the family interpret, clarify, and continue cohesive discussions regarding the patient's medical illness and treatments.

Q What should the nurse do if the patient has repeated the story about the traumatic event several times during the shift?

A Listen.

A step toward acceptance of a traumatic event is to verbally reconstruct the event. Allow the patient to reconstruct the event of the trauma. They may repeat the story or talk about the event repetitively, but the nurse should actively listen each time to assist with validation of the event.

HINT

Posttraumatic stress disorder (PTSD) has been found to ease the more the person involved in the traumatic event tells the story of the event.

Q What has been found to be the number one need of the family during the hospitalization of their loved one?

A Information

The number one identified need of the family of a hospitalized loved one is the need for information. The family frequently wants to know everything that is going on with their loved one and often ask for lab results and vital signs or watch the monitors. There are three information-seeking reactions by family: monitoring, vigilance, and learning (Table 10.1).

Table 10.1 Information-seeking reactions

Monitoring	Asks general questions about their loved ones.
Vigilance	Seeks information to ensure necessary tasks are being carried out ("I thought they were going to do CT this morning." "Has she had her dinner yet?").
Learning	Uses the information to understand aspects of care.

HINT

Family commonly fixate or focus on certain things about their loved ones such as the blood pressure, heart rate, or temperature.

Q What is the primary benefit of assigning the same nurse to the patient every day when possible?

A Continuity of care

Continuity of nursing assignments provides consistency for patient and family. The nurse is more aware of family needs and is better able to reinforce teaching already provided to the family.

HINT

Family and patient's comfort level increases when they know who is providing the care.

Q What type of visitation in the ICU has been shown to be more effective for the patient and family?

A Open visitation

Families allowed to remain at the bedside with their loved one express feeling more assured about the care their loved one is receiving. They are more aware of any changes being made in the patient's care and this provides a sense of control for the family.

HINT

Not knowing what is happening on the "other side" of the doors when not allowed to visit produces anxiety.

Q What is an advantage of allowing a family member to remain at the bedside during the trauma resuscitation?

A Family knows everything possible has been done for their loved one

Currently, many institutions allow a family member to remain with their loved ones during the trauma resuscitation in the ED or during major invasive procedures. One of the most frequently found advantages to this is that the family is able to see the resuscitation and know that everything possible has been done for their loved one (Box 10.6).

Box 10.6 Advantages of family presence during resuscitation

Bonding between patients' family members and healthcare clinicians is facilitated.
Family members observe the efforts of the healthcare clinicians.
Family members can provide comfort and words of encouragement to the patient.
The family is able to have closure.
Acceptance of the outcome is facilitated.
Families perceive they are actively involved in the resuscitation of their loved one.
Family members can touch the patient while the patient is still "alive" or warm to say their goodbyes.
Staff can view the patient as part of a loving family; the patient is perceived as a "real" person.
The mystery of the activities that occur behind "closed doors" during a resuscitation is reduced.
Assists the family's comprehension of the seriousness of the condition.
Allows the family to become a part of the decision-making on when to stop a resuscitation.
Reminds staff that the patient is a person.
Encourages professional behavior of the healthcare team.

HINT

An important aspect of the success of family presence during resuscitation is the identification of a support person to be with the family member to explain the events during the resuscitation and provide clear family guidelines.

Q What approach is used to improve the quality of life at the time of a life-threatening illness?

A Palliative care

Palliative care is an approach that improves the quality of life of patients and families facing problems associated with life-threatening illness (Box 10.7). It involves the integration of physical, psychological, spiritual, cultural, and social needs of all those involved. It takes a significant role at end of life but may be administered concurrently with curative therapy.

Box 10.7 Measures provided by palliative care

Humanity
Dignity
Respect
Good communication
Clear information
Comfort
Pain management

HINT

Palliative care uses a multidisciplinary approach.

Q What is the ethical principle that is used to justify the administration of medication to relieve pain even though it may lead to the unintended, although foreseen, consequence of hastening death by causing respiratory depression?

A Principle of double effect

The principle of double effect provides that an action with both a good and a bad effect is ethically permissible if the following conditions are met:

1. The action itself must be morally good or at least indifferent.
2. Only the good effect must be intended (even though the bad or secondary effect is foreseen).
3. The good effect must not be achieved by way of the bad effect.
4. The good result must outweigh the bad result.

HINT

There is no debate among specialists in palliative care regarding pain control, and the belief is that it is unethical to withhold pain medication at the end of life.

Q A patient has recovered from a gunshot wound and is discharged home. At the 3-month follow-up clinic visit, the patient states they are beginning to experience nightmares and the family reports the person is easily angered and has heightened sensitivity. What is the most likely diagnosis?

A PTSD

PTSD occurs when an individual witnesses, experiences, or learns indirectly about a life-threatening event that endangers self or others. Trauma and critically ill patients can experience PTSD after the event and subsequent hospitalization. The onset of nightmares and being easily angered coupled with heightened sensitivity are all signs of PTSD (Table 10.2).

Table 10.2 Symptoms of posttraumatic stress disorder

Hyperarousal	Anger, irritability, hypervigilance, difficulty concentrating, heightened startle response
Intrusive recollection	Intrusive thoughts, nightmares, feelings and imagery, dissociative-like reexperiencing of trauma
Avoidance	Numbing of responsiveness; avoidance of feelings, situations, and ideas
Reliving the event	Mentally and emotionally
Flashbacks	
Avoiding people and situations	
Developing heightened sensitivity to changes in environment	Constantly on guard, "jumpy," easily startled
Severe anxiety	
Nightmares	
Intense emotions	Guilt, helplessness, hopelessness, or shame
Anhedonia	Loss of interest in former enjoyable activities

HINT

Following a critical care illness, patients may develop PTSD 3 to 6 months after discharge.

Q What is the underlying issue that can lead to PTSD in an ICU?

A Experiencing a traumatic event

Critical illness is a traumatic event and can lead to PTSD. Critical illness and the critical care environment can lead survivors to experience the symptoms of PTSD after hospital discharge. PTSD is a mental health disorder. It can be defined as the development of characteristic symptoms following exposure to extreme traumatic stressor and the person's response to the event involves intense fear, helplessness, or terror (Table 10.3).

Table 10.3 Critical care stressors for posttraumatic stress disorder

Isolation	Sedation
Painful procedures	Sleep deprivation
Feelings of helplessness	Fear of dying/imminent threat of death
Loss of control	

HINT

Cognitive processing at the time of the critical illness is important for the development of PTSD.

Q What is an identified risk factor for the traumatically injured patient to develop PTSD after hospital discharge?

A Delusional memories

The patient's recall of delusional events rather than the factual events has been found to be linked to greater incidence of PTSD after hospitalization (Table 10.4). Amnesia for the period of critical care is related to the severity of the PTSD. Some studies have found that patients who are more awake while on mechanical ventilation had less incidence and severity of PTSD. Fractions of memory and memory of events that did not occur increase the difficulty for patients to understand what happened to them during that time period.

Table 10.4 Risks for developing posttraumatic stress disorder in critically ill patients

Delusional memories	Fractional memory
Hallucinations	Delirium
History of depression and mental health issues	Minimizing sedation
Coping skills	ICU length of stay
Sepsis and MSOD	Lack of social support
Intubation and mechanical ventilation	Physical restraints
Sleep deprivation	Intraoperative recall of events

MSOD, multisystem organ dysfunction.

Q Which sleep disorder is most commonly found in posttrauma patients with PTSD?

A Nightmares

Nightmares are a common sleep abnormality that is a sign of PTSD. These nightmares can lead to the fear of sleeping and eventually sleep deprivation.

Q What nursing intervention can potentially improve and lower the PTSD after a traumatic event?

A Improve the patient's understanding of events

One area that can potentially lower the incidence and severity of PTSD is implementing interventions that improve the patient's understanding and recollection of true events (Table 10.5). ICU diaries are being used more often for hospital staff and family to write down events that happened for the patient to read after improvement. This provides factual information about their stay in the ICU, which allows the patient to reconstruct their memory on more factual recollections.

Table 10.5 Interventions to improve memory of critically ill patients

Explain all procedures to the patient.	Reorient the patient frequently.
Allow open family visitation.	Maintain ICU diaries.
Provide counseling sessions after discharge.	Allow patient to talk about their memories.

HINT

Even patients who are sedated or unresponsive can develop delusional memory and should be managed the same as lightly sedated patients.

Q What is a potential sequela of depression and PTSD after a traumatic injury?

A Suicide is associated with PTSD and depression (Table 10.6)

Table 10.6 Complications of posttraumatic stress disorder

Suicide	Drug and alcohol abuse
Loss of self-identity	Decreased quality of life

KNOWLEDGE CHECK: CHAPTER 10

1. Following a trauma, the patient is experiencing sleep deprivation, anxiety, and frequently complains of pain. Which of the following phases best describes these symptoms?

   A. Resuscitative phase
   B. Critical care phase
   C. Recovery phase
   D. Community phase

2. It is important that the trauma nurse understands the stages of grief and the grieving process to better recognize a trauma patient's behavior in grief. Which of the following is considered a stage of grief?

   A. Guilt
   B. Fear
   C. Bargaining
   D. Frustration

3. The family members of trauma patients may be afraid to leave and miss seeing the physician. The nurse can perform several interventions to aid the family in this process. Which intervention is most effective in dealing with this situation?

   A. Obtain their phone numbers to keep at bedside for the physician when they come to the bedside or when an emergency arises.
   B. Encourage family to take breaks and rest to conserve their energy for when the patient leaves the ICU.
   C. Promise them that they will not miss anything and encourage them to leave and take a break.
   D. Set up family/physician visits.

4. Which of the following is most commonly found in posttraumatic stress disorder (PTSD) following a traumatic injury?

   A. Reexperiencing the traumatic event
   B. Hallucinations
   C. Denial of the event
   D. Early-onset dementia

5. A 5-year-old patient was witness to a domestic dispute between their mother and father. The event concluded with the father physically attacking the mother. Which of the following is a common behavior of a child who is suffering from posttraumatic stress disorder (PTSD)?

   A. Bed-wetting
   B. Being disrespectful
   C. Turning to alcohol and drugs
   D. Feeling guilty for the situation

(*See answers next page.*)

1. B) Critical care phase

The resuscitative phase occurs early following the trauma and the patient experiences fear of death or disability, loss of self-control, severe pain, avoidance behaviors, agitation, hostility, and overall negativity. The second phase is the critical care phase, which includes fear of altered function rather than fear of death, severe pain, sleep deprivation, and anxiety, which the patient is currently experiencing. The last phase is the recovery phase, and it includes the patient dealing with loss, feeling "powerless," experiencing stages of grief, and relying on a support system. Community phase is not an identified phase of psychological progression in trauma care.

2. C) Bargaining

Although a trauma patient will frequently exhibit feelings of frustration, fear, and guilt, they are not identified as a part of the grieving process. The most widely accepted process of grieving includes denial, anger, bargaining, depression, and acceptance. Understanding the grieving process is important for nurses so they can recognize symptoms of grief and manage the behaviors of patients and their families during this time.

3. D) Set up family/physician visits.

Setting up physician/family meetings to keep everyone on the same page with the plan of care is the most effective way to improve comfort of the family. Promising the family that they "won't miss anything" is unreliable. The nurse should not "promise" that the patient's status will not change, or that a physician might not come in during time frame when they are gone. Keeping contact numbers visible and obtainable at bedside is important but does not solve the issue of the family wanting to speak to the physicians. The nurses should encourage families to take a break and conserve energy for when the patient leaves the ICU, but this does not solve the issue of worrying about missing speaking with the physician.

4. A) Reexperiencing the traumatic event

Reexperiencing the traumatic event commonly occurs and may include upsetting memories, flashbacks, and nightmares. PTSD may also present with difficulty concentrating, feeling jumpy, irritable, and hypervigilant. Denial of the event and hallucinations are not typically a normal response with PTSD. Early-onset dementia is not a risk with PTSD.

5. A) Bed-wetting

Children can have extreme reactions to trauma and children younger than 6 years of age can develop bed-wetting habits after being potty-trained. Forgetting how to or being unable to talk, acting out the scary event during playtime, and being unusually clingy are other signs of PTSD. Older children and teens are more likely to develop disruptive, disrespectful, or destructive behaviors. Older children and teens may feel guilty for not preventing the injury or death or turn to alcohol and drugs.

Shock

ANAPHYLAXIS

Q How is anaphylaxis different than anaphylactoid reaction?

A It is mediated by immunoglobulin E (IgE)

Anaphylaxis and anaphylactoid reactions are both acute life-threatening hypersensitivity reactions, but anaphylaxis is immune related, whereas anaphylactoid reaction is not. Anaphylaxis involves antibodies binding to an antigen to which the person was previously exposed. Anaphylactoid reactions do not have the immune component but are similar in assessment, diagnosis, and treatment.

HINT

Anaphylaxis and anaphylactoid reactions are called *life-threatening hypersensitivity reactions*.

Q How quickly can symptoms of hypersensitivity reactions occur following exposure to the provoking agent?

A Within minutes

Onset of symptoms can occur within minutes to hours. Typically, symptoms will peak in severity within 5 to 30 minutes. The episode frequently lasts less than 24 hours but can be protracted or reoccur after an initial resolution.

HINT

Rapid intervention to hypersensitivity reactions is required to maintain airway and circulation.

Q In both hypersensitivity reactions, what is triggered causing the release of chemical mediators?

A Mast cells

Mast cells are activated in both anaphylaxis and anaphylactoid reactions, releasing several chemical mediators (Box 11.1). Overall, the mediators increase capillary permeability and cause peripheral vasodilation. The increased capillary permeability can cause airway swelling and angioedema. Peripheral vasodilation results in hypotension, which is considered a distributive shock.

Box 11.1 Chemical mediators

Bradykinin
Platelet-activating factor
Prostaglandins
Leukotrienes

HINT

The most life-threatening component of a hypersensitivity reaction is angioedema.

Q What are the two most common causes of anaphylaxis?
A Food allergies and insect stings

Food allergies (Box 11.2), insect stings, and antibiotics are the most common causes of an IgE-mediated anaphylactic reaction (Box 11.3). These occur after previous exposure to the provoking agent. Stinging insects, such as bees, wasps, and fire ants, contain a substance in their venom that initiates the IgE antibody response. Penicillin is the most common antibiotic to cause an anaphylaxis reaction. Other common antibiotics include cephalosporin and sulfonamides (Box 11.4).

Box 11.2 Common food allergies causing anaphylaxis

Peanuts
Shellfish
Fish
Tree nuts
Milk
Eggs
Seeds

Box 11.3 Causes of immunoglobulin E-mediated hypersensitivity reactions

Food allergies
Insect stings
Pollen
Antibiotics
Muscle relaxants
Latex
Snake bites

Box 11.4 Causes of nonimmunologic hypersensitivity

- Contrast media
- Opioids
- ASA and NSAIDs

ASA, acetylsalicylic acid; NSAIDs, nonsteroidal anti-inflammatory drugs.

HINT

Some food allergens are so severe that just touching or inhaling the odor of the food can cause the hypersensitivity reaction.

Q What is the most life-threatening symptom of anaphylaxis reactions?

A Angioedema

Angioedema can cause the loss of airway from edema and is the most life-threatening symptom of anaphylaxis. Symptoms include wheezing and dyspnea. Urticaria is a common associated symptom. Sudden loss of consciousness can also be an initial sign and patients may report a feeling of "impending" doom (Box 11.5).

Box 11.5 Symptoms of anaphylaxis

- Airway swelling
- Urticaria and pruritus
- Dyspnea
- Wheezing
- Shortness of breath
- Tachypnea
- Nausea and vomiting
- Diarrhea
- Abdominal pain
- Hypotension
- Dizziness and syncope
- Chest tightness and pain
- Headache
- Seizure
- Flushing

HINT

Airway issues should be considered the most life-threatening complication of an anaphylactic reaction.

Q What is the initial drug used to treat an anaphylaxis reaction?

A Epinephrine (adrenergic agonist)

Epinephrine is administered in a 1:1,000 dilution 0.2- to 0.5-mg dose subcutaneously or intramuscularly. If severe hypotension exists, administer epinephrine via continuous infusion. It is an alpha and beta agonist but will also decrease release of mast cells. Hypotension is treated with fluid resuscitation and vasopressors, and supplemental oxygen is applied. Steroids and antihistamines (Benadryl) sometimes provide even greater relief of symptoms.

HINT

Antihistamines block the H1 receptor; adding an H2 receptor blocker (Famotidine) can enhance effectiveness.

Q What drug can limit effectiveness of epinephrine?

A Beta-blockers

Patients taking beta-blockers may be resistant to epinephrine, demonstrating continued hypotension and bradycardia. Atropine may be required to manage the bradycardia.

HINT

Other drugs that may interfere with the effectiveness of epinephrine include angiotensin-converting enzyme (ACE) inhibitors and monoamine oxidase (MAO) inhibitors.

Q If a patient states that they have had an allergic reaction to contrast dye but still requires the diagnostic procedure, what can be given prior to the administration of contrast dye to decrease its allergic reaction?

A Steroids and antihistamines

Pretreatment can be performed with steroid and antihistamine prior to giving contrast dye in a sensitive patient requiring a diagnostic procedure.

HINT

Pretreatment with steroids and antihistamines does not guarantee that the patient will not have hypersensitivity reactions; therefore, the patient requires close monitoring.

CARDIOGENIC SHOCK

Q What type of shock is the most severe form of heart failure?

A Cardiogenic shock

Cardiogenic shock is the most severe form of heart failure and requires emergency management. It is a life-threatening condition.

HINT

Cardiac tamponade can also result in shock and is called an *obstructive shock*.

Q What is the primary cause of cardiogenic shock?

A Ischemia

Acute coronary syndromes (ACSs) result in myocardial ischemia and loss of myocardial muscle. This can lead to abnormal contractility and dilated cardiomyopathy. Ischemic cardiomyopathies are the primary causes of cardiogenic shock (Box 11.6). *Cardiogenic shock* is defined as hypoperfusion caused by cardiac failure (Box 11.7).

Box 11.6 Other causes of cardiogenic shock

Box 11.6 Other causes of cardiogenic shock
Hypertrophied cardiomyopathy
Aortic dissection with aortic insufficiency
Aortic or mitral stenosis (increases myocardial stress)
Acute myopericarditis
Stress-induced cardiomyopathy (Takotsubo cardiomyopathy)
Acute valvular regurgitation (endocarditis or chordal rupture)
Cardiac tamponade
Massive pulmonary embolism

Box 11.7 Definition of cardiogenic shock

Presence of at least two of the following:
Hypotension with SBP <90 or need for inotropes to maintain pressure >90 mmHg
Evidence of end organ hypoperfusion
Cardiac index <2.2 L/min/m^2

SBP, systolic blood pressure.

HINT

Blunt trauma to the chest can cause myocardial contusion, which can also result in cardiogenic shock.

Q What are the characteristic hemodynamic parameters of cardiogenic shock?

A Low cardiac index (CI), high systemic vascular resistance (SVR), and high filling pressures

Cardiogenic shock demonstrates persistent hypotension with severe reduction in CI and adequate or elevated filling pressures (Box 11.8). Compensatory mechanisms for low CI include vasoconstriction (elevates SVR) and tachycardia, which actually worsen the CI because of the decreased filling and increased workload of the heart, causing a vicious cycle to develop.

Box 11.8 Other symptoms of cardiogenic shock

Tachycardia
Cool, clammy skin
Pale nail beds with delayed capillary refill
Decreased urine output
Altered mental status
Tachypnea
Presence of arrhythmias

HINT

Severe reduction of the CI is defined as less than 1.8 L/min/m² without support, and less than 2.0 to 2.2 L/min/m² with support.

Q What monitoring device may be used to assist with the diagnosis of cardiogenic shock?

A Pulmonary artery catheter (PAC)

The PAC provides information on the CI, filling pressures, and is used to calculate the SVR. These readings can be used to define and recognize cardiogenic shock. Newer hemodynamic monitors that are minimally invasive and use the arterial waveform may also be used to assist with the diagnosis.

HINT

Echocardiogram may be used to confirm the diagnosis of high filling pressures and rule out other causes of hypotension following blunt chest trauma.

Q What is an early treatment method used to manage acute myocardial ischemic cardiogenic shock (AMICS)?

A Mechanical circulatory support (MCS)

MCS has been found to improve outcomes when applied early in the shock process. Current MCS includes intra-aortic balloon pumps (IABP), Impella, and venoarterial extra-corporeal membrane oxygenation (VA-ECMO).

HINT

Early percutaneous coronary intervention (PCI) for management of acute myocardial ischemia (AMI) is recommended as treatment for cardiogenic shock.

Q What is the greatest concern when administering an inotropic agent to a patient in cardiogenic shock?

A Increased myocardial workload and oxygen consumption

Inotropic agents are frequently needed to increase CI and reduce filling pressures in the right and left ventricles, but they can increase the oxygen demand in the heart with limited oxygen supply. This may increase the ischemic injuries to the myocardium. Inotropes are recommended in hypoperfusion states with or without pulmonary congestion but may be initiated at a lower dose in cardiogenic shock to limit complications.

> **HINT**
>
> **Inotropes can also induce arrhythmias in ischemic hearts and should be closely monitored.**

Q What is a first-line intervention in managing hypotension in cardiogenic shock?

A Inotropes

Vasoconstrictors (i.e., norepinephrine) should not be used initially to treat hypotension in cardiogenic shock because of the presence of increased SVR. Other interventions for managing hypotension in cardiogenic shock include a combination of inotropic agents with vasodilators, fluid challenges with inotropic agents, and MCS.

> **HINT**
>
> **If vasoconstrictors are needed, norepinephrine and dopamine may be used.**

HEMORRHAGIC/HYPOVOLEMIC SHOCK

Q What is the major component in defining shock?

A Hypoperfusion

Shock is the pathophysiologic state in which there is defective vascular perfusion of tissues and organs. It is a state of inadequacies between delivery of oxygen and the removal of end products of metabolism from peripheral tissues. This results in widespread reduction in tissue perfusion, hypoxia, and conversion of cellular respiration to an anaerobic form of metabolism that produces lactate as a by-product. Rapid restoration of oxygen delivery can be a major factor in preventing the development of end-organ ischemia.

> **HINT**
>
> **Remember, shock is defined by hypoperfusion, not hypotension.**

Q During hypovolemic shock, which compensatory mechanism decreases urine output in an attempt to restore circulating blood volume?

A Renin–angiotensin system

During periods of hypovolemia and hypoperfusion, the kidneys release renin, which converts angiotensin I to angiotensin II. Angiotensin II is a potent vasoconstrictor that shunts blood away from nonvital organs. Angiotensin II stimulates the release of aldosterone, which results in sodium and water reabsorption. This decreases the urine output while increasing vascular volume. The sympathetic nervous system is another compensatory system activated during hypovolemic shock. It results in tachycardia, increased myocardial contractility, and vasoconstriction.

HINT

Vasoconstriction may maintain a mean arterial pressure (MAP) during hypovolemic shock. Vital signs may not reflect the presence or severity of shock.

Q What are the hemodynamic findings of hypovolemic shock that differentiate it from other types of shock?

A Low filling pressures and high SVR

Hypovolemic shock is caused by a decrease in circulating blood volume, causing a low stroke volume (SV) and cardiac output (CO). Hypovolemia can be caused by blood loss (trauma), poor intake, increased fluid losses, or redistribution of fluid (third-spacing).

HINT

Both the central venous pressure (CVP) and pulmonary capillary wedge pressure (PCWP) are low in hypovolemic shock.

Q What compensatory compartmental fluid shift occurs with hemorrhagic shock?

A Fluid shifts from extravascular space into intravascular space

In hemorrhagic shock, fluid shifts from the extravascular spaces into the intravascular space to compensate for the blood loss. In disease states in which plasma volume is lost, fluid shifts from the intravascular to the interstitial space (burn injuries).

HINT

The shift into extravascular space is frequently called *third-spacing* and can result in hypovolemic shock. Examples include peritonitis, burns, and crush injuries.

Q Following a trauma, the patient presents with the following vital signs on admission:
Heart rate (HR): 124 beats per minute
Respiration rate: 32 breaths per minute
Blood pressure (BP): 94/60 mmHg
Urinary output: 15 mL/hr
Based on these vital signs, what is the class of hemorrhagic shock?

A Class III hemorrhagic shock

The American College of Surgeons (ACS) has developed a classification of hemorrhagic shock based on vital signs to indicate the severity of blood loss. This is not exact and patient presentation can vary.

HINT

Older adults patients may not become tachycardic because of limited response to catecholamines.

Q A class III hemorrhagic shock would indicate what percentage of blood loss?

A About 30% to 40%

The classification is based on the percentage of total blood volume (TBV) loss. The estimated amount of blood volume loss is based on a 70-kg male who has approximately 5 L TBV. A 30% to 40% TBV loss (class III) would be approximately 1,500 to 2,000 mL (Table 11.1).

Table 11.1 American College of Surgeons classification of hemorrhage

	Class I	Class II	Class III	Class IV
Blood loss (mL)	<750	750–1,500	1,500–2,000	>2,000
Blood loss (%)	<15	15–30	30–40	>40
Systolic BP	Normal	Normal	Decreased	Decreased
Heart rate (beats/min)	<100	>100	>120	>140
Respiratory rate (breaths/min)	14–20	20–30	30–40	>35
Mental status	Anxious	Agitated	Confused	Lethargic

BP, blood pressure.

HINT

Because of the effectiveness of their compensatory mechanisms, young patients may have a normal BP and HR even in the presence of significant blood loss. Older adults patients may be hypotensive even with minimal blood loss.

Q What classification of drugs limits the tachycardic response that occurs during hemorrhagic shock?

A Beta-blockers

Blocking the beta-receptors of the heart results in limited ability to respond to the sympathetic nervous system with tachycardia. The lack of tachycardia does not rule out hemorrhagic shock in patients taking beta-blockers. Other signs of hypovolemic shock include pale, cool, and clammy skin. The urine output will progressively decrease as shock worsens.

HINT

Hypovolemic or hemorrhagic shock patients may narrow the pulse pressure before decreasing systolic BP.

Q Which laboratory studies may be used to identify the presence of shock in a normotensive patient?

A Lactate and base deficit

Vital signs are not reliable in identifying all patients in shock. Cellular metabolism is limited by inadequate tissue perfusion and results in mandatory changes from an aerobic to an anaerobic metabolism. In anaerobic metabolism, the production of lactic acid is an end product that creates lactic acidosis.

HINT

Elevated lactate levels and presence of a base deficit are used to identify hypoperfusion.

Q What is a base deficit?

A Amount of base needed to titrate 1 L of whole blood to pH of 7.40

The base deficit reflects the extent of anaerobic metabolism and severity of the metabolic acidosis. This value is obtained from an arterial blood gas. The normal base is +2 to −2 mEq/L, with positive numbers indicating a base excess and negative numbers indicating a base deficit.

HINT

Base deficit is used as an end point of resuscitation (Table 11.2).

Table 11.2 Base deficit determines severity of hypovolemia

Severity of Hypovolemia	Base Deficit
Mild	−3 to −5
Moderate	−6 to −14
Severe	> −15

Q Why does the hemoglobin (Hgb)/hematocrit (Hct) not accurately reflect the red blood cell (RBC) mass during an acute hemorrhage?

A Because of equal loss of all blood components

Hct and Hgb concentrations are indices of balance between loss of blood and movement of extravascular fluid to intravascular space. During an acute hemorrhage, a loss of whole blood occurs and all blood components decrease in a similar ratio. If the initial Hgb is low, it is caused by fluid administration and hemodilution. The rate of change in Hgb over time is more predictive of the severity of bleeding.

HINT

A normal Hgb and Hct does not rule out active bleeding.

Q What is the primary treatment for hemorrhagic shock?

A Intravenous (IV) fluids

IV fluids are the mainstay treatment for hypovolemia. In the case of trauma or acute bleeding, finding the source of blood loss and stopping the bleeding surgically may be required. If the patient is hypothermic, the resuscitation fluids should be warmed prior to or during infusion.

HINT

Remember that airway and breathing are still priorities of care in a hemorrhagic shock patient.

Q What is the greatest disadvantage of resuscitating with crystalloids?

A Fluid shifts from intravascular to interstitial space

Crystalloids are electrolyte solutions with small molecules, which can shift across the spaces. A large amount of infused crystalloids will shift from the intravascular to the interstitial space within minutes of administration. This requires larger volumes of fluids to be administered to replace the vascular losses. Frequently used crystalloids for resuscitation include isotonic solutions such as lactated Ringer's and normal saline (NS).

HINT

A 3:1 replacement rule has been used to determine the amount required for crystalloid resuscitation.

Q Large-volume infusions of NS can cause which acid–base imbalance?

A Metabolic acidosis

A 1-L bag of NS contains 154 mEq/L of sodium and chloride. Large amounts of NS administered during resuscitation can cause a hyperchloremic metabolic acidosis. Lactated Ringer's solution is a more balanced salt solution and may be used in large-volume resuscitations to prevent metabolic acidosis (Table 11.3).

Table 11.3 Crystalloids versus colloids

	Crystalloids	Colloids
Advantages	Replaces interstitial fluid losses that may have occurred Cheaper Easier to store	Use less fluid to resuscitate May draw fluid into the vascular space from interstitial Albumin may have anti-inflammatory effects
Disadvantages	Uses larger amounts of fluid to resuscitate	During altered capillary permeability, albumin shifts can shift interstitial Synthetic colloids (i.e., dextran) activate immune response May cause hypersensitivity reaction Synthetic colloids increase bleeding tendencies More expensive Difficult to store

HINT

Patient's respiratory rate may be rapid to compensate for metabolic acidosis.

Q Which crystalloid is used to increase serum osmolality and rapidly expands the intravascular space?

A Hypertonic saline

Small amounts of hypertonic saline (4–5 mL/kg) can decrease the total amount of crystalloids used during resuscitation. Hypertonic saline increases serum osmolality and draws fluid from the extravascular into the intravascular space. It may improve blood flow to organs and has been found to lower intracranial pressure (Box 11.9).

Box 11.9 Hypertonic saline

Na+ (sodium) in 3% saline is 513 mEq/L with Cl– (chloride) of 513 mEq/L
Na+ in 7.5% saline is 1,283 mEq/L with Cl– of 1,283 mEq/L

HINT

Metabolic acidosis and hypernatremia are complications of hypertonic saline caused by the large amount of chloride, even greater than in NS.

Q When giving multiple units of packed red blood cells (PRBCs), what other blood products need to be administered?

A Fresh frozen plasma (FFP) and platelets

Administering PRBCs and fluid causes a dilutional coagulopathy. PRBCs are void of clotting factors and platelets. Hemostatic resuscitation pushed for early use of blood transfusions and not as much crystalloid. Currently, a 1:1:1 rule of plasma, platelets, and PRBC is followed. For every one unit of blood, administer plasma and platelets.

HINT

Whole blood does have platelets and clotting factors and can be used instead of PRBCs to resuscitate a trauma patient.

Q What is a benefit of hypotensive resuscitation in a bleeding patient?

A It limits blood loss

Avoiding aggressive fluid resuscitation to increase the BP may limit the amount of blood volume loss in a bleeding patient prior to surgery. Hypotensive resuscitation aims to maintain the systolic BP between 80 to 90 mmHg with smaller boluses of fluid (200 mL bolus). Higher systolic BP increases intravascular hydrostatic pressure, worsening blood loss in a bleeding patient. The risk of this strategy is hypoperfusion.

HINT

Maintain the systolic BP greater than 90 mmHg for those with traumatic brain injury.

Q What is the lethal triad complication following severe traumatic injury with significant blood loss?

A Acidosis, hypothermia, coagulopathy

The acute loss of blood can result in decreased perfusion contributing to metabolic acidosis. Trauma-induced coagulopathy can occur in absence of fluid resuscitation.

KNOWLEDGE CHECK: CHAPTER 11

1. A shock patient experiences vasoconstriction, tachycardia, and increased myocardial contractility. This is a result of which system being activated?

   A. Parasympathetic nervous system
   B. Sympathetic nervous system
   C. Renin–angiotensin system (RAS)
   D. Brain natriuretic peptide (BNP)

2. What is the fluid shift that occurs with hemorrhagic shock?

   A. Fluid shifts from the extravascular to the intravascular space.
   B. Fluid shifts from the intravascular to the extravascular space.
   C. Fluid shifts into the brain parenchyma.
   D. Fluid shifts into the kidney's parenchyma.

3. A patient comes into the ED after an accidental saw injury to the right arm. The patient is anxious and confused about the time and situation. The following vital signs are obtained:
   Respiratory rate is 33 breaths per minute.
   Heart rate is 135 beats per minute (bpm).
   Blood pressure is 92/56 mmHg.
   Oxygen saturation is 92% on 2 L via nasal cannula.
   What classification of hemorrhagic shock is the patient most likely experiencing?

   A. Class I
   B. Class II
   C. Class III
   D. Class IV

4. A bleeding patient comes into the ED. The healthcare team is administering blood products. There is no crossmatch so this patient will receive the universal donor blood, O negative, until a crossmatch can be obtained. Which of the following statements is most correct?

   A. A new crossmatch needs to be sent after multiple universal blood transfusions.
   B. The universal donor blood type is AB negative.
   C. Massive transfusion patients are defined as 5 units or more in a 24-hour period.
   D. O-positive blood can be administered to a female patient of childbearing age as uncrossmatched blood.

5. Which of the following differentiates anaphylaxis from anaphylactoid reaction?

   A. Angioedema is always related to anaphylaxis.
   B. Anaphylactoid reactions occur after the second exposure to an antigen.
   C. Anaphylaxis involves the immune system.
   D. Anaphylactoid reactions are not life-threatening.

(See answers next page.)

1. B) Sympathetic nervous system

When activated, the sympathetic nervous system, also known as the *fight-or-flight response*, results in tachycardia, vasoconstriction, and increased myocardial contractility. The vasoconstriction shunts blood to vital organs such as the heart and brain. The parasympathetic nervous system would do the exact opposite; it causes vasodilation and bradycardia. The RAS is activated in a state of shock and releases angiotensin II and aldosterone. This also causes vasoconstriction but does not increase myocardial contractility or tachycardia, but does decrease renal output. BNP are released when the heart becomes over stretched. It works similar to the RAS.

2. A) Fluid shifts from the extravascular to the intravascular space.

In hemorrhagic shock, there is a shift of fluid from the extravascular to intravascular space in order to compensate for the low circulation. This results in both interstitial and intravascular depletion of fluid. Fluid shifts from the organs (brain and kidneys) during hemorrhagic shock, not into the organ parenchyma.

3. C) Class III

Class III hemorrhagic shock is experienced when a patient loses 30% to 40% of total blood volume (TBV), which is approximately 1,500 to 2,000 mL. This results in hypotension, a respiratory rate in the 30s, a heart rate greater than 120 bpm, urine output of 5 to 10 mL/hr, and the patient is usually confused and anxious. Class I is a 15% TBV loss, approximately 800 mL; a respiratory rate in the 20s; heart rate is greater than 100 bpm; and the patient is slightly anxious. In class II, the patient loses 15% to 30% TBV, approximately 800 to 1,500 mL; respiratory rate is 20 to 30; heart rate is greater than 100 but less than 120 bpm; and urine output is 20 to 30 mL/hr, with decreased capillary refill, and mild anxiety. Class IV hemorrhagic shock occurs when there is greater than 40% TBV loss, which is greater than 2,000 mL; respiratory rate is 30 to 40; heart rate is greater than 140 bpm; there is no urine output; and patient is hypotensive and lethargic.

4. A) A new crossmatch needs to be sent after multiple universal blood transfusions.

A new crossmatch is recommended after multiple uncrossmatched blood transfusions to reduce error in the type and screen. The universal blood donor type is O negative. Male patients, not females of childbearing age, may receive O positive as uncrossmatched blood, whereas women within childbearing age require the negative. Massive transfusions are typically defined as infusions of 10 units of blood or more in a 24-hour period.

5. C) Anaphylaxis involves the immune system.

Anaphylaxis and anaphylactoid reactions are both acute life-threatening hypersensitivity reactions but anaphylaxis is immune related, whereas anaphylactoid reaction is not. Anaphylaxis involves immunoglobulin E (IgE) binding to an antigen to which the person was previously exposed. Anaphylactoid reactions do not have the immune component but are similar in assessment, diagnosis, and treatment. Angioedema, even with involvement of the tongue and pharynx with no systemic features, is not anaphylaxis although frequently erroneously so labeled in accidents, EDs, and medical admissions units. Angioedema is not accompanied by systemic features.

12 Systemic Inflammatory Response Syndrome

Q What is the presence of bacteria in the bloodstream called?

A Bacteremia

Bacteremia is the viable presence of bacteria in the bloodstream as determined by blood cultures being positive for bacteria. Fungemia is the presence of a fungus in the bloodstream. A positive culture is one of the signs of an infection. An infection initiates the inflammatory response and the onset of sepsis (Box 12.1).

Box 12.1 Signs of an infection

Presence of white blood cells in normally sterile body fluid
Positive culture (urine, blood, sputum)
Perforated viscous
Radiographic evidence of pneumonia in association with purulent sputum

Q What is the white blood cell (WBC) criterion used to define sepsis?

A WBC count of more than 12,000, or less than 4,000, or band cells of more than 10%

Sepsis is the inflammatory response to a known infection. *Sepsis* is defined as the presence of two or more of the stipulated criteria (Box 12.2). Systemic inflammatory response syndrome (SIRS) is a systemic inflammatory response to a variety of severe clinical insults. SIRS is defined by the same criteria used to determine sepsis, but without signs of infection and a negative blood culture.

Box 12.2 Criteria that defines sepsis

Temperature >38.3°C (101°F) or <36°C
Heart rate >90 beats/min
Respiratory rate >20 breaths/min or $PaCO_2$ <32 mmHg
WBC >12,000 cells/mm^3 or <4,000 mm^3, or >10% immature granulocytes (bands)

WBC, white blood cells.

▶ HINT

Sepsis is a disease process managed in all areas of the hospital and is not exclusive to critical care.

HINT

SIRS frequently has negative blood cultures.

Q What are the hemodynamic complications in septic shock?

A Hypotension and hypoperfusion

Septic shock is accompanied hemodynamically by profound hypotension and hypoperfusion. Hypotension is defined as a systolic blood pressure (SBP) less than 90 mmHg, mean arterial pressure (MAP) less than 65 mmHg, or a decrease in blood pressure (BP) by greater than 40 mmHg from baseline. Hypoperfusion may include but is not limited to oliguria, increased lactate levels, or acute alteration in mental status (Box 12.3). The sepsis bundles use a lactate level greater than 2 mmol/L to recognize hypoperfusion.

Box 12.3 Signs of hypoperfusion

Acute altered mental status
Blood glucose >140 mg/dL in patients without diabetes
Arterial hypoxemia (PaO_2/FiO_2 ratio <300)
Acute oliguria (<0.5 mL/kg/hr for at least 2 hours)
Creatinine increase >0.5 mg/dL above baseline
Coagulation abnormalities (INR >1.5 or a PTT >60 sec)
Ileus
Thrombocytopenia (platelet count <100,000)
Hyperbilirubinemia (total bilirubin >2 mg/dL)

INR, international normalized ratio; PTT, partial thromboplastin time.

HINT

The goal or therapeutic threshold is to maintain an MAP greater than 65 mmHg.

HINT

Septic shock is hypotension and hypoperfusion despite adequate resuscitation.

Q What is multiple organ dysfunction syndrome (MODS) in sepsis caused by?

A Hypoperfusion

MODS is the presence of altered organ function in two or more organs in an acutely ill patient such that homeostasis cannot be maintained without intervention. It is progressive but potentially reversible and is a result of hypoperfusion and injury to the organs (Table 12.1).

Table 12.1 Signs of organ dysfunction

System	Major Sign
Pulmonary	PaO_2/FiO_2 ratio <300
Renal	Increased serum creatinine >2.0 or creatinine increase >0.5 mg/dL or 44.2 mmol/L

(*continued*)

Table 12.1 Signs of organ dysfunction (*continued*)

System	Major Sign
Hepatic	Increased bilirubin levels >4 mg/dL
Hematology	Decreased platelet counts <100,000/μL INR >1.5 PTT >60 seconds
Central nervous system	Altered GCS

GCS, Glasgow Coma Scale; INR, international normalized ratio; PTT, partial thromboplastin time.

HINT

Mortality is related to the number of organs involved and the severity of organ dysfunction.

Q What is the most common microorganism that causes sepsis?

A Gram-positive bacteria

Gram-positive bacteria have surpassed the gram-negative bacteria in causing sepsis (Box 12.4). A common gram-positive bacteria is methicillin-resistant *Staphylococcus aureus* (MRSA; Box 12.5).

Box 12.4 Types of gram-negative bacteria

Escherichia coli
Klebsiella pneumonia
Pseudomonas aeruginosa
Enterobacter
Serratia
Proteus

Box 12.5 Types of gram-positive bacteria

Staphylococcus
Streptococcus

HINT

Gram-negative bacteria colonize the gastrointestinal (GI) tract and oral secretions.

HINT

Central-line sepsis is caused by gram-positive bacteremia.

Q Which microorganism is the most common cause of a secondary infection?

A Fungus (*Candida*)

Fungal infections are found to cause a second episode of infection. This is due to use of antibiotics in treating the first infection, which alters the normal flora, thereby allowing opportunistic infections to develop. Immunosuppressed patients are also at high risk for secondary infections. Fungal sepsis (fungemia) has a higher mortality than bacteremia and is harder to diagnose. Presence of fungemia may not result in a positive blood culture. Management is typically based on presumptive therapy, which is to "presume" fungemia is present and treat it with antifungal medication.

Q An increase in bands greater than what percentage indicates severe sepsis?

A Greater than 10%

Bands are immature WBCs. When more than 10% of the circulating WBCs are bands, an overwhelming infection and sepsis are indicated. Other WBC changes that potentially indicate sepsis are a WBC count greater than 12,000 or less than 4,000.

HINT

For example, if a complete blood count (CBC) differential finds 45% bands, this indicates 45% of the circulating WBCs are immature and nonfunctional.

Q In severe sepsis or septic shock, does the left ventricle (LV) ejection fraction (EF) increase or decrease?

A Decrease

Proinflammatory cytokine and tumor necrosis factor (TNF) are released following the presence of a microorganism and initiation of the inflammatory response. Sepsis has a negative contractility effect on the myocardium and results in a decrease in EF. The cardiac output is usually high in sepsis because systemic vasodilation lowers the vascular resistance (Box 12.6).

Box 12.6 Symptoms of sepsis or septic shock

Tachycardia
Tachypnea
Leukocytosis or leukopenia
Increase in bands
Fever
Decreased SVR
Hypotension (vasodilation)
Increased cardiac output
Decreased ejection fraction
Left ventricular dilation
Metabolic acidosis
Respiratory alkalosis
Pulmonary artery hypertension
Altered mental status
Edema or positive fluid balance
Hyperglycemia (>140 mg/dL or 7.7 mmol/L) in nondiabetic patients
Signs of organ dysfunction

SVR, systemic vascular resistance.

▶ HINT

Use of a right ventricular ejection fraction (RVEF) pulmonary artery catheter in sepsis patients has shown a decrease in EF even during periods of high cardiac output. RVEF commonly ranges between 30% and 40% during early sepsis.

▶ HINT

A significant positive fluid balance is defined as greater than 20 mL/kg over 24 hours.

Q What is used to determine the microorganism(s) involved in causing the infection and the best antibiotics needed to treat the infection?

A Culture and sensitivity

Once sepsis is recognized, cultures are sent for testing to determine the causative microorganisms and their susceptibility to certain antibiotics. Recommendation is to test at least two sets of blood cultures (both anaerobic and aerobic bottles) with at least one drawn percutaneously. One can be drawn from a vascular access device if the device was inserted greater than 48 hours prior. Both blood cultures can be drawn at the same time if obtained from two different sites. Cultures from other potential sites of infection (urine, sputum, cerebrospinal fluid [CSF], wounds) should also be obtained and sent with blood cultures.

▶ HINT

If the same organism is recovered from both samples, there is a better likelihood that the organism is responsible for the sepsis.

Q What other lab tests besides the CBC can be used to determine the presence of an infection?

A Plasma C-reactive protein and prolactin

Plasma C-reactive proteins and prolactin are biomarkers for diagnosis of infection. They may be used as additional information but at this time are not shown to distinguish from infection and other causes of inflammation.

▶ HINT

Procalcitonin levels may be beneficial in determining when to discontinue the antibiotics but are not recommended to determine when to start the antibiotics.

Q What is the overall best management goal for sepsis?

A Prevention

Prevention of an infection or sepsis is still the best management. Handwashing is the main area of prevention found to lower incidence of infections across the continuum of patient types and ages (Box 12.7).

Box 12.7 Sources of hospital-associated infections

Catheter-associated urinary tract infection
Central line-associated bloodstream infections
Ventilator-associated pneumonia
Hospital-acquired pneumonia
Intra-abdominal source

Q What is the current recommendation to prevent a catheter-associated urinary tract infection (CAUTI)?

A Minimize use and duration of a urinary catheter

CAUTIs are the most common type of healthcare-associated infection. Current practice is to avoid insertion of a bladder catheter, if possible. If a bladder catheter is required in surgery, the goal is to discontinue it within 24 hours. Removing the indwelling catheter as soon as possible lowers the incidence of CAUTIs (Box 12.8). The most common causative microorganisms are *E. coli* and *Candida* (Box 12.9).

Box 12.8 Appropriate reasons for urinary catheter use

Obtain accurate I & O in critically ill patients
- Need to monitor urine output

Unable to use bedpan or urinal
- Coma
- Sedation and paralytics

Large volume of fluid infusions or diuretics
Urologic surgery patients
Urinary retention or obstruction

I & O, input and output.

Box 12.9 Prevention of catheter-associated urinary tract infections

Use aseptic insertion technique and sterile equipment.
Keep urine collection bag off the floor.
Keep urine collection bag lower than the bladder.
Properly secure the collecting bag to prevent movement in the bladder.
Maintain a closed drainage system.
Empty collecting bag regularly.
Use catheters impregnated with antiseptic or antimicrobial agents.
Use alternative external devices for urine collection.

▶ HINT

Remember all lines and tubes in the patient are a source of infection and should be removed as soon as possible if a suspected source of the infection.

▶ HINT

Changing bags or indwelling catheters on a routine basis is not recommended.

Q What is a nursing intervention found to lower the incidence of ventilator-associated pneumonia (VAP)?

A Oral decontamination

Oropharyngeal decontamination with chlorhexidine gluconate is recommended to lower the incidence of VAP (Box 12.10).

Box 12.10 Methods of preventing ventilator-associated pneumonia

Proper handwashing
Oral decontamination
Digestive decontamination
Elevated HOB
Prevent unplanned extubations/reintubations
Avoid saline lavages

HOB, head of bed.

Q How quickly should antibiotics be started following the diagnosis of sepsis?

A Within 1 hour

Antibiotics are the main treatment of sepsis and may halt the progression of sepsis and improve outcomes if administered early in the course of sepsis. Cultures should be obtained before the administration of antibiotics unless this causes a significant delay in the administration of antibiotics. Antibiotics can result in sterilization of the cultures within a few hours, making identification of the causative organism more difficult. Broad-spectrum antibiotics should be used to be effective against all likely organisms. Once culture results are obtained, antibiotics should be changed to be more specific to the organism's susceptibility (within 3–5 days). If patient is at high risk for MRSA, add antibiotic coverage for MRSA.

▶ HINT

The recommendation is to maintain a 5- to 7-day course of antibiotic therapy. The number of days may increase if there is a slow clinical response or continued presence of infection.

Q In early goal-directed therapy of severe sepsis, what is the central venous pressure (CVP) goal of the initial fluid resuscitation in a spontaneously breathing patient?

A CVP of 8 to 12 mmHg

Severe sepsis is persistent hypotension or hypoperfusion after an initial bolus of fluid. An early goal-directed strategy includes monitoring CVP and central venous oxygen saturation ($ScvO_2$) to determine the adequacy of resuscitation. CVP of 8 to 12 mmHg is recommended for spontaneously breathing patients, and slightly higher on ventilated patients (12–15 mmHg) because of the positive pressure effects in the chest. The $ScvO_2$ can be monitored intermittently or continuously (Box 12.11).

Box 12.11 Goals of resuscitation of severe sepsis

CVP 8–12 mmHg in spontaneously breathing pateint
CVP 12–15 mmHg in ventilated patient
MAP ≥65 mmHg
Urine output ≥0.5 mL/kg/hr
$ScvO_2$ of 70% or SvO_2 of 65%

CVP, central venous pressure; MAP, mean arterial pressure; $ScvO_2$, central venous oxygen saturation; SvO_2, mixed venous oxygen saturation.

▶ HINT

These are static methods used to monitor hemodynamics with the trend moving to adding dynamic monitoring technologies, such as pulse pressure or stroke volume variations, for improved hemodynamic monitoring.

Q What is the recommended time period from recognition of sepsis to completion of interventions to manage sepsis?

A 6 hours

The goals should be obtained within 6 hours on recognition of sepsis. Goals can be obtained with fluid administration, blood products, dobutamine infusion, or lower oxygen demands with sedation or paralysis.

▶ HINT

Lactate levels may also be monitored with the goal to normalize serum lactate.

▶ HINT

A lowering of the heart rate is also a good indication of successful resuscitation.

Q What fluids are recommended for the initial resuscitation in sepsis?

A Crystalloids

The current recommendation for fluid resuscitation in severe sepsis or sepsis-induced hypoperfusion is crystalloids. Balanced crystalloids, such as lactated Ringer's, is recommended over normal saline. If the patient requires a substantial amount of fluid to meet the goals of volume resuscitation, then albumin administration is recommended with crystalloids. Initially, the fluid challenge should be a minimum of 30 mL/kg bolus of crystalloids within 3 hours of resuscitation.

▶ HINT

Hydroxyethyl starches (hetastarch) are not recommended in resuscitation of sepsis patients because of the worsening effect on kidneys.

Q What vasopressor is considered the first choice to maintain MAP more than 65 mmHg?

A Norepinephrine (Levophed)

Vasopressor therapy is recommended to maintain the MAP at 65 mmHg or greater following initial fluid resuscitation. Below this perfusion pressure, the autoregulation in the critical vascular beds is lost. Norepinephrine is the recommended first-line vasopressor. If an additional vasopressor therapy is required, vasopressin may be added to increase MAP instead of increasing the dosing of norepinephrine. Epinephrine is considered the third-line vasopressor that may be added to improve MAP greater than 65 mmHg. Vasopressin is not recommended as a single first-line vasopressor in sepsis.

▶ HINT

An arterial line is recommended for continuous and more accurate BP readings. Vasopressor therapy can be initiated in a peripheral intravenous (IV) line until a central line is obtained.

Q When should corticosteroid therapy be considered in a patient with sepsis?

A When requiring ongoing vasopressor therapy

A patient who responds to fluids or vasopressor therapy by improving hemodynamic parameters and lactate levels does not require corticosteroid treatment. If hemodynamic stability cannot be achieved, even after resuscitation and vasopressor administration, 200 mg/d of hydrocortisone as a continuous infusion is recommended. Continuous infusions may control blood glucose more effectively than intermittent boluses with less significant hyperglycemia. Once vasopressors are not required, hydrocortisone may be tapered and discontinued. The adrenocorticotropic hormone (ACTH) test is not recommended to determine an indication for corticosteroid therapy.

▶ HINT

Side effects of hydrocortisone are hypernatremia and hyperglycemia.

Q According to the Surviving Sepsis Campaign guidelines, when should the insulin protocol be initiated in a sepsis patient?

A When two consecutive blood glucose levels are greater than 180 mg/dL

The current recommendation for glucose control is to treat with sliding-scale insulin if blood glucose levels are greater than 180 mg/dL for two consecutive glucose checks. Maintain glucose less than 180 mg/dL while avoiding hypoglycemia. Blood glucose levels may be checked every 4 hours when stable and every 1 to 2 hours while elevated. Maintaining strict glucose levels of less than 110 mg/dL is not recommended because of the frequent incidence of hypoglycemia.

▶ HINT

Point-of-care glucose tests may not be as accurate as plasma glucose levels from the laboratory and should be interpreted cautiously.

Q At what serum pH would sodium bicarbonate therapy be administered in septic shock patients with lactic acidosis?

A Less than 7.20

There is no benefit tof treating a pH with sodium bicarbonate until pH decreases to less than 7.20 and acute kidney injury (AKI) exists. The side effects of sodium bicarbonate cause the risks of administration to be greater than the benefit (Box 12.12).

Box 12.12 Complications of sodium bicarbonate

Fluid overload
Hypernatremia
Increased lactate levels
Hypercarbia
Decreased serum ionized calcium
Greater affinity of Hgb to RBCs

Hgb, hemoglobin; RBCs, red blood cells.

Q What is the best management if there is a known source of infection?

A Remove the source of infection

Radiograph studies are frequently used to find the location of the infection. If the infectious source is amendable to line removal, drainage, percutaneous drainage, or surgical excision (Box 12.13) may be required. Source control as rapid as possible (within 12 hours) can lower the incidence of mortality.

Box 12.13 Surgically amendable focal infections

Abscesses (including intra-abdominal)
Gastrointestinal perforation
Cholangitis
Pyelonephritis
Intestinal ischemia
Necrotizing soft tissue
Empyema
Septic arthritis

HINT

If the source is determined to be an IV access source, the catheter needs to be removed promptly after obtaining other access.

Q What is the primary physiology for the hypoperfused state in sepsis?

A Inability of cells to utilize oxygen

Initial hypoperfusion is a result of distributive shock (vasodilation) and hypovolemia (due to increased vascular permeability). Even after vascular volume is restored, hypoperfusion may continue to persist. This is largely attributed to an inability of the cells to utilize the oxygen delivered to the tissues. Another major contributing factor is that maldistribution of blood flow occurs at the regional level (splanchnic, renal, and mesenteric) as well as the microvascular level (Box 12.14).

Box 12.14 Causes for inadequate tissue oxygenation

Decreased oxygen delivery
Inability to extract oxygen
Blockage of normal cellular metabolism
Greater distance between vessels and tissue (edema)
Inability to offload O_2 from Hgb
Arteriovenous shunt
Endothelial injury
Loss of vascular tone

Hgb, hemoglobin.

HINT

Remember the saying, "You can lead a horse to water but you can't make it drink." In sepsis, you can optimize delivery of oxygen to the tissues or cells, but you can't make them take the oxygen.

Q What is a GI complication that occurs because of the use of multiple antibiotics in treating sepsis?

A *Clostridium difficile*

C. difficile is a superinfection that may occur as a result of using multiple, broad-spectrum antibiotics for a prolonged period of treatment. Narrowing the spectrum and shortening the time of antibiotic therapy may lower the risk of acquiring opportunistic infections such as *Candida*, or superinfections such as *C. difficile*, and resistant bacteria (vancomycin-resistant *Enterococcus faecium*).

HINT

Antibiotics can change the normal GI flora. Probiotics may be used to prevent this altered flora.

Q What is the most common cause of death in septic shock?

A MODS

MODS is a complication of the tissue and organ hypoperfusion that occurs in severe sepsis and septic shock. MODS is defined as the presence of altered organ function in acutely ill patients such that homeostasis cannot be obtained without intervention (Box 12.15). The number of organs affected predicts mortality. Any organ can be affected by sepsis-induced hypoperfusion.

Box 12.15 Common types or organ failures

Acute respiratory distress syndrome
Acute kidney injury
Hepatic failure
Gastrointestinal tract
Septic encephalopathy
Systolic and diastolic dysfunction myocardium
Disseminated intravascular coagulation
Metabolic dysfunction with hyperglycemia

HINT

This is also commonly called *multisystem organ failure (MSOF).*

Q What plays a central role when microvascular dysfunction occurs in MODS?

A Endothelium

The endothelium regulates vasomotor tone, coagulation, vascular permeability, and balance between pro- and anti-inflammatory cytokines. Biomarkers that measure endothelial activity (plasminogen activator inhibitor-1) demonstrate increased levels following activation of the inflammatory system and correlate with the severity of MODS.

Q What tool can be used to determine the rate and extent of organ failure?

A Sequential organ failure assessment (SOFA)

The SOFA scoring system is used to determine the extent of organ function or rate of failure (Tables 12.2–12.7).

Table 12.2 Sequential organ failure assessment scoring: Respiratory system

PaO_2/FiO_2	SOFA Score
<400	1
<300	2
<200 and mechanically ventilated	3
<100 and mechanically ventilated	4

SOFA, sequential organ failure assessment.

Table 12.3 Sequential organ failure assessment scoring: Nervous system

Glasgow Coma Scale	SOFA Score
13–14	1
10–12	2
6–9	3
<6	4

SOFA, sequential organ failure assessment.

Table 12.4 Sequential organ failure assessment scoring: Cardiovascular system

MAP or Vasopressor Requirement	SOFA Score
MAP <70 mmHg	1
Dopamine <5 OR dobutamine (any dose)	2
Dopamine >5 OR epi ≤0.1 OR norepi ≤0.1	3
Dopamine >15 OR epi >0.1 OR norepi >0.1	4

Epi, epinephrine; MAP, mean arterial pressure; norepi, norepinephrine; SOFA, sequential organ failure assessment.

Table 12.5 Sequential organ failure assessment scoring: Liver

Bilirubin	SOFA Score
1.2–1.9	1
2.0–5.9	2
6.0–11.9	3
>12	4

SOFA, sequential organ failure assessment.

Table 12.6 Sequential organ failure assessment scoring: Coagulation

Platelets × 103	SOFA Score
<150	1
<100	2
<50	3
<20	4

SOFA, sequential organ failure assessment.

Table 12.7 Sequential organ failure assessment scoring: Renal system

Creatinine or Urine Output	SOFA Score
1.2–1.9	1
2.0–3.4	2
3.5–4.9	3
>5	4

SOFA, sequential organ failure assessment.

▶ HINT

When scoring, if none match the patient, the score is 0 for that organ. If more than one item matches, use the highest score.

Q What type of pulmonary edema occurs with acute respiratory distress syndrome (ARDS)?

A Noncardiogenic pulmonary edema

ARDS is defined as a noncardiac pulmonary edema characterized by an increase in capillary permeability with interstitial and alveolar edema of the lungs.

▶ HINT

A patient with congestive heart failure (CHF) can be diagnosed with ARDS if the clinical condition cannot be fully explained by cardiac failure or fluid overload.

Q What role does a surfactant have in the lungs?

A ecreases alveolar surface tension

A surfactant decreases surface tension in the alveoli, thus allowing the alveoli to inflate more readily and increase lung compliance. The surfactant "splints" alveoli open and allows for recruitment of alveoli, thus improving the functional residual capacity (FRC) in the lungs. This correlates to work of breathing (WOB).

▶ HINT

Balloon analogy: Take a balloon that is already filled with air, empty some of the air out, and then blow it back up. It is easy because of the FRC or "splinting" of the balloon walls, which open with the remaining air. This is how alveoli act with a normal surfactant. Now, take a new balloon and blow it up. It is much harder to inflate because of the surface tension within the balloon without air. This is how alveoli act without a normal functioning surfactant.

Q What are the initial symptoms in a patient during the early stages of ARDS?

A Hypoxemia, tachypnea, and dyspnea

The symptoms usually have a quick onset, within hours to days after the initial injury or insult to the lungs. The initial presentation is hypoxemia with tachypnea and dyspnea. Chest x-ray (CXR) changes may also be an early sign of ARDS and can occur within 4 to 24 hours of the initial insult (Table 12.8).

Table 12.8 Early signs of acute respiratory distress syndrome

Use of Accessory Muscles	Course Crackles
Shallow, rapid breathing	Restlessness
Respiratory alkalosis	Increased work of breathing

▶ HINT

A cardinal sign of ARDS is hypoxemia refractory to supplemental oxygen.

Q What is the primary issue with ventilating a patient in the later stages of ARDS?

A Decreased lung compliance

The lung is considered a "baby lung" with only about one third of the lung being ventilated during the later stages of ARDS. The lung is filled with fluid and alveoli have collapsed, signaling the onset of pulmonary fibrosis. The characteristic problem associated with ventilating ARDS patients is decreased lung compliance (Table 12.9).

Table 12.9 Symptoms of acute respiratory distress syndrome at later stages

Increase PIP	Tachycardia
Course crackles and rhonchi bilateral	Severe hypoxemia
Metabolic acidosis due to elevated lactate levels	Pallor and cyanosis
Respiratory acidosis due to hypercarbia	Bilateral pulmonary infiltrates
Use of accessory muscles and nasal flaring	Increased work of breathing

PIP, peaked inspiratory pressures.

HINT

Peak inspiratory and plateau pressures increase on the ventilator due to decrease in lung compliance.

Q What are the primary CXR criteria used to diagnose ARDS?

A Bilateral fluffy infiltrates

ARDS is a bilateral lung disease characterized by pulmonary infiltrates. It is commonly seen as "white out" on CXR. A CT scan may also be used to determine the presence of bilateral fluffy infiltrates (Table 12.10).

Table 12.10 Berlin definition of acute respiratory distress syndrome

Acute onset	Within 7 days of a defined event
Impaired oxygenation	Abnormal PaO_2/FiO_2 ratio (PF ratio <200)
Bilateral fluffy infiltrates	CXR or CT scan
Not fully explained by cardiac failure or fluid overload	

CXR, chest x-ray.

Q Severe ARDS is defined by what PaO_2/FiO_2 ratio?

A Less than 100

The Berlin definition of ARDS includes categories of severity based on the PaO_2/FiO_2 ratio (also called the *PF ratio*). To calculate, use the PaO_2 from the blood gas and divide by the FiO_2 the patient was on when the blood gas was drawn. The normal PF ratio is greater than 350.

HINT

Remember, when calculating the PaO_2/FiO_2 ratio, use the decimal point (40% is 0.40; Table 12.11).

For example:

If a patient's PaO_2 is 80 on 50% FiO_2,

$80 \div 0.50 = 160$

Table 12.11 Severity of acute respiratory distress syndrome

Severity of ARDS	PaO_2/FiO_2 Ratio
Mild	200–300
Moderate	100–200
Severe	<100

ARDS, acute respiratory distress syndrome.

HINT

A normal PaO_2 is only normal on room air. If on a higher FiO_2, a normal PaO_2 (80–100 mmHg) may actually be abnormal. PF ratio calculation is used to determine severity of impaired oxygenation.

Q What is the most common indirect injury to the lungs that can result in the development of ARDS?

A Sepsis

The development of respiratory failure following a clinical injury to the lungs, either directly or indirectly, leads to the diagnosis of ARDS. An indirect injury is usually the result of an inflammatory reaction to a certain disease or clinical state. Direct injury to the alveoli or lung parenchyma results in a loss of integrity of the alveolar–capillary membrane, leading to ARDS (Tables 12.12 and 12.13).

Table 12.12 Indirect lung injury

Sepsis/septic shock	DKA
Pancreatitis	Drug or alcohol overdose
Massive trauma	Cardiopulmonary bypass
Multiple blood transfusions	Amniotic fluid embolus
Prolonged severe shock	Tissue necrosis

DKA, diabetic ketoacidosis.

Table 12.13 Direct lung injury

Excessive fluid resuscitation	Pneumonitis
Inhalation injuries (smoke or toxic gases)	Drug inhalation
Oxygen toxicity	Pulmonary contusions
Aspiration	Pneumonia
Near drowning	Pulmonary embolism

Q What is the recommended tidal volume (TV) for a patient with ARDS?

A 4 to 6 mL/kg

ARDS patients have been found to benefit from small TVs with lower plateau pressures (PLPs) with improved outcomes. The recommendation is TV of 4 to 6 mL/kg with PLP less than 30 to 35 cm H_2O. The high inspiratory pressure required to deliver traditional TVs (8–10 mL/kg) to the remaining normal lung tissue causes significant overdistension, barotrauma, and diffuse alveolar damage. Low TVs have also been associated with less release of intra-alveolar cytokines.

HINT

Use ideal body weight (in kg), not actual body weight, to calculate TV (Table 12.14).

Table 12.14 Goals of ventilation

Oxygenation	Maintain >88%–90%
FiO_2	<60%–70%
PIP	<40–45 cm H_2O
PLP	<30 cm H_2O
TV	6 mL/kg ideal body weight
RR	Up to 35 bpm (breaths per minute; MV 7–9 L/min)

MV, minute ventilation; PIP, peak inspiratory pressure; PLP, lower plateau pressures; RR, respiratory rate; TV, tidal volume.

Q Which mode of ventilation is used to control peak inspiratory pressures?

A Pressure-controlled ventilation (PCV)

PCV sets an upper pressure limit on the ventilator (pressure control) that determines the end of the inspiratory cycle and inspiratory volume. The TV varies per breath, depending on the compliance of the airway and lungs. This method of ventilation is used to limit excessive airway pressures and improve mean airway pressure. Inverse inspiratory to expiratory (I:E) ratios may be used in this mode of ventilation.

HINT

The flow waveform used to deliver a breath in PCV is a decelerating waveform (volume control uses a square waveform).

Q A patient with ARDS demonstrating problems with maintaining saturations can be placed in what position?

A Prone

In ARDS, lung infiltrates and damaged lung units are not uniformly distributed. CT scans have found that dependent portions of the lungs are more affected and less dependent areas remain normal with normal compliance. The prone position can improve oxygenation by improving ventilation perfusion ratios in the dependent regions. The use of the intermittent prone position can improve oxygenation. It is recommended in refractory hypoxemic patients (Table 12.15).

Table 12.15 Risks of prone position

Inadvertent dislodgement of the endotracheal tube	Initial worsening in respiratory status
Inadvertent dislodgement of lines or tubes	Facial edema
Development of pressure ulcerations	Hemodynamic instability

Q What is the first pharmacologic intervention for ventilator dyssynchrony ("bucking the ventilator")?

A Sedation

Sedation is the first step to improve ventilator–patient synchrony. Neuromuscular blocking agents (NMBAs) can be used but are considered to be the last resort. If the patient continues to "fight" the ventilator, and ventilatory pressures remain elevated with sedation and analgesics alone, then adding an NMBA would be appropriate.

▶ HINT

Ensure adequate sedation and pain management before initiating NMBA.

Q How are NMBAs monitored?

A Peripheral nerve stimulation using the train-of-four (TOF)

Patients receiving NMBAs should be monitored with both observation and TOF. The peripheral nerve stimulator is used to assess neuromuscular blockade, and the most common stimulation is called *TOF*. Frequently used sites for peripheral nerve stimulation include the ulnar and facial nerves. Count the number of twitches. If stimulating the ulnar nerve, observe the thumb and the facial nerve, watch the muscle above the eyebrow.

▶ HINT

The goal for adjusting NMBA is typically to achieve one or two twitches (Table 12.16); 0/4 twitches indicate the need to lower the infusion rate to prevent prolonged paralysis.

Table 12.16 Train-of-four twitches

Number of Twitches	Amount of Blockade
4/4	0%–75% receptors blocked
3/4	At least 75% receptors blocked
2/4	80% receptors blocked
1/4	90% receptors blocked
0/4	100% receptors blocked

KNOWLEDGE CHECK: CHAPTER 12

1. A trauma patient has been on a ventilator in the ICU for 2 weeks. The patient is tachycardic, has been spiking fevers, and now has decreased urine output. The nurse notes that the white blood cell (WBC) count is 25,000 and the sputum cultures reveal gram-positive cocci. Which of the following is responsible for this systemic inflammatory response?

   A. Cytokines
   B. Interleukins
   C. Procalcitonin
   D. Lactate

2. A patient came into the ED 48 hours ago presenting with tachycardia, hypotension, vomiting, and a large foot wound with purulent drainage. The patient's lactate level on arrival was 3.1. The patient was diagnosed with sepsis and has been started on antibiotics, fluid resuscitation, and vasopressors. The repeat lactate today is 1.8. What statement would be most accurate about this patient's plan of care?

   A. The patient's lactate level is now normal.
   B. The patient is demonstrating signs of improvement.
   C. The lactate level is not used to predict outcomes.
   D. The patient has a high predictive mortality risk.

3. Which of the following hemodynamic monitoring parameters utilized in a septic shock patient would be considered a dynamic parameter?

   A. Central venous oxygen saturation ($ScvO_2$)
   B. Central venous pressure (CVP)
   C. Urine output
   D. Stroke volume variance (SVV)

4. A septic trauma patient remains in the ICU on a ventilator. The sepsis management bundle is in progress. The patient is on hydrocortisone 200 mg/dL and plateau pressures are being maintained less than 30 cm H_2O on the ventilator. Which of these treatment modalities would most likely be recommended for this patient?

   A. Keep plateau pressures >30 cm H_2O
   B. Glucose control of 80 to 110 mg/dL
   C. Recommended tidal volume of 10 mL/kg
   D. Maintain glucose <180 mg/dL

5. A trauma patient who was involved in a motor vehicle collision has been in intensive care on a ventilator for 3 days. The patient is hypoxic despite increasing FiO_2 levels, tachycardic, and chest x-rays (CXR) showing bilateral infiltrates. The nurse should have a high suspicion that the patient is experiencing symptoms of:

   A. Pulmonary embolism (PE)
   B. Tension pneumothorax
   C. Cardiac tamponade
   D. Acute respiratory distress syndrome (ARDS)

(See answers next page.)

1. A) Cytokines

Systemic inflammatory response syndrome (SIRS) is a condition of systemic inflammation, organ dysfunction, and organ failure. Proinflammatory cytokines initiate the inflammatory process such as elevation of WBC and initiation of the complement system. Interleukins function directly on tissue or work by secondary mediators to activate the coagulation cascade and fever. Other cytokines stimulate the release of acute-phase reactants such as C-reactive protein and procalcitonin. Lactate elevates when SIRS is present, it is not a cellular response.

2. B) The patient is demonstrating signs of improvement.

The normal lactate level is 0.5 to 1.0 mEq/L and is considered elevated if greater than 2.0 mEq/L. The average initial lactate level for survivors is 2.8 mEq/L versus nonsurvivors' initial lactate level of 4.0 mEq/L. The lactate level has been shown to predict survivability following sepsis. There is a significantly increased chance of survival if lactate levels normalize within 24 hours. The survival rate is improved if lactate levels normalize within 48 hours but if greater than 48 hours the risk of mortality significantly increases.

3. D) Stroke volume variance (SVV)

SVV is considered a dynamic parameter that may be used to monitor the hemodynamic status of a septic patient. CVP and $ScvO_2$ are often used in monitoring septic patients but are considered to be static parameters. Urine output is also used but is a physical assessment for hemodynamic monitoring.

4. D) Maintain glucose <180 mg/dL

Glucose management would be indicated due to sepsis and administration of hydrocortisone. The recommended goal for glucose management is <180 mg/dL. Maintaining a level between 80 to 110 mg/dL is considered strict glycemic control and is not recommended due to increased incidences of hypoglycemia. Maintaining the plateau pressure on the ventilator <30 cm H_2O is recommended. Tidal volumes should be set at 4 to 6 ml/kg.

5. D) Acute respiratory distress syndrome (ARDS)

This patient is showing signs of ARDS with hypoxia despite administering increased levels of oxygen, tachycardia, and bilateral infiltrates on CXR. Trauma patients are at risk for both PE and ARDS but in this scenario the bilateral infiltrates lead toward the suspicion of ARDS. Tension pneumothorax would have a deviated trachea and collapsed lung on CXR. Cardiac tamponade presents with hypotension and distant heart sounds.

Special Populations

13

PEDIATRIC TRAUMA

MECHANISM OF INJURY

Q What is the narrowest part of the trachea in a child?

A Cricoid cartilage

Airway is a major concern in pediatric trauma patients. The trachea is smaller and shorter than in an adult and the narrowest part of the trachea in a child is the cricoid cartilage; in an adult the narrowest part is at the level of the vocal cords. With children under the age of 8 years old, use uncuffed endotracheal tubes as cuffed tubes can cause vocal cord injury, subglottic edema, and pressure necrosis.

HINT

Because of the size of the airway, a small amount of blood or the presence of a foreign body, edema, mucus, or the tongue can lead to airway obstruction (oral cavity is small compared to tongue size as well).

Q Would rib fractures in a child indicate greater or less severe injury?

A Greater

In children, the rib cage and sternum are less ossified and more compliant. Rib and sternal fractures are rare and, if present, indicate an ominous sign. Significant thoracic injuries frequently occur without the presence of rib fractures.

HINT

Traumatic asphyxiation can occur with direct compression of the chest wall in a child.

Q What is a common mechanism of injury for abdominal trauma in a child?

A Seat belt injury

Children tend to wear the lap belt over their abdomen instead of the iliac crest. The liver and spleen are not well protected by the rib cage, so are at a greater risk for injury. The jejunum lies in the umbilical region and the ileum is in the hypogastric and pelvic region, which makes them more susceptible to injury with a lap belt.

HINT

Measure the abdominal girth at the level of the umbilicus to detect subtle abdominal distention.

Q What is a major risk of a child with developmental disabilities?

A Abuse

Children with developmental disabilities have been found to have a significant increase in risk of being victims of a crime compared to nondisabled children. The risk of abuse, both sexual and physical, is higher in special needs children and adults. Children with developmental disabilities are at risk due to their limited knowledge and social skills.

HINT

Children with developmental disabilities are less likely to tell someone about the abuse. If exposed to an abusive situation, they may demonstrate trauma-related behaviors.

TRAUMATIC INJURIES

Q A child in a motor vehicle collision (MVC) is more prone to what type of injury due to disproportionate body parts?

A Head injury

Children are prone to head injuries because their heads are larger in proportion to the rest of their bodies. The cranial bones are thinner and cranial sutures are not closed until 16 to 18 months of age. Children are prone to longer periods of unconsciousness but can still have a good outcome.

HINT

Significant intracranial bleeds in infants can lead to hypotension and shock.

Q What type of spinal cord injury is more commonly seen in pediatric patients compared to adults?

A Spinal cord injuries without radiographic abnormalities (SCIWRAs)

SCIWRAs, such as vertebral fractures, are more common in pediatrics due to the size of the head, increased flexibility between C1 and C2, and poor musculoskeletal support. C-spine x-rays identify vertebral fractures but do not visualize ligaments or the spinal cord.

HINT

MRI may be required to clear a c-spine on a child due to its ability to identify cord injuries.

ASSESSMENT AND DIAGNOSIS

Q What assessment is unreliable in pediatric patients in identifying a significant amount of blood loss?

A Hypotension

A normal blood volume for a child is 80 mL/kg so a small amount of blood loss can result in significant shock, but children may not become hypotensive until 40% of their blood volume is lost. Hearts rates can significantly elevate to rates of 180 to 200 beats per minute (bpm) to compensate.

▶ HINT

Bradycardia is a late and dangerous sign of shock in the pediatric population.

MEDICAL/SURGICAL INTERVENTION

Q What is a common problem that occurs during intubation of a child?

A Intubation of right mainstem

Intubation often results in right mainstem intubation because the bronchus is shorter. When inserting oral airways, do not rotate with insertion as with adults due to possible trauma to the soft tissue of the palate and hypopharynx. It is recommended to use a forward motion with the tongue depressed outward.

▶ HINT

If using a bag mask to ventilate, be careful not to push your fingers on the submandibular tissue, occluding the airway.

NURSING INTERVENTIONS

Q You are caring for a 30-kg child with a chest tube that was placed for a hemothorax. This last hour there was 200 mL output from the CT. What do you think will be the plan of care for this patient?

A Surgical repair

Drainage from a chest tube may indicate the need for surgical control. If output is greater than 30 mL/kg initially or 2 to 3 mL/kg/hr, the patient may require a thoracotomy.

COMPLICATIONS

Q What type of fracture can interfere with growth and cause limb length discrepancy?

A Fracture at the growth plate

Fractures occurring at the growth plate can interfere with growth under the age of 16 for boys and 14 for girls. The majority of growth is completed by the time a girl is 14 years old and a boy is 16 years of age. A growth plate fracture can result in limb length discrepancies.

▶ HINT

Limb length discrepancies in the lower extremities can adversely affect the child's gait.

Q A child is most susceptible to which element of the trauma triad (hypothermia, coagulopathy, and metabolic acidosis)?

A Hypothermia

Heat loss and hypothermia occur more rapidly in children, and they are more sensitive to hypothermia. Children younger than 6 months of age lack a layer of subcutaneous tissue and in a coma will lack the shivering mechanism.

HINT

Children have a large body surface and high metabolic rate, which can lead to dehydration.

GERIATRIC TRAUMA

MECHANISM OF INJURY

Q What is the most common cause of injury in the older adult population?

A Falls

Falls are the most common cause of injury in older adults and are a leading cause of trauma-related deaths. Overall weakness, gait instability, and sensory changes (e.g., sight and hearing) place this population at the greater risk for falls. MVC are the second most common cause of trauma in older adults.

HINT

Falls can be complicated by widespread use of anticoagulants and antiplatelet medications in this age group.

Q What frequently contributes to the mortality in older adult trauma patients?

A Comorbidities

Advancing age is frequently associated with multiple comorbidities and will increase the mortality rates following trauma. Older trauma patients experience higher mortality than the younger population following trauma regardless the mechanism of injury.

HINT

When determining risk of morbidity and mortality, it is important to take into account the patient's comorbidities along with their age.

TRAUMATIC INJURIES

Q What injury is commonly associated with falls in older adults?

A Hip fractures

Older adult patients frequently experience osteoporosis and are prone to fractures. As bones weaken, sometimes the hip fracture occurs prior to the actual fall. Osteoporosis is more common in women.

HINT

Aging bones with increasing osteoporosis easily fracture, even with minor trauma.

Q What injury is more common in older adult patients with osteoarthritic changes in their spine?

A Type II odontoid fracture

An odontoid fracture is the fracture of the odontoid bone on C2 in which C1 rotates. A Hangman's fracture may also be seen and is the bilateral fracture of C2 and is commonly associated with "stiffening" of C1 and C2 due to osteoarthritic and degenerative changes.

▶ HINT

Cervical injuries are greater with degenerative changes due to the limited movement of C1 and C2.

Q An older adult patient sustained a fall and hit their head on the kitchen cabinets about 2 weeks prior. The patient now presents with confusion and altered mentation. What is the most likely cause?

A Chronic subdural hematoma (SDH)

Chronic SDH occurs more often in the older adult population. The most frequent presentation is a history of head injury several weeks prior to presentation to the ED with altered neurologic status. Due to brain atrophy and slower bleeding rate in the subdural space (venous injury), the older adult patient has a delayed presentation following the trauma.

▶ HINT

Acute on chronic SDH may also be present and can contribute to the new onset of neurologic changes.

ASSESSMENT AND DIAGNOSIS

Q What classification of cardiac medication commonly prescribed to older adults can mask hemodynamic compromise following trauma?

A Beta-blockers

Beta-blockers will limit the heart rate response that would normally occur following a trauma and hemorrhagic shock. Older adult patients on beta-blockers may not develop tachycardia thus interfering with the ability to recognize signs of hypovolemia. This can also contribute to undertriage in older adult patients.

▶ HINT

Older adult patients also have impaired sensitivity or response to catecholamines even without being on beta-blockers (Box 13.1).

Box 13.1 Physiologic changes in older adult patients

Decreased GFR
Decreased vital capacity, forced expiratory volume, and functional residual capacity
Blunted responses to hypoxia and hypercarbia (less tachypneic responses)
Impaired sensitivity to catecholamines (less tachycardic responses)
Greater incidence of hypertension
Brain atrophy
Osteoporosis
Increased incidence of atrial fibrillation
Cardiac arrhythmias
Decreased contractility, stroke volume, and cardiac output
Preexisting neurologic impairments
Hearing and visual impairments
Loss of subcutaneous tissue
Reduced immunity and increased risk of infections

GFR, glomerular filtration rate.

Q What is the most common triage issue with assessing severity of injuries with older adults?

A Undertriaging

Undertriaging (Box 13.2) can occur with older adults due to physiologic changes, reduced lresponsiveness to catecholamines, respiratory complications, comorbidities, and medications that mask the severity of injuries. There are limitations to the trauma scores used to gauge severity of trauma patients in older adults (such as heart rate and blood pressure [BP]) and these may underestimate the injuries. Older adult trauma patients who are treated at a trauma center have shown lower mortality rates.

Box 13.2 Causes of undertriaging in older adult patients

Symptoms masked due to medications
Low energy mechanism of injuries
Unreliability of vital signs
Age bias (conscious or unconscious)
History of altered mentation (i.e., dementia)
Comorbidities increase mortality in less severe injuries

HINT

Serious injuries should be suspected in geriatric trauma patients even with normal vital signs.

▶ **HINT**

Advanced age may be a sole criterion for transfer to a trauma center to avoid undertriaging.

Q What assessment finding is more indicative of hemorrhagic shock in older adult trauma patients?

A Altered mentation

Altered mentation, decreased urine output, and diminished capillary refill are findings of hemorrhagic shock in older adult trauma patients. Tachycardia and hypotension are not commonly found in older adults with shock and their absence should not be used to rule out shock.

▶ **HINT**

Use of ultrasound to identify injuries that would cause hemorrhagic shock is recommended to prevent missing greater severity of injuries.

MEDICAL/SURGICAL INTERVENTION

Q An older adult patient on warfarin with an elevated international normalized ratio (INR) sustained a traumatic brain injury (TBI). What medication should be considered in this situation?

A Prothrombin precipitate complex (KCentra)/vitamin K

Early reversal of the INR should be considered in older adult patients on warfarin who sustain TBI. Serial brain CT scans are recommended to evaluate for hemorrhagic complications of TBI in anticoagulated older adult patients. KCentra and vitamin K are used to reverse INR in patients taking warfarin.

▶ **HINT**

Glasgow Coma Scale (GCS) is not as reliable in the older adult patient due to brain atrophy and more space available to bleed into the cranium before increased intracranial pressure (ICP) occurs.

Q What lab finding can be used to assess for hypoperfusion in an older adult trauma patient who may not be showing signs of shock?

A Lactic acid and base deficits

To identify occult injuries, lactic acid and base deficits can be useful in the management of older adult trauma patientsto identify occult injuries. These lab markers are sensitive for identifying hypoperfusion even with normal vital signs.

▶ **HINT**

Serial lactic acid findings should be used to identify response to resuscitation and persistent hypoperfusion (if they remain elevated).

NURSING INTERVENTIONS

Q A geriatric trauma patient requires bag-mask ventilation. It is noted they have dentures. What should you do with the dentures while performing bag-mask ventilation?

A Ventilate with dentures in place

Ventilation with bag mask is more difficult with the dentures out. The dentures should be kept in place, if intact, for ventilation.

▶ HINT

Early administration of high-flow oxygen is recommended in geriatric trauma patients because of low respiratory reserve and diminished response to hypoxia and hypercarbia.

Q What potential complication of fluid resuscitation should the trauma team be assessing during the resuscitation of an older adult trauma patient?

A Congestive heart failure (CHF)

Older adult trauma patients may require aggressive fluid resuscitation but the trauma team should be assessing breath sounds for crackles to prevent volume overload. Older adults may have compromised myocardial contractility, cardiomyopathies, and valvular disorders and cannot tolerate large volumes of fluid.

▶ HINT

Rapid infusions of boluses should be followed with assessment of patient's response to the fluid.

COMPLICATIONS

Q What are the physiologic changes in older adult patients that increase the risk of contrast-induced nephropathy?

A Decreased glomerular filtration rate (GFR)

There is a decrease in GFR and renal function in the older adult population. This leads to increased risk of acute kidney injury (AKI) and contrast-induced nephropathy (CIN). Trauma patients typically require frequent contrast procedures to identify injuries.

▶ HINT

Older adult patients may not be able to handle large volumes of fluid resuscitation due to impaired renal function.

Q Following chest trauma and rib fractures, what is a common complication found in the older adult population?

A Pneumonia

Pneumonia can occur due to limited pulmonary function in older adults. Those with advancing age will experience decreased functional residual capacity, vital capacity, and forced expiratory volume. This complication can increase mortality in older adults.

HINT

Good pain management is necessary to prevent the complication of pneumonia following rib fractures.

BARIATRIC TRAUMA PATIENTS

MECHANISM OF INJURY

Q What is the obesity classification of a trauma patient presenting with body mass index (BMI) of 36 kg/m²?

A Class II obesity

Obesity is defined as an abnormally high percentage of the body weight that is fat. Class II obesity (formerly called *morbid obesity*) is defined as a BMI of 35 to 39.9 kg/m² (Box 13.3).

Box 13.3 Classification of obesity

Overweight: BMI greater than or equal to 25 to 29.9 kg/m²
Class I obesity: BMI of 30 to 34.9 kg/m²
Class II obesity: BMI of 35 to 39.9 kg/m²
Class III obesity: BMI of > or = to 40 kg/m²

BMI, body mass index.

HINT

Anatomical and physiologic changes that occur in obese patients can affect trauma management and outcomes.

Q What are the metabolic changes seen in obese patients?

A Increased oxygen consumption and carbon dioxide production

Increased body weight increases oxygen consumption and carbon dioxide production. This occurs due to the increased metabolic rates in adipose tissue.

HINT

Desaturation times during rapid sequence intubation is decreased with obese patients.

Q What is the major contributing factor for the increased work of breathing (WOB) that occurs when an obese patient is supine?

A Abnormally high diaphragm

The obese patient has an elevated diaphragm due to the abdominal fat pressing up against the diaphragm when in a supine position. This will contribute to the increased WOB. Class II and III obese patients also experience increased airway resistance.

▶ HINT

These alterations in ventilatory effort result in shallow, rapid breathing and limited ventilatory reserve, especially in the supine position.

TRAUMATIC INJURIES

Q Which mechanism is less likely to cause serious injuries in obese patients?

A Abdominal stab wounds

With stab wounds to the abdomen, the anterior fat in an obese patient protects the internal organs from injury with stab wounds to abdomen and lowers the rates of exploratory laparotomies.

▶ HINT

Obese patients have been shown to experience fewer TBIs and a greater number of chest and lower extremity injuries.

Q What mechanism of injury is common in obese patients due to carrying the extra weight?

A Falls

The extra weight the obese patient carries affects the gait and stability, leading to increased risk of falls. Obese patients are prone to developing osteoarthritis and joint problems, which contribute to falls. Nonambulatory obese patients are at a higher risk for burns and inhalation injuries in house fires.

▶ HINT

Lower extremity fractures are commonly associated with falls in obese patients.

Q What safety feature is commonly not used by obese people and can increase the severity of injury?

A Seat belts

Seat belts are not designed for obese people and frequently are not utilized because of discomfort. This can increase the severity of injuries following an MVC.

▶ HINT

Obese patients in MVC with the impact on the same side door are at high risk for diaphragm injury.

ASSESSMENT AND DIAGNOSIS

Q What is the concern with secondary diagnostic imaging (i.e., CT or MRI) in obese patients?

A Image quality

The excessive amount of adipose tissue can interfere with the beam penetration and image quality in CT and MRI imaging. The patient's size may also prevent the use of CT or MRI and may require use of other diagnostic studies.

▶ HINT

When obtaining BP, make sure to use appropriately fitting cuffs to improve accuracy of BP measurements.

Q What finding on an arterial blood gas is commonly found with an obese patient?

A Hypercapnia

CO_2 retention is common in obese patients due to decreased tidal volumes (TVs) and chest wall compliance. It is also common to find oxygen saturation levels on the lower end of normal.

MEDICAL AND SURGICAL INTERVENTIONS

Q What puts the obese patient at a high risk for obtaining an artificial airway?

A Short, large necks

Short, large necks place an obese patient at a high risk for airway management, including difficult intubations and bag-mask ventilation. Cricothyroidotomy may also be difficult due to the short neck and deeper trachea. Obstructive sleep apnea (OSA), common in obese patients, is another risk factor for difficult airways.

▶ HINT

The short, large neck can make the cervical collar more difficult to fit appropriately to secure the cervical spine.

Q After intubation, when calculating the TV, would the actual or ideal weight be used in an obese patient?

A Ideal

TVs should be calculated on ideal weight based on the patient's height. This prevents overdistension and barotrauma of the alveoli during ventilation, especially in obese patients.

▶ HINT

Remember the abdominal fat will increase abdominal pressures, which decreases the ability to expand the thoracic cavity with ventilation.

NURSING INTERVENTIONS

Q A bariatric trauma patient is brought into the ED supine on a stretcher. What is a nursing intervention to improve ventilation?

A Elevate head of bed

The primary respiratory problem of an obese patient is a reduction in the expiratory reserve volume. This is due to decreased chest wall expansion and elevated diaphragm. Obese patients usually experience dyspnea and orthopnea. The chest wall compliance decreases to one third that of normal-weight people. Obese patients are also more likely to experience OSA. Lying flat will increase the risk of airway obstruction and aspiration.

HINT

Increased WOB is caused by elevated diaphragm and decreased lung expansion.

Q What is the potential problem during the exposure phase of resuscitation in morbidly obese patients?

A Missing posterior injury

During exposure, log rolling an obese patient is difficult and posterior injuries could potentially be missed. Additional staff may be required for the safety of the patient and staff.

HINT

Mobilizing obese patients as soon as possible is important to prevent complications. This may require mobilizing devices such as hoists.

Q What should be avoided if possible or placed with caution in a trauma patient with a history of bariatric surgery?

A Gastric tube

Gastric feeding tubes can cause injury during placement in patients following bariatric surgery. Nutritional assessment is important due to high risk of nutritional deficiency with bariatric surgeries.

HINT

Obese patients will break down their muscle for energy during critical illness and will accelerate loss of protein.

COMPLICATIONS

Q Obese patients are prone to increased abdominal pressure. Which organ is at high risk for failure?

A Kidneys

Obesity is a high-risk factor for the development of acute and chronic renal failure with elevated blood urea nitrogen (BUN) and creatinine levels (Box 13.4).

Box 13.4 Higher risk complications in obese patients

Decubitus
VTE
Infections
Delayed wound healing
Wound dehiscence
Rhabdomyolysis

VTE, venous thromboembolism.

HINT

The increased intra-abdominal pressure causes poor perfusion to the kidneys.

KNOWLEDGE CHECK: CHAPTER 13

1. Which of the following is a true statement regarding the airway of a child?

   A. Children under the age of 8 years old should use an uncuffed endotracheal tube.
   B. The narrowest part of the trachea is the vocal cords.
   C. Airway obstruction is not a common injury.
   D. The trachea is disproportionately long for the body size.

2. Which of the following traumatic injuries would best indicate a greater severity of injury for children?

   A. Abdominal bruising
   B. Spiral fracture of arm
   C. Rib fractures
   D. Ankle sprain

3. An 85-year-old female sustains liver and splenic lacerations after being T-boned by a truck. The following are her admission vital signs:

   Heart rate (HR) = 78
   Blood pressure (BP) = 96/67 mmHg
   Respiratory rate (RR) = 34

   Which of the following medications is the patient more likely to be taking prior to the motor vehicle collision (MVC)?

   A. Loop diuretic
   B. Beta-blocker
   C. Angiotensin-converting enzyme (ACE) inhibitor
   D. Insulin

4. Which of the following is considered a reason for the undertriaging that can occur in older adult trauma patients?

   A. Experience less fractures
   B. Less pain response to injuries
   C. Poor historian by the patient
   D. Age bias

5. An older adult patient sustained a fall and hit their head on the kitchen cabinets about 2 weeks prior. The patient now presents with confusion and altered mentation. What is the most likely cause?

   A. Acute subdural hematoma (SDH)
   B. Chronic SDH
   C. Epidural hematoma
   D. Intracerebral hemorrhage

(See answers next page.)

1. A) Children under the age of 8 years old should use an uncuffed endotracheal tube.

Airway is a major concern in pediatric trauma patients. In children under the age of 8 years old, use uncuffed endotracheal tubes since cuffed tubes can cause vocal cord injury, subglottic edema, and pressure necrosis. The trachea is smaller and shorter than in an adult and the narrowest part of the trachea in a child is the cricoid cartilage, whereas in an adult it is at the level of the vocal cords. Due to the size of the airway, a small amount of blood or the presence of a foreign body, edema, mucus, or the tongue can lead to airway obstruction.

2. C) Rib fractures

The rib cage and sternum are less ossified and more compliant in children. Rib and sternal fractures are rare and, if present, indicate an ominous sign. Significant thoracic injuries frequently occur without the presence of rib fractures. Spiral fracture may indicate abuse but not necessarily greater severity of injury. Ankle sprain is not indicative of a severe injury.

3. B) Beta-blocker

Following liver and splenic lacerations, patients will typically experience hemorrhagic shock from the injuries. Expected vital sign findings would be tachycardia and hypotension. In the preceding scenario, the patient did not have a significant increase in HR. Beta-blockers can mask hemorrhagic shock by limiting the tachycardic response.

4. D) Age bias

Age bias can occur and may be conscious or unconscious. Patients may not be considered as "viable" as a younger trauma patient. Older adult patients may be poor historians but this should not affect the triage process in a trauma patient. Older adult patients can be less responsive to pain, but this is not typically the main reason for undertriaging. Older adults experience greater number of fractures frequently due to presence of osteoporosis.

5. B) Chronic SDH

Chronic SDH occurs more often in the older adult population. The most frequent presentation is a history of head injury several weeks prior to presentation to the ED with altered neurologic status. Due to brain atrophy and slower bleeding rate in the subdural space (venous injury), the older adult patient has a delayed presentation following the trauma. Acute subdural, epidural, and intracerebral hemorrhages would present earlier with neurologic deficits.

PART V

Continuum of Care for Trauma

Injury Prevention and Public Education

Q What is the first step of trauma prevention?

A Identify risks

When risks for trauma or injury are identified, then prediction of an injury and prevention are possible. Injuries follow patterns, therefore they are frequently preventable. Analysis of risk factors leads toward identifying steps that may be used to prevent the injury. Injury surveillance systems may be used on the national level to determine trends of injuries (Box 14.1).

Box 14.1 Steps to injury-prevention programs

Collect data.
Analyze data.
Identify specific concerns or problems.
Identify the population at risk.
Develop preventive strategies or countermeasures.
Implement the prevention plan.
Evaluate the effectiveness of the plan.

HINT

The word *accident* is no longer recommended when referring to a trauma because an accident is not preventable.

HINT

Identifying risk factors includes answering the questions of where, who, and with whom.

Q What does the physical damage caused by the transfer of energy cause?

A Injury

Injury is physical damage caused by the transfer of energy, which can include kinetic, chemical, thermal, or electrical energy. Linking the mechanism of injury to the trauma is one step in identifying potential prevention strategies.

HINT

The word *injury* has replaced *accident* because most injuries are preventable and an accident, by definition, is not preventable.

Q When identifying the biomechanics of a trauma, a commonly used physics law states that force equals mass multiplied by what?

A Acceleration

Force is mass multiplied by the rate of acceleration or deceleration. A mechanism of injury is the transfer of energy from an external source to the human body. Energy is defined in trauma as the source of the physical injury (Table 14.1).

Table 14.1 Agents of trauma

Mechanical	Blunt trauma Penetrating trauma Bites Assault and battery Machines Falls
Chemical	Poisons Snake bites Gases Drugs
Thermal	Burns
Lack of oxygen	Drowning Smoke inhalation Carbon monoxide poisoning Asphyxiation
Electrical	Electrical burns Lightning
Radiant	Sunburn Explosions X-ray exposures Radiation Nuclear exposure

HINT

Kinematics **refers to motion and is used to study trauma mechanisms by looking primarily at the motion involved.**

Q What level of injury prevention actually prevents the trauma from occurring?

A Primary prevention

Primary prevention is the least commonly used and most difficult form of prevention to accomplish. It is designed to prevent the occurrence of the injury. The goal is to reduce the number of traumas, or totally eliminate the incident from occurring.

HINT

An example of primary prevention is the placement of a stoplight at a dangerous intersection. The goal is to prevent collisions.

Q What does secondary injury prevention focus on?

A Decreasing the severity of injury

Secondary prevention is designed to reduce the severity of the injury once the trauma has occurred. This is the most common form of prevention (Table 14.2).

Table 14.2 Examples of primary and secondary prevention

Primary Prevention	Secondary Prevention
DUI checkpoints	Use of safety belts
Stoplights at dangerous intersections	Airbags
Limited access to weapons	Wearing helmets
Rumble strips on side and center of road	
Bike paths	
Animal barriers along highways	

DUI, driving under the influence.

HINT

An example of secondary prevention is the use of seat belts and airbags. They do not prevent collisions, but if a collision occurs, they decrease the severity of the injury.

Q When one initiates a bundle of care to improve outcomes following a trauma, what level of injury prevention is this?

A Tertiary

Tertiary prevention is the improvement in outcomes after a trauma has occurred.

HINT

An example of tertiary prevention is the initiation of a sepsis protocol for early recognition and treatment of sepsis. This lowers the risk of mortality, improving outcomes.

Q What type of injury-prevention strategy is being used when a bicycle helmet safety talk is being given to young children?

A Education

Education is one of the most common methods of trauma prevention. Education can be targeted at high-risk populations or general populations.

HINT

The education method typically relies heavily on behavior modification to prevent trauma.

Q What type of injury-prevention strategy is being used when a person is ticketed for texting while driving?

A Enforcement

Enforcement strategies are injury-prevention techniques that can be legally mandated or legislated to protect the people. These involve laws or regulations.

▶ **HINT**

Seat belt laws are an example of enforcement.

Q The placement of airbags in car doors in response to the high morbidity and mortality of lateral impacts is what type of injury-prevention strategy?

A Engineering

Engineering is an effective way to reduce the degree of injury from a traumatic event. It involves redesigning products and vehicles to improve safety. This involves modification of the environment or of products. In this case, engineering was used to determine how to reduce the impact of energy.

▶ **HINT**

The development of airbags for car doors to lower the severity of injury in a lateral impact is an example of using engineering for prevention.

Q When a person is speeding and is ticketed, what type of injury-prevention strategy is being used?

A Economic

This uses money as an impetus for behavioral modification. Therefore, economic prevention involves a financial impact, such as paying fines for speeding, to discourage certain behaviors (Table 14.3).

Table 14.3 Examples of the four Es of injury-prevention strategies

Engineering	Airbags Seat belts Automated collision notification Athletic safety gear
Enforcement	Laws (local)—seat belts, helmets, DUI, no cell phones while driving, no texting while driving Legislation (federal)—gun safety
Education	School-based injury-prevention programs Multimedia—newspapers, internet, billboards, commercials Education for healthcare clinicians
Economic	Fines Loss of license to drive

DUI, driving under the influence.

Q Are preventive interventions that occur automatically and do not require an action from an individual an active or passive approach?

A Passive

Preventive measures are categorized as either passive or active approaches. Passive approaches are interventions that occur automatically without an individual having to do anything. An active approach involves an individual having to make a choice for a particular action for the intervention to be effective (Table 14.4).

Table 14.4 Examples of active and passive interventions

Active Intervention	Passive Intervention
Seat belt	Airbag
Life vest	Smoke detector
Child car seats	Antilock brakes
Helmet	Guardrail
Safety glasses	Antiscald device

HINT

The most successful intervention for prevention is one that requires a minimal amount of effort. Airbags are an example. They deploy automatically and do not require any effort as compared to putting on a seat belt, which requires effort.

HINT

Engineering and environmental strategies to prevent trauma tend to be passive interventions, whereas education usually involves an active intervention.

Q When developing a countermeasure to prevent an identified risk for injury, what should be determined about the intervention before initiating it?

A Proven effectiveness

This is based on the concept of evidence-based practice. When developing an intervention in an attempt to prevent an injury, the data on effectiveness of the intervention should be reviewed. A countermeasure should either have already been proven to be successful or have a reasonable potential to be effective at preventing the identified injury.

HINT

The countermeasure needs to have acceptable side effects and be cost-effective.

Q A person drinks at a party and then while driving home becomes involved in a collision. What is identified as the risk factor for this injury?

A Human factor

The human factor was the person drinking alcohol before driving a motor vehicle. When considering risk factors for an injury, there are several factors to be considered, including the human factor. This is usually the behavior that needs to be modified to prevent an injury (Box 14.2).

Box 14.2 Considerations in identifying risk factors

Human factor contributes to the event or injury
Agent involved in the injury
Environmental factors
Social factors

Q Which of the following would be considered a priority for developing a countermeasure to prevent the injury: high frequency or low mortality?

A High frequency

The highest priority for developing injury-prevention programs is for those injuries that have either a high frequency or a high mortality.

HINT

A data analysis finds that out of four intersections with stop signs, one has had 10 crashes within a month. That intersection would be the priority for placement of a traffic light, as it has a higher frequency of injury.

KNOWLEDGE CHECK: CHAPTER 14

1. Which of the following injury-prevention programs best describes seat belt laws being reinforced with fines?

   A. Economic
   B. Education
   C. Enforcement
   D. Engineering

2. Which is the best example of enforcement of an injury-prevention program?

   A. Mandatory seat belt law
   B. Fines for infractions of laws
   C. Development of airbags
   D. Instruction in high school regarding drunk driving

3. A pediatric patient in the ED is suspected of being abused. Notifying child protective services is which type of prevention?

   A. Primary trauma prevention
   B. Secondary trauma prevention
   C. Educational trauma prevention
   D. Engineering trauma prevention

4. The utilization of best practices and guidelines when managing trauma patients in the acute care setting is which of the following type of prevention?

   A. Educational prevention
   B. Secondary prevention
   C. Tertiary prevention
   D. Enforcement prevention

5. Which of the following trauma-prevention techniques is the least successful technique for preventing trauma?

   A. Engineering
   B. Education
   C. Enforcement
   D. Ergonomics

(See answers next page.)

1. A) Economic

Injury-prevention programs may use one of these four Es: education, enforcement, engineering, or economic incentives. Education in injury prevention should be targeted toward high-risk groups. Enforcement of injury-prevention programs can be accomplished through the passing of laws and legislation. Engineering is the design and development of better protective gear. Economic incentives involve the use of money to change behavior.

2. A) Mandatory seat belt law

A mandatory seat belt law is an example of injury prevention by enforcement. Enforcement includes the passing of laws and legislation. The fine for infractions of the law is an example of an economic incentive. The development of airbags in vehicles is an example of engineering, which includes the designing of protective vehicles or gear. A class provided in high school regarding drunk driving is education for trauma prevention.

3. B) Secondary trauma prevention

A pediatric patient in the ED is suspected of being abused. Notifying child protective services is a type of secondary prevention. Primary prevention would have been an intervention to prevent the initial occurrence of abuse. Secondary prevention is an intervention to decrease the injury or prevent it from occurring again. Educational trauma prevention involves education to the public regarding prevention of trauma. Engineering trauma prevention is the change of the design of a product or vehicle so that it will decrease injury.

4. C) Tertiary prevention

Tertiary prevention involves efforts following the incident that will optimize the outcome from injury, regardless of the severity of injury (after the event). This includes utilizing best practices and guidelines to improve the outcomes of trauma patients. Educational prevention is the use of public intervention with education to prevent trauma. Secondary prevention does not prevent trauma but is an intervention that may lessen its injuries. Enforcement involves fines or fees that are used to enforce changes that will prevent trauma.

5. B) Education

Education is the least effective injury-prevention strategy and requires the most amount of time to produce the desired effect. Engineering is the most effective because the change in design can provide primary prevention without involvement from a person. Enforcement can be more effective in some situations but still requires decision-making from the individual. Ergonomics is not a type of trauma prevention.

Prehospital Care

Q **A patient has a fall from second-floor balcony. Which one of the four recommendations for field triage by prehospital personnel would be considered in transporting this patient to a level 1 trauma center?**

A **Mechanism of injury**

The recommendation for field triage of a trauma patient utilizes a four-step process to evaluate the severity of injury in the field. The four components are physiologic, anatomical, mechanism of injury, and special considerations.

▶ HINT

In rural areas, it is not always possible to transport trauma patients to level 1 or 2 trauma centers because of the distance, and level 3 or 4 trauma centers must be used until air transport can be arranged.

Q **What is considered a hemodynamic criterion used by emergency medical services (EMS) to triage a trauma patient to a level 1 trauma center?**

A **Systolic blood pressure (SBP) less than 90 mmHg**

EMS attempts to identify the most seriously injured patient in the field to ensure transportation to the most appropriate level of care. An SBP less than 90 mmHg is one criteria used by the prehospital emergency personnel to decide to transport a trauma patient to a specialized trauma center such as a level 1or 2 trauma center. Physiologic criteria have been found to be a good predictor of severity of injury and mortality (Box 15.1).

Box 15.1 Examples of physiologic criteria

GCS <13
SBP <90 mmHg
Respiratory rate >29 or <10
Cool, diaphoretic skin

GCS, Glasgow Coma Scale; SBP, systolic blood pressure.

▶ HINT

A trauma patient with an SBP less than 90 mmHg with tachycardia has typically lost approximately 30% to 40% of their blood volume.

HINT

If the patient is younger than 15 years of age, the EMS is usually directed to transport the patient to a pediatric unit designated as level 1 or 2.

Q What type of trauma is more likely to be transported to a level 1 or 2 trauma facility, blunt or penetrating?

A Penetrating

All penetrating trauma to the head, neck, torso, or proximal extremities should be transported to a level 1 or 2 trauma center, if available. High-impact blunt trauma also requires a higher level of trauma care, but some blunt trauma is considered low impact and less likely to incur injuries (Box 15.2).

Box 15.2 Examples of anatomical criteria for higher level of trauma care

Penetrating injury to head, neck, torso, and proximal extremities
Flail chest
Pelvic fractures
Paralysis
Open or depressed skull fractures
Two or more proximal long bone fractures
Amputation
Crushed or mangled extremity
Severe facial injuries

HINT

Burn patients may require transportation to designated burn centers depending on the degree and location of the burn.

HINT

Some patients with lethal injuries may have normal vital signs, therefore, using physiologic criteria only may result in undertriage.

Q What type of impact is involved if the patient was an unrestrained passenger in a 45-mile-per-hour motor vehicle collision (MVC)?

A High-energy impact

A high-impact event is described as a rapid acceleration–deceleration event in which the patient absorbs large amounts of energy. Determinants of high- versus low-energy impact include direction, velocity of impact, and the use of personal protective devices. Following a high-energy impact, the trauma victim is considered severely injured until proven otherwise.

HINT

Use of personal protective devices can lower the energy of the impact by dissipating the energy. The previous scenario involved an unrestrained person, so the impact would be considered one with high energy.

Q What mechanism of injury in an MVC requires transporting the patient to a level 1 trauma center if available?

A Ejection

There are certain mechanisms of injury that are associated with greater injury severity and require a higher level of care. High-speed MVCs and ejection from the vehicle are two types of mechanisms that indicate the need for a higher level of trauma care (Box 15.3).

Box 15.3 Examples of mechanism of injury criteria

Significant intrusion of doors (>12″ occupant side and >18″ any side)
Ejection (complete or incomplete) from the vehicle
Vehicle rollover
Death at the scene
Automobile versus pedestrian
High-speed MVC (>40 mph)
Automobile versus bicycle, especially if victim is thrown or run over
Falls (>20 ft in adults)
Burns >10%

MVC, motor vehicle collision.

HINT

The goal of prehospital triage is to get the right patient to the right place in the right amount of time.

Q Following a low-speed MVC, the patient is determined to be on Coumadin for atrial fibrillation. Which is the more appropriate center to transport the patient, level 2 or level 3 trauma center?

A Level 2

A level 2 trauma center is more equipped to care for a complicated trauma patient. Although this patient was involved in a low-speed MVC, the patient is on Coumadin, an anticoagulant. The anticoagulant places the patient at a higher risk for bleeding and would increase this patient's potential for a greater severity of injury (Box 15.4).

Box 15.4 Examples of special considerations

Anticoagulation therapy or bleeding disorders
Older adults (age >55 years)
Pediatrics (age <15 years)
Burns
End-stage renal disease needing dialysis
Pregnancy >20 weeks
Insulin-dependent diabetes
Morbid obesity
Immunosuppression

HINT

The clinical judgment of the EMS personnel on the predicted severity of injury is also considered.

HINT

Geriatric patients commonly have occult injuries that are more difficult to recognize, and rapid deterioration can occur unexpectedly.

Q When EMS transports a large number of patients to a level 1 trauma center that could have been easily managed in a level 3 trauma center, what is this called?

A Overtriage

When looking at the patients transported to trauma centers, their acuity level and appropriateness of the facility are reviewed. Overtriage occurs when a large number of patients who could have been treated in outlying hospitals are transported to a level 1 or 2 trauma center. This causes overcrowding of those centers and can adversely affect the care of those with higher acuity levels. Undertriage occurs when patients who do require a higher level of trauma care are not transported to level 1 or 2 trauma centers.

HINT

Undertriage of potentially severe trauma patients to facilities unable to provide appropriate interventions can result in greater morbidity and mortality.

Q What is the goal for transport from the time of arrival on the scene?

A Less than 10 minutes

The goal of EMS, from the time of arrival at the scene to initiation of transport, is 10 minutes. This is frequently called *scoop and run* to facilitate getting the patient to definitive care quickly, but some effort toward stabilization is recommended at the scene (following Prehospital Trauma Life Support protocol). Transportation should be to the nearest most appropriate facility. A notification to the receiving hospital of the estimated time of arrival facilitates the care of the trauma patient on arrival at the ED (Box 15.5).

Box 15.5 Interventions performed at the scene

Airway control
Oxygen or ventilatory support
Hemorrhage control
Spinal immobilization

HINT

Trauma injuries are time sensitive. Trauma has always used the "golden hour" to stress the need for early intervention.

HINT

Intravenous (IV) catheters may be placed en route to the trauma facility.

Q Should a trauma patient always be transported to the nearest hospital for stabilization because of the time factor?

A No

Trauma centers are designed to recognize, stabilize, and provide definitive care to the trauma patient in the shortest amount of time. Therefore, even if the transport of the trauma patient might take 10 minutes longer for a designated trauma center, the overall time to definitive treatment may still be lower.

HINT

Prehospital personnel should match the needs of the injured patients to the closest hospital with the capability to provide definitive care within an appropriate time frame.

Q What would be the best mode of transportation to a trauma center in an MVC occurring in a rural area with a prolonged extrication?

A Air transport

In prolonged extrications with serious injuries, especially in a rural area, air transportation should be considered to reduce transport time as more ground transports are able to administer blood now.

HINT

Air transport may be limited in bad weather conditions.

Q EMS arrives at the scene of an MVC involving two vehicles. What important information should the prehospital personnel obtain regarding the collision?

A Speed and details of the collision

Mechanism of injury can guide the care provided for a trauma patient, both in appropriate diagnostic testing and interventions. Information deemed important about an MVC includes the speed of vehicles at time of impact and the details (front- or rear-end collision, or lateral impact; Table 15.1).

Table 15.1 Pertinent information emergency medical services obtain at the scene

MVC	Falls	Gunshot Wounds	Knife Wounds
Speed of impact	Height of fall	Distance from perpetrator	Type of weapon
Damage to vehicle	Which body part impacted first	Caliber of weapon	Angle of penetration
Type of impact	Surface of impact		
Death within vehicle			
Ejection (complete or partial)			
Rollover			
Restraints or airbag deployed			

MVC, motor vehicle collision.

HINT

Photographs of the involved vehicle at the scene have been found to assist the emergency care clinicians in the trauma center with understanding the mechanism of injury.

Q A patient is noted to have a wood sliver impaled in their eye. What would be the best intervention by the EMS in the field?

A Eye shield

The prehospital care of a patient with an impaled object in the eye is to place an eye shied to protect the eye. The removal of the object should not be attempted in the field.

HINT

Chemical injuries to the eye require copious irrigation of the eye prehospital.

Q The EMS arrive at the scene to find a complete amputation of the patient's hand. What would be the best intervention for the amputated part?

A Place it on ice

The ice cools the extremity and allows for a greater time to reimplant it. The limb should not be buried in the ice because of the tissue damage that occurs when frozen and during the defrosting of the limb.

HINT

Do not clean, scrub, or apply an antiseptic to the wound or amputated extremity part in the prehospital setting.

Q What type of injury should have limited fluids provided in the prehospital setting?

A Penetrating injury to torso

IV fluids should be limited or withheld in the prehospital setting for patients with penetrating trauma to the torso, chest, and abdomen. Administration of IV fluids before definitive treatment of the injuries may increase the blood loss, and the patient may require more blood transfusions. Limiting fluid intake until active bleeding is controlled is recommended. IV fluids administered in the prehospital setting should be titrated for palpable radial pulse using small boluses of fluid (250 mL). Aggressive rapid fluid resuscitation should not be used in the prehospital setting.

HINT

This practice of administering minimal to no fluids before definitive care is sometimes referred to as *permissive hypotension* or *delayed fluid resuscitation*.

KNOWLEDGE CHECK: CHAPTER 15

1. Which of the following is the most accurate statement regarding time of emergency response at the scene of trauma to a patient?

   A. Emergency medical services (EMS) should remain at the scene until the trauma patient is stabilized.
   B. Rapid transport to the nearest appropriate trauma center is needed with minimal interventions except basic ABCs (airway, breathing, circulation) performed in the field.
   C. The trauma patient should be transported immediately to the nearest hospital for stabilization.
   D. All trauma patients should be taken to a level 1 trauma center.

2. A family member wants to follow the ambulance from the scene to the hospital. Which of the following would be the best response by the paramedic?

   A. "Yes, stay right behind us all the way to the hospital."
   B. "The police can provide you a lead through the intersections."
   C. "Please do not try to follow the ambulance. You need to obey all speed limits and traffic lights."
   D. "There is no hurry to get to the hospital since the patient will need to be stabilized in the ED first before you can visit."

3. What is the optimal time for emergency medical services (EMS) to remain at the trauma scene before transport?

   A. 30 minutes
   B. 1 hour
   C. 10 minutes or less
   D. Less than 2 minutes

4. Which of the following would indicate the need for emergency medical services (EMS) transport to a level 1 or 2 trauma center?

   A. Glasgow Coma Scale (GCS) of 14
   B. Fall from a second-floor balcony
   C. All motor vehicle collisions
   D. Blunt trauma

5. Which of the following is considered a physiologic indication for a higher level of trauma care in a level 1 to 2 trauma center?

   A. Low-speed impact motor vehicle collision
   B. Pelvic fracture
   C. Flail chest
   D. Systolic blood pressure (SBP) <90 mmHg

(See answers next page.)

1. B) Rapid transport to the nearest appropriate trauma center is needed with minimal interventions except basic ABCs (airway, breathing, circulation) performed in the field.

The *scoop and run* concept is defined as rapid transport to the nearest appropriate trauma center with minimal interventions except basic ABCs performed in the prehospital setting. If the transport time to the nearest trauma center is short, limited time should be spent at the scene. Delays at the scene to "stabilize" a patient beyond airway and breathing can increase morbidity and mortality. The nearest hospital may not actually be the most appropriate trauma center for definitive care of a trauma patient. Not all trauma patients require a level 1 trauma center for quality care.

2. C) "Please do not try to follow the ambulance. You need to obey all speed limits and traffic lights."

Prehospital personnel should instruct families not to try to follow the ambulance during transport because of the need to obey traffic laws and protect the family from injury.

3. C) 10 minutes or less

Optimal time on the scene for major trauma patients is 10 minutes. Performing interventions delays the transport of the patient to definitive care. A primary survey should be completed, which includes securing an airway and stopping blood loss. The primary survey typically takes longer than 2 minutes. Obtaining intravenous (IV) fluids and initiating fluid resuscitation can occur during transport and should not delay transport.

4. B) Fall from a second-floor balcony

The recommendation for field triage of a trauma patient utilizes a four-step process to evaluate the severity of injury in the field. The four components are physiology, anatomy, mechanism of injury, and special considerations. A fall from a second-floor balcony requires higher level of trauma care (level 1–2) due to the mechanism of injury. Not all motor vehicle collisions require a higher level of trauma care, which depends upon several factors such as speed and impact. GCS is a component of physiology, but a GCS of 14 would not require level 1 or 2 trauma care. Not all blunt trauma requires a higher level of care. A low-impact motor vehicle collision does not require level 1 or 2 trauma centers.

5. D) SBP <90 mmHg

Physiologic criteria for emergency medical services (EMS) to transport a patient to a facility offering a high level of trauma care involves the level of consciousness (GCS), hemodynamic stability (SBP <90 mmHg), respiratory insufficiency, and signs of shock. Pelvic fracture and flail chest are anatomical indications for transporting to a higher level of trauma care. Low-speed impact in a motor vehicle collision is not an indication to transport to a higher level of trauma care and is a component of the mechanism-of-injury criteria.

Hemostatic Resuscitation

16

Q What is a major and preventable cause of death in trauma?

A Hemorrhage

Death from hemorrhaging following trauma occurs typically within the first several hours of the trauma. These deaths are due to exsanguination and uncontrolled blood loss.

HINT

Major hemorrhage can be defined as a loss of more than one blood volume in 24 hours (>5 liters in 70 kg males; Box 16.1).

Box 16.1 Severe hemorrhage definitions

Loss of 50% of TBV in less than 3 hours
Blood loss in excess of 15 mL/hr
30%–40% of blood loss

TBV, total blood volume.

Q What can decrease the mortality and overall blood product use in the trauma center?

A Massive transfusion protocol (MTP)

MTP has been found to decrease mortality and overall use of blood products. It should be a written document available to all members of the trauma team. The content should be based on the principle of damage control.

HINT

Competencies and regular drills should be performed to improve the success of the MTP (Box 16.2).

Box 16.2 Components of masssive transfusion protocol

Triggers to initiate MTP
Ensure MTP blood product availability
Identify MTP blood product delivery flow
Process of MTP blood product administration
Continual MTP infusion throughout transitions of care (ED, OR, ICU)
Establish targets for endpoint of MTP
Use adjuncts for massive transfusions
Establishing improvement monitoring

MTP, massive transfusion protocols; OR, operating room.

Q What is the potential complication of activating the MTP if the patient did not require this volume of resuscitation with blood products?

A Unnecessary exposure to blood products

Exposure to blood products can place the patient at risk for volume overload and all blood transfusion complications. One of the most common complications of massive transfusions is volume overload, or transfusion-associated circulatory overload (TACO).

HINT

The pulmonary complication of blood transfusion is transfusion-related acute lung injury (TRALI; Box 16.3).

Box 16.3 Blood transfusion complications

TRALI
TACO
Febrile nonhemolytic transfusion reactions
Acute hemolytic transfusion reaction
Transfusion related sepsis
Hypocalcemia
Transfusion-related hypokalemia

TACO, transfusion-associated circulatory overload; TRALI, transfusion-related acute lung injury.

Q What is a tool that can be used to determine the need for blood product transfusions in trauma patients?

A Assessment of Blood Consumption (ABC) score

The ABC score (Box 16.4) can be used to determine the need for blood product administration. It is a validated tool used to score the need for MTP. Each finding is assigned one point. A score of two or more requires the initiation of MTP.

Box 16.4 Assessment of blood consumption score

Heart rate >120
SBP <90
FAST
Penetrating torso injury

FAST, focused abdominal sonography for trauma; SBP, systolic blood pressure.

HINT

Other triggers initiate MTP include persistent hemodynamic instability and active bleeding requiring surgery following a trauma.

Q If MTP is triggered based on the established criteria, which is administered first, fluids or blood products?

A Blood products

Administering universal blood products is the initial resuscitation recommended in MTP over crystalloids and colloid fluids. In MTP, rapid delivery and transfusion of the blood products should continue in appropriate ratios until the patient is stabilized or transferred to the operating room (OR) for definitive management (Box 16.5).

Box 16.5 Key components of massive transfusion protocol resuscitation

Transfuse RBC and plasma in 1:1 or 1:2 ratio (plasma to RBC)
Utilization of universal donor blood products
Transfuse platelets for each six units RBCs
Transfusion service should automatically send correct ratio
Subsequent blood products should be delivered at 15 minute intervals
Universal donor blood products maintained in the trauma bay

RBC, red blood cells.

HINT

Large volumes of crystalloids contribute to third-spacing and volume overload complications.

HINT

The goal is to keep the next set of blood products available in the resuscitation area for the duration of the resuscitation.

Q When would it be appropriate to utilize laboratory results to make decisions regarding blood product transfusions?

A Once major bleeding is controlled.

MTP should be continued as long as the patient has an ongoing blood loss. Once the bleeding is controlled or patient is hemodynamically stable, the transfusion process may be changed to one determined by the patient's lab values. MTP may also be discontinued when care is determined to be futile.

HINT

Lab findings based on point of care (POC) may be used for faster turnaround times for decision-making (Table 16.1).

Table 16.1 Laboratory findings to monitor resuscitation

Lab	Results
Hgb	>10 g/dL
PT	<18 seconds
aPTT	<35 seconds
Fibrinogen	>180 g/L
Platelets	<150,000

aPTT, activated partial thromboplastin time; Hgb, hemoglobin; PT, prothrombin time.

Q What is the blood type that is considered to be a "universal donor" blood?

A O Rh negative

O Rh negative is the universally compatible blood type used in transfusions when patients are not stable enough to wait for the type and crossmatch. O Rh positive can also be used as universal donor blood except in women of childbearing age and should be used in male trauma patients. Crossmatched blood should be administered as soon as available.

HINT

Trauma centers should have O Rh negative blood and thawed plasma readily available for resuscitation.

Q What blood type is the ideal universal plasma donor?

A AB plasma

The ideal universal plasma donor is AB. This is a rare blood type and is not always available. A large proportion of type A donors are low in anti-B titers and their blood can be used as a universal donor plasma.

HINT

Plasma transfusion should be changed to type-specific plasmas as soon as the blood type has been determined.

Q What blood products contain fibrinogen and are needed to replace fibrinogen losses?

A Fresh frozen plasma (FFP) and cryoprecipitate

Fibrinogen levels will fall after 1 to 1.5 blood volumes are replaced with packed red blood cells (PRBC). This can occur even earlier in trauma patients with coagulopathies. FFP, fibrinogen concentrate, and cryoprecipitate can be used to replace the fibrinogen. Cryoprecipitate also contains coagulation factors.

HINT

Fibrinogen is the precursor to fibrin and is required to form a stable clot.

Q What electrolyte abnormality commonly occurs with multiple blood transfusions?

A Hypocalcemia

Citrate is used in in stored blood as a preservative and an anticoagulant. Citrate binds and lowers the ionized calcium levels.

HINT

Hypocalcemia is associated with cardiac dysfunction and contributes to worsening of bleeding.

Q What is the recommended technique for infusion of RBCs and plasma?

A Rapid transfuser with blood warmer

One of the principles of damage control resuscitation (DCR) is prevention of hypothermia associated with trauma and trauma resuscitation. Administering large volumes of fluid and blood can lower the patient's body temperature so fluids should be administered through a blood warmer. RBCs and plasma are administered quickly to restore homeostasis by a rapid transfuser.

HINT

Platelets and cryoprecipitate should not be administered through a blood warmer.

Q What is one of the techniques used to maintain permissive hypotension?

A Restrict crystalloids.

Permissive hypotension limits secondary blood loss until hemostasis is obtained. It delays the resuscitation and limits the volume used in resuscitation. It is one of the techniques utilized to maintain a lower blood pressure to avoid secondary blood loss and the need for large amounts of fluid resuscitation with crystalloids. Typically, permissive hypotension will target an MAP of 50 or a systolic blood pressure (SBP) of 80 to 90 mmHg.

HINT

Large volumes of crystalloids can cause multiple complications, including abdominal compartment syndrome (ACS).

Q What are the three components considered to make up the "lethal triad" following a major trauma?

A Coagulopathy, hypothermia, acidosis

These are three complications that are considered to be a major contributor to death following a trauma. These are all considered to be life-threatening complications and can complicate resuscitation by increasing the bleeding (Box 16.6).

Box 16.6 Hemostatic disturbances following trauma

Fibrinogen depletion
Impaired platelets
Inadequate thrombin generation
Fibrinolytic dysregulation
Hyperfibrinolysis

HINT

Coagulation also becomes further impaired with hypothermia, coagulopathies, and acidosis.

Q What is the purpose of DCR in trauma resuscitation?

A Strategies to correct the lethal triad

DCR's goal is prevention and rapid management. DCR includes the surgical management that occurs at the same time as resuscitation (Box 16.7).

Box 16.7 Techniques of damage control resuscitation

Permissive hypotensive resuscitation
Early airway control
Early use of blood and blood products in a 1:1 ratio
Limit use of crystalloids
Utilization of hemostatic products
Rapid diagnosis and management

HINT

DCR attempts to prevent rather than treat a coagulopathy.

Q What can exacerbate the metabolic acidosis present in trauma shock patients?

A Overuse of normal saline (NS)

NS contains higher amounts of chloride (Cl-) than normal serum Cl- levels and can lead to hyperchloremic metabolic acidosis following large-volume resuscitation with NS. Acidosis can further contribute to decease in coagulation leading to an increase in bleeding. The degree of acidosis may correlate to a trauma patient's mortality.

HINT

Lactated Ringer's (LR) does not increase Cl- levels or metabolic acidosis and may be used if large volumes of crystalloids are required.

Q What is the standard for reversing the metabolic acidosis that occurs with hemorrhagic shock?

A Aggressive blood and blood product administration

Metabolic acidosis is a result of anaerobic metabolism in hemorrhagic shock. Aggressive administration of blood and blood products is recommended in an attempt to reverse the shock and improve organ perfusion until surgical intervention can control hemorrhage. Direct management of the metabolic acidosis is not recommended unless pH decreases below 7.0.

HINT

Tris-hydroxymethyl aminomethane (THAM) may be preferred to bicarbonate therapy if patient is hypernatremic or in concurrent respiratory acidosis.

Q What is the adverse effect of hypothermia in a trauma patient?

A Increased bleeding

Hypothermia can worsen the coagulopathy in the trauma patient. Hypothermia increases bleeding by several factors, including interference with platelet aggregation, interference with coagulation factors, and interference with fibrinolysis (Box 16.8).

Box 16.8 Causes of hypothermia in trauma patients

Environmental cold exposure
Exposure in ED
Administration of cold fluids
Anesthesia/sedatives

HINT

Preventing hypothermia is better than reversing hypothermia (Box 16.9).

Box 16.9 Rewarming techniques

Severity of Hypothermia	Interventions
Mild	Passive external warming • Remove wet clothing. • Apply warm blankets. • Keep room temperature warm.
Moderate	Active external rewarming • Forced air warming devices
Severe	Active internal core rewarming • Fluid warmers • Humidified and warmed oxygen • Body cavity warming with lavage • Endovascular warming

HINT

Rewarming the torso before the extremities will prevent worsening of hypotension and acidosis due to peripheral vasodilation.

Q Besides surgical management, what other less invasive technique may be utilized to control bleeding?

A Interventional embolization

Interventional embolization, a less invasive technique than open surgeries, can be used to rapidly limit blood loss with arterial injuries. Rapidly controlling blood loss will allow more conservative volume resuscitation.

HINT

Pelvic fractures can result in a significant blood loss. Embolization is frequently utilized to control the blood loss.

Q What minimally invasive device may be used to control blood loss in noncompressible areas?

A Resuscitative endovascular balloon occlusion of the aorta (REBOA)

REBOA is a minimally invasive device used to "cross clamp" the aorta and limit blood loss.

Q What is the main priority in damage control surgery?

A Find the source of blood loss and control it.

Damage control surgery controls major blood loss, contains contamination, and applies temporary closure devices. These techniques include abdominal packing and use of hemostatic agents until patient is more stable for definitive repair.

HINT

Once the patient's body temperature is normalized and coagulopathy reversed, definitive surgery may be indicated.

Q What is an antifibrinolytic medication that has been used to reverse bleeding in trauma patients?

A Tranexamic acid (TXA)

Plasminogen is the precursor to plasmin, which degrades fibrin and breaks down the clot. TXA andr aminocaproic acid are antifibrinolytic medications that inhibit plasminogen activation and plasmin activity which stabilizes a clot.

HINT

Early administration, within 3 hours, of an antifibrinolytic agent may improve survival following major traumatic hemorrhage.

Q What product contains concentrated levels of three to four coagulation factors?

A Prothrombin complex concentrate (PCC)

Prothrombin concentrates contain concentrated levels of coagulation factors. These concentrates contain either three or four factors (II, IV, V) or (II, IV, IX, X).

HINT

PCC is similar to PRBC when compared to whole blood. PCC is considered a concentrated "FFP."

Q What laboratory test can be used to quantify the coagulation state of the trauma patient?

A Thromboelastography (TEG)

TEG can be used to measure hemostasis and quantify the coagulation state of the patient. It measures the strength and elasticity of the clot. TEG can identify hypercoagulable, hypocoagulable, and hyperfibrinolytic states.

HINT

TEG can be used in real time management decisions regarding blood product administration.

Q What is the initial time metric monitored during MTP infusions?

A Time from calling for MTP to initial transfusion

Time metrics are used to evaluate the trauma's center performance and can be used to identify areas of needed improvement. Rapid initiation of MTP will decrease morbidity and mortality.

HINT

Speed of initiating MTP affects stabilization of the bleeding trauma patient and outcomes (Box 16.10).

Box 16.10 Quality metrics in massive trasfusion protocol

Time from calling for MTP to initial transfusion
Time from calling for MTP to infusion of first unit of plasma
Adherence to predetermined ratio of blood products after MTP is initiated
Initiation of deactivation of MTP within 1 hour of termination of protocol
Track wastage rates of blood products

MTP, massive transfusion protocol.

Q What is a laboratory value that can be used as an endpoint to resuscitation?

A Base deficit

Base deficit and lactate levels are two serum lab values that can be used as endpoints to resuscitation. They are reliable indices to determine tissue hypoperfusion and reperfusion. The values trended over time during the resuscitation.

▶ HINT

Base deficit levels can guide trauma resuscitations.

KNOWLEDGE CHECK: CHAPTER 16

1. A trauma patient in the ICU is being monitored following repair of the liver. The central venous pressure (CVP) is found to be 2 mmHg. The nurse notifies the physician and anticipates the physician will order which of the following?

   A. Levophed
   B. Lasix
   C. Intravenous fluids
   D. Zosyn

2. The nurse receives a trauma patient in the ED who was unable to be resuscitated after a drowning incident and is unable to be resuscitated. The family is asking for all the patient's belongings. Which of the following would be the most appropriate response by the trauma nurse?

   A. This was clearly an accidental drowning, and all the patient's belongings should be returned to the family.
   B. Do not give the family anything and instruct them that the belongings and valuables need to be kept at this time for evidence purposes.
   C. The nurse instructs the family that they can have the valuable items, but all other belongings need to stay with the patient for evidence.
   D. Because the patient has expired, the family can have all the personal items that were with the patient.

3. FA patient ollowing a motor pedestrian injury, a patient received eight units of packed red blood cells during resuscitation. Two hours later in the ICU, the patient became hyperthermic, oxygen saturations decreased to 90%, and the patient developed a cough and required intubation. What is the most likely cause of this complication?

   A. Hemolytic blood transfusion reaction
   B. Exacerbation of chronic obstructive pulmonary disease (COPD)
   C. Pneumothorax
   D. Transfusion-related acute lung injury (TRALI)

4. A patient was admitted after being hit by a train. The patient received massive transfusion protocol. Which of the following is one component of the triad of complications in trauma?

   A. Hyperthermia
   B. Metabolic acidosis
   C. Decreased hemoglobin level
   D. Hypotension

(See answers next page.)

1. C) Intravenous fluids

A normal CVP reading is 3 to 8 mmHg. A low CVP, especially following a liver repair, indicates hypovolemia. The first-line treatment is to administer intravenous fluids. Sometimes antibiotics, such as Zosyn, are given when there is a low CVP and an infection, or sepsis involvement, but the first-line treatment is fluid hydration. The same is true for vasoconstricting medications; they are ordered for hypotensive patients, but if the tank is dry, we need to fill it before we can squeeze it. When the CVP reading is high diuretics are given to extract the extra fluid load.

2. C) The nurse instructs the family that they can have the valuable items, but all other belongings need to stay with the patient for evidence.

The family should not take personal items except for the valuable items, such as jewelry, because all trauma patients are potential forensic cases until completely ruled out. Items, such as personal clothing, need to be carefully packed and kept with the body as potential evidence. Trauma deaths need to be handled with special consideration for forensic evidence. Nurses need to be aware of the environment around them and the belongings that came with the patient because they can be used as potential evidence.

3. D) Transfusion-related acute lung injury (TRALI)

TRALI is a "two hit" insult to the patient's lungs. The first hit is the stressful situation, in this case the trauma, which causes neutrophils to adhere to the pulmonary endothelial bed. The second hit is the actual blood transfusion, which contains donor antibodies that activate the neutrophils, resulting in increased capillary permeability and noncardiogenic pulmonary edema. This causes a sudden onset of fever, cough, and hypoxia. Most patients require intubation but will usually recover within 96 hours. The patient did not present with any signs of hemolytic blood transfusion reaction, including shock state and disseminated intravascular coagulation. The patient has no identified risks or presence of COPD. Pneumothorax presents with dyspnea, tracheal shift, and diminished or absent breath sounds on the affected side.

4. B) Metabolic acidosis

The triad of complications following a trauma with massive hemorrhage includes hypothermia (not hyperthermia), coagulopathy, and metabolic acidosis. Hypotension and decreased hemoglobin are commonly experienced with blood loss, however, it is not considered a component of the triad.

5. A patient presents with a scalp laceration from blunt trauma. The wound is bleeding profusely but the amount of blood loss is unknown. The patient's vital signs indicate hypotension and tachycardia. A fluid challenge of 2 L is administered to the patient. What would be the expected response if the blood loss was less than 20% of the total blood volume?

   A. Vital signs stabilize after the bolus but deteriorate when the fluids are stopped.

   B. Vital signs stabilize after administration of the fluids without further deterioration of status.

   C. Vital signs fail to stabilize with the fluid bolus.

   D. Vital signs stabilize after a second fluid challenge.

(*See answers next page.*)

5. B) Vital signs stabilize after administration of the fluids without further deterioration of status.

A 2-L fluid challenge is commonly used in resuscitation to assist with determining the amount of blood loss. If the vital signs stabilize after the fluid administration without further deterioration in status, the patient probably has had a blood loss less than 20%. If the vital signs stabilize after the bolus, but deteriorate when the infusion is stopped, the patient probably has blood loss greater than 30%. If the vital signs fail to stabilize with the fluid bolus, then the blood loss is probably greater than 40% and may require immediate surgery to control the hemorrhage.

Regulations and Patient Safety

17

Q What does *EMTALA* stand for?

A Emergency Medical Treatment and Active Labor Act

EMTALA is a statute that governs when and how a patient may be refused treatment or transferred from one hospital to another when in an unstable medical condition. This was passed as part of the Consolidated Omnibus Budget Reconciliation Act (COBRA). The purpose of EMTALA is to ensure that patients with an emergency condition are assessed and treated at any hospital providing emergency services without any consideration for the ability to pay.

HINT

This statute is intended to prevent hospitals from refusing emergency care to patients who are unable to pay for their care.

Q What does EMTALA require the hospital to provide for a patient seeking medical assistance?

A Medical screening examination

Any patient who comes to the ED seeking medical assistance must be provided with an appropriate medical screening examination to determine whether the patient is suffering from an emergency medical condition. If they are, the hospital is obligated to provide treatment until stable, or provide transfer to another hospital in accordance with the statute.

HINT

The person doing the medical screening must be a qualified healthcare worker as determined by the hospital's bylaws.

Q When should a hospital inquire about the patient's ability to pay for the ED services?

A After the screening examination

The patient should not be asked to pay for or the hospital should not try to elicit payment for services before the medical screening. The ED staff should be trained to respond to the patient's questions about costs in an effort to make sure the patient realizes the extent to which EMTALA procedures are available without cost.

HINT

The ability to pay should not interfere with the medical screening of the patient presenting for an emergency condition.

Q When can a patient be transferred to another facility that provides a higher level of care?

A After being stabilized

When the patient is stabilized, or the emergency medical condition is resolved, then the patient can be transferred to another facility. A patient can be transferred to a facility with a higher level of care before they are stabilized only if the patient meets certain standards and the transfer is appropriate.

HINT

A hospital that does not specialize in trauma may transfer a trauma patient to a trauma facility if the hospital is unable to provide the care necessary to stabilize the patient.

Q What is the best description of the patient's condition if their condition is unlikely to deteriorate as a result of the transfer?

A Stabilized

A stabilized condition allows for the patient to be transferred and is often considered a clinical judgment. The definition frequently used is that no deterioration in the patient's condition is likely to result from the transfer or to occur during the transfer.

HINT

If the trauma patient is in active labor, they are stabilized only after the baby and placenta are delivered.

Q When would it be appropriate to transfer a trauma patient who is unstable to a level 1 trauma center?

A When the patient requires treatment only the receiving hospital can provide

If a patient requires a treatment that can only be provided by the receiving trauma center and the medical benefits outweigh the risks, then a transfer would be appropriate even if the patient is deemed unstable. The transferring hospital stabilizes the patient as best as possible within its limits. Transfer of the patient for definitive care in a trauma center should occur as early as possible. If the patient is deemed to need a higher level of trauma care, the transferring hospital should not complete all the diagnostic studies.

HINT

All trauma patients should have a chest x-ray (CXR) before transfer to identify presence of pneumothorax or hemothorax.

Q What is the priority of care for the referring hospital before transporting a patient to a trauma center?

A Airway management

The primary role of the referring hospital is to ensure that the patient's airway, breathing, and circulation (ABCs) are checked before the transfer. Obtaining and securing the airway is the priority of the transferring hospital. If the patient has a pneumo- or hemothorax, a chest tube should be placed before transfer. Adequate intravenous (IV) fluids should be obtained, and fluid resuscitation initiated, including administering blood transfusions if required. Bleeding should be controlled before transfer.

HINT

When in doubt, secure the airway before transport. A lower threshold for intubation should be used when transporting a trauma patient from one facility to another.

Q Which hospital is responsible for arranging transportation, the transferring or receiving hospital?

A Transferring

The transferring hospital is responsible for securing the appropriate transportation based on the acuity of the patient. The transferring hospital must ensure the transport is with qualified personnel and equipment as required by the patient's circumstances, including appropriate life-support measures during transfer. The transferring hospital is ultimately responsible for decisions made in modes of transfer.

HINT

A copy of the medical records and a summary of the treatment that was provided by the transferring hospital must accompany the patient to the receiving hospital.

Q A patient in the ED following a motor vehicle collision (MVC) is refusing care and wants to leave the hospital without care. What does EMTALA require the hospital to document?

A Discussion of risks

If a patient is refusing treatment or transfer, EMTALA requires certain documentation, which includes that the patient was properly informed of the risks of leaving and the benefits of the treatment or transfer.

HINT

If an emergency medical condition is recognized by the hospital, it is required to provide transfer to another hospital if unable to provide the care required by the patient's condition or document appropriately the patient's refusal.

Q What is the risk or penalty if a hospital is found to have violated EMTALA?

A The Medicare clinician agreement is revoked

The regulation of the EMTALA statute is enforced in hospitals even if individual physicians may be making the decisions in the ED. The Medicare clinician agreement can be revoked by the Centers for Medicare & Medicaid Services (CMS) as a penalty for violation of the EMTALA statute. Smaller penalties, typically monetary, may also be utilized for violations of the statute.

HINT

A transfer of the patient from the ED to another hospital cannot be based on the patient's inability to pay for services.

Q What is the primary obligation of a burn center or a level 3 or 4 trauma center?

A Accept the transfer

Most of the responsibilities for a transfer belong to the transferring hospital, and not the burn centers or trauma centers. The primary obligation of these advanced centers is to accept the transfer if they have the capacity to treat the patient. In most cases, if the receiving hospital's capabilities exceed the transferring hospital's capabilities, the specialized center is obligated to accept the transfer.

HINT

This obligation may stand even if there is a temporary overcrowding or staff are unavailable.

Q A patient is brought to the ED in a rural hospital without a trauma designation and is noted to have a widened mediastinum on CXR. What would be the most appropriate intervention?

A Transfer to a trauma center

A patient with a widened mediastinum on CXR is likely to have an aortic injury. This would be an indication for a rural hospital to transfer the patient to a designated trauma center after initial stabilization (Box 17.1).

Box 17.1 Examples of indications for transfer to trauma center

Major vessel injuries (e.g., carotid or vertebral dissection)
Thoracic aortic dissection
Severe traumatic brain injuries
Spinal cord injuries
Severe facial injuries
Pelvic ring disruption (unstable pelvis)
Extremity injury with loss of pulse
Multiple traumatic injuries
Severe single-organ injury
Hemodynamic instability
Abdominal trauma patient requiring multiple blood transfusions
Serious eye injury
Degloving injuries
Bilateral pneumothoraces

HINT

Patients with severe injuries or multiple traumatic injuries may require stabilization and transportation to a designated trauma center.

Q What is an anatomical scoring system that provides an overall score for patients with multiple traumatic injuries?

A Injury Severity Score (ISS)

The ISS is used to determine the severity of injury in patients with multiple traumas. The ISS can be used to determine the need to transfer to a higher level of trauma care or determine predicted outcomes. The ISS uses six body regions and the Abbreviated Injury Scale (AIS) in each region (Box 17.2).

Box 17.2 Six regions of the Injury Severity Score

Head and neck
Face
Chest
Abdomen
Extremity
External

HINT

The ISS cannot be calculated in a prehospital setting and is used in the hospital primarily for MVCs.

Q What is the highest score a patient can get on the ISS?

A 75

The scoring system uses a range of 0 to 75. A higher number correlates to a greater severity of injury. This scoring system correlates with mortality, morbidity, length of hospital stay, and other severity scores (Box 17.3).

Box 17.3 Other trauma scores

Trauma index
Trauma score or revised trauma score
CRAMS scale
Prehospital index

CRAMS, circulation, respiration, abdomen, motor, speech.

HINT

A patient who scores a 6 on the AIS for a body region (indicates nonsurvivable injury) automatically scores 75 on the ISS.

Q How is a hospital declared a trauma center by the state: designation or verification?

A Designation

Trauma center designation is a process that is developed at the state or local level. The process and requirements vary from state to state, although the verification is a process performed by the American College of Surgeons (ACS). The ACS verifies the presence of resources outlined by the ACS, including the hospital's commitment, readiness, resources, policies, and performance improvements. This occurs at a national level and is standardized.

HINT

The verification by ACS lasts for 3 years, and then the trauma center needs to be reverified.

Q A trauma center that has 24-hour in-house coverage by general surgeons and prompt availability of specialized services meets which level of trauma designation or verification?

A Level 1

A level 1 trauma center has the general surgeons in-house 24-hours a day, whereas the level 2 trauma center has 24-hour immediate coverage by general surgeons (but not in-house). The level 1 trauma centers are able to provide comprehensive trauma care from prevention through rehabilitation.

HINT

Transferring high-severity trauma patients to a level 1 trauma center from level 2 is shown to improve outcomes and lower mortality.

Q How many levels of trauma designation or verifications are there?

A Four (ACS verification)

The trauma center verification by ACS has four levels. Some state-designated systems have five levels. Level 1 is the most specialized trauma center, going all the way to level 4 or 5 in which the hospital wants to provide the best trauma care but does not have the capabilities to provide complete trauma care (Table 17.1).

Table 17.1 Coverage in the designated or verified levels

Level 1	Level 2	Level 3	Level 4
24-hour in-house coverage by general surgeon	24-hour immediate coverage by general surgeon	24-hour immediate coverage by ED physician with prompt availability of general surgeon	Basic ED coverage with ED physician and nurse available on patient's arrival
In-house OR and SICU service	24-hour OR availability desirable	24-hour x-ray, CT scan, and PACU required	24-hour ED and lab; does not need 24-hour emergency medicine
Level 2 requirements plus cardiac and microvascular surgery	Level 3 requirements plus hand, neurosurgery, OB/GYN, ophthalmic, thoracic care	Orthopedics, plastic surgery, radiology, and anesthesia staff available 24 hours	
Teaching center and research	Injury-prevention outreach		

OR, operation room; PACU, postanesthesia care unit; SICU, surgical intensive care unit.

HINT

Severely injured trauma patients are frequently transported by emergency medical services (EMS) or air transport to a level 1 or 2 trauma center for definitive care.

HINT

A level 3 hospital may be able to provide emergency surgery to stabilize the patient before transfer (e.g., splenic rupture).

Q What does *HIPAA* stand for?

A Health Insurance Portability and Accountability Act

HIPAA was developed to provide standards to address the privacy of an individual's health information. This protected health information allows people to control who and how their health information is used. A major goal of HIPAA is to ensure that individuals' health information is properly protected. Yet still allowing health information to provide and promote high-quality healthcare and to protect the public's health and well-being. HIPAA ensures patients receive information about the way their health data are used and disclosed.

HINT

The standard developed by HIPAA is called the *Privacy Rule*.

Q What does the Privacy Rule call individually identifiable health information?

A Protected health information (PHI)

Individually identifiable health information is information, such as demographics, that can identify the person and their health records or health payments. HIPAA defines and limits the situations in which the health information can be used.

HINT

The key to HIPAA is determining whether the health information can be identified as belonging to a certain individual.

Q Can you use a picture of an x-ray without permission from the individual who was x-rayed in a presentation if there are no individual identifiers on the x-ray?

A Yes

There are no restrictions to the use of health information if it has been de-identified. De-identified health information does not have any identifiers and does not provide a reasonable basis on which to identify an individual.

HINT

The use of patient cases and x-rays for education does not require permission from the patient if there are no identifiers used during the educational event.

Q When can a hospital provide information about a patient to another person?

A When the patient gives permission

Patients can determine to whom they want to have their individual health information disclosed. This needs to be in writing before the hospital or hospital personnel can disclose the health information to that identified person.

HINT

The patient has the right to change or amend the list of people who are able to access their individual health information at any time.

Q A physician is asked to consult on a trauma patient. Does the patient need to give written permission to the consulting physician to review their individual healthcare information?

A No

The hospital may disclose individual healthcare information for treatment activities to any other healthcare clinician. This includes physicians, nurses, therapists, and so on, who are involved in the patient's healthcare. There are also situations involving the overall public interest in which the individual health information may be shared without permission from the individual (Box 17.4).

HINT

This does not allow a healthcare clinician to review a patient's chart if the clinician does not have any direct or indirect professional involvement with the patient.

HINT

Obtaining consent from the patient for healthcare operations and third-party payers is optional under the HIPAA Privacy Rule.

Box 17.4 Routine disclosures

Treatment by healthcare clinicians
Payment activities of insurance companies
Healthcare operations (e.g., quality management)
Required by law
Public health activities:
- FDA
- CDC

Victims of abuse, neglect, or domestic violence
Health oversight activities:
- Hospital audits

Judicial and administrative proceedings
Law enforcement purposes

(*continued*)

Box 17.4 Routine disclosures (*continued*)

Decedents:
- Medical examiners
- Funeral directors

Cadaveric organ, eye, or tissue donation
Research
Serious threat to health or safety
Essential government functions
Worker's compensation

CDC, Centers for Disease Control and Prevention; FDA, Food and Drug Administration.

Q What is the assurance HIPAA provides patients about their own medical records?

A Access to the records

A component of HIPAA is the assurance that patients can have access to their own medical records. Patients have the right to review and obtain a copy of their individual medical records.

HINT

There are exceptions to this; patients are denied access to certain healthcare information (Box 17.5).

Box 17.5 Exceptions to right of access

Psychotherapy notes
Information compiled for legal proceedings
Laboratory results that CLIA prohibits
Information from certain research laboratories

CLIA, Clinical Laboratory Improvement Amendments.

KNOWLEDGE CHECK: CHAPTER 17

1. Which of the following best describes Emergency Medical Treatment and Active Labor Act (EMTLA)?
   A. Provides guidelines for insurance to continue coverage after change in employment.
   B. Defines how a patient may be refused treatment or transferred from one hospital to another.
   C. Identifies patients who are unable to pay for services.
   D. Identifies criteria for admission to a nontrauma hospital.

2. A trauma facility receives a burn patient in the ED. Upon assessment of the patient, it is noted that this patient would be a candidate for transfer to a burn center. Which of the following criteria supports this assessment as correct?
   A. Partial-thickness burn to less than 20% total body surface area (TBSA)
   B. Partial-thickness burns to the thighs
   C. Inhalation injuries
   D. Full-thickness burns on 3% TBSA

3. Which of the following is the most accurate statement regarding discharge planning?
   A. All patients are candidates for rehabilitation following a trauma.
   B. Discharge planning should occur once the patient is stabilized.
   C. Arranging for transportation is the final step in transfer to a rehabilitation center.
   D. Discharge planning should involve both the patient and family and include completion of tests before transfer.

4. A nurse on the trauma floor is providing discharge instructions for a patient being discharged home. The patient primarily speaks Spanish with limited English. Which of the following is the most correct statement regarding the discharge instructions?
   A. Provide the patient with written discharge instructions in Spanish in place of the English discharge instructions.
   B. The patient is able to understand some English and should be okay with English instructions.
   C. The nurse can use a family member to assist with the translation.
   D. The nurse should use a hospital-provided translator.

5. Which of the following would be indicated before transfer from the initial hospital to a trauma center?
   A. Chest tube placed for pneumothorax
   B. MRI of brain if unresponsive
   C. Central line placed for resuscitation
   D. Full set of radiographs

(See answers next page.)

1. B) Defines how a patient may be refused treatment or transferred from one hospital to another.

EMTALA is a statute that governs when and how a patient may be refused treatment or transferred from one hospital to another when in an unstable medical condition. This was passed as a part of the Consolidated Omnibus Budget Reconciliation Act (COBRA). The purpose of EMTALA is to ensure that patients with an emergency condition are assessed and treated at any hospital providing emergency services without any consideration for the ability to pay. It does not provide guidelines for insurance or identifying patients who cannot pay for services or criteria for admission in a nontrauma hospital.

2. C) Inhalation injuries

Stabilization of the patient in the initial receiving center is required. Inhalation injuries or large body surface area burns need to be transferred to a burn center. Transfers are usually for full-thickness burns greater than 5% TBSA and greater than 20% TBSA for partial-thickness burns. Partial- or full-thickness burns to hands, feet, face, genitalia, or major joints should be transferred to a burn center.

3. D) Discharge planning should involve both the patient and family and include completion of tests before transfer.

Discharge planning involves an evaluation of the patient, discussing options with the patient and/or family, planning the actual transfer, and arranging any tests or procedures required before leaving. Not all patients are candidates for rehabilitation and this depends on the patient's ability to participate in the rehabilitation. Discharges and transfers are frequently delayed because the accommodation or transportation is either unavailable or late; there should not be any delay in the final step of transfer.

4. D) The nurse should use a hospital-provided translator.

The nurse providing discharge instruction to a Spanish-speaking patient should use an official hospital-approved translator. It is not recommended to use family members for interpretation, even if they are bilingual. The patient may not understand enough English, so a translator is recommended. The patient should have both verbal and written discharge instructions.

5. A) Chest tube placed for pneumothorax

A pneumothorax can be life-threatening and should be managed with chest tube placement in the ED prior to transfer. All interventions used to stabilize the trauma patient should be initiated before transfer. A full set of radiographs, brain MRI, and central-line placements are best performed at the trauma center and should not delay the transfer.

Forensic Issues

Q Following a violent crime, who is a candidate for evidence collection, the victim or the perpetrator?

A Both

Both the victims and perpetrators of violent crimes or accidental injuries should have evidence collected in the ED. It is essential for trauma nurses to have basic skills in the preservation of evidence. During resuscitation or treatment, evidence can be overlooked, lost, or destroyed.

HINT

Trauma nurses need to be aware of potential cases for the forensic and medical examiner (Box 18.1).

Box 18.1 Examples of medical examiner cases

Domestic violence (child, spouse, partner, elder abuse)
Trauma (nonaccidental or suspicious and accidental injuries)
Motor/vehicle pedestrian injury
Substance abuse
Attempted suicide or homicide
Environmental hazard incidents (fire, smoke, toxins, chemicals)
Occupational injuries
Victims of terrorism or violent crimes
Illegal abortion practices
Supervised care injuries

Q What type of trauma should be considered a potential forensic case with the need for evidence collection?

A All trauma

All trauma cases are potential forensic cases until ruled out. All nonvehicular trauma should be considered abuse until ruled out.

HINT

For evidence to be used in court, the evidence must be properly collected and preserved (Box 18.2).

Box 18.2 Types of evidence

Clothing
Hair
Nails
Bullets
Lacerations
Contusions
Any wounds

Q What belongings can the trauma nurse give to the family following a traumatic death in the ED?

A Only valuables

In any trauma death, whether dead on arrival or death in ED or hospital, the patient's belongings, except for valuables, should not be returned to the family in case the death may require investigation by the medical examiner (Box 18.3).

Box 18.3 Care of trauma death

Do not wash the body.
Do not remove any lines or tubes.
All appliances should be left in place.
Personal clothing should be carefully packaged and retained with the body.
Do not return belongings to the family (except valuables).

HINT

The valuables returned should be accurately documented in the medical records.

Q Evidence collected from a trauma patient should be placed in what type of bag?

A Paper bag

Place evidence collected from a trauma patient in a paper bag or an envelope. Always use paper to prevent breakdown of biological evidence (semen, blood, or saliva). If evidence is placed in plastic containers, it may decay or mildew because of moisture inherent in the plastic, so holes would need to be punched in the lid. If an envelope is used, seal the envelope with evidence tape and initial, indicating the date and time on the patient label. Do not use gummed envelopes or staple to seal (Table 18.1).

Table 18.1 Method for folding paper containing evidence

Step 1	Place evidence on a white piece of paper while wearing gloves.
Step 2	Fold the paper in thirds with evidence in the center.
Step 3	Turn paper 90°.

(*continued*)

Table 18.1 Method for folding paper containing evidence (*continued*)

Step 4	Fold the paper again into thirds.
Step 5	Tuck the upper third into the lower third of the second folding.
Step 6	Place paper in an envelope.
Step 7	Tape the envelope and label.

HINT

The hands of a patient with a potential self-inflicted gunshot wound should be covered with paper bags to preserve residue.

Q When cutting the clothing off a gunshot or stabbing victim, what does the trauma nurse need to avoid?

A Avoid defects in clothing

When cutting clothes, do not cut through defects in clothing such as bullet holes, tears, or stab entry. Cutting through a tear in the clothing can destroy evidence.

HINT

Document the description of all defects in the clothing, including defects such as tears, holes, residue, burns, or stains.

Q How can gunpowder around a wound best be preserved?

A With tape

The gunpowder can be preserved from around a wound with tape pressed on the wound then placed on a glass slide. This is then preserved in an envelope in the appropriate manner.

HINT

If gunpowder is present on a wound, photograph the wound prior to cleansing it.

Q A bullet is found in the clothing of a trauma patient during resuscitation. What is the best method to use to handle the bullet?

A Rubber-tipped forceps

Rubber-tipped forceps are used to handle a bullet in a trauma patient. The use of metal forceps can alter the markings on the outside of the bullet, thereby damaging evidence. The bullet should then be wrapped in gauze and secured in a container.

HINT

Do not shake clothing after removal from a patient. This can potentially cause loss of evidence.

Q What is the priority when a victim of an intentional trauma is being resuscitated?

A The patient

The collection of evidence should never take priority over lifesaving interventions.

Q What should be placed on the floor when removing the clothing of a victim of an intentional trauma?

A A clean, white sheet

Place a clean, white sheet on the floor, under the gurney or for the patient to stand on while undressing. This sheet will collect any evidence that may be shed from the clothing or victim's body. Once the clothing is removed, place the clothing on the sheet away from traffic. After the crisis, take the clothing from the sheet and place each garment in a paper bag and label appropriately.

HINT

Never just throw clothes on the ED floor because this may lead to gross contamination of critical evidence.

Q How is evidence collected from under the fingernails?

A Scraping

Scraping or swabbing under the fingernails can preserve evidence. The scrapings should be allowed to fall on clean, white paper. Any broken nails should be clipped.

HINT

Separate evidence and nail clippings by right and left hand.

Q When handling clothing of a patient that requires forensic management, what should the nurse change frequently?

A Gloves

Frequently changing the gloves during the handling of the clothing prevents cross-contamination of the evidence being handled. The trauma nurse should also use powder-free gloves when handling the evidence.

HINT

Minimizing the handling of the evidence also helps prevent contaminating the evidence.

Q What should be obtained to document a wound prior to suturing the wound of victims in a potential crime?

A Photographs

Good-quality photos should be taken of the location of injury or traumatic wounds in victims of a potential crime. The photo of the injury should be with and without a scale to judge the size of the wounds. If possible, photographs should be obtained before suturing or other procedures are performed in the area of injury.

HINT

Bruises and bite marks may require the use of ultraviolet or infrared photos, if available.

Q When should body fluids be obtained for forensics on a trauma victim?

A As early as possible

The earlier the fluids are drawn or obtained, the greater the forensic value of the fluids. Blood work includes sending one red-, purple-, and gray-topped tube, each for a different lab. Do not use alcohol to prepare a venipuncture site if blood alcohol levels are being obtained. Cleanse with povidone–iodine followed by saline. Place evidence tape across the top of the tubes, label and initial them, then wrap the tubes with protective material and package, label, seal, and store in a secure location.

HINT

Body fluids that may be obtained include blood, urine, gastric secretion, peritoneal fluid, or spinal fluid.

Q How should a gunshot wound be described in the medical records?

A Exact description

All physical findings should be precisely documented using correct terminology. Traumatic wounds, such as gunshot and stab wounds, should be described using exact location, size, and character of the wound. To be most accurate, the use of both narrative descriptions and body diagrams are recommended.

HINT

Refrain from using forensic statements, such as "entry" or "exit" wound, when documenting in the medical record.

Q What needs to be generated every time evidence changes hands?

A A receipt

There needs to be a documented trail of who handled the evidence and where the evidence was located. Minimizing the number of people handling the evidence assists with securing the evidence and minimizes tampering or destroying the evidence. Each time the evidence changes hands, a receipt should be generated and signed by both people involved in the transfer of the evidence.

HINT

Ensure the evidence is well secured to prevent tampering.

KNOWLEDGE CHECK: CHAPTER 18

1. The trauma nurse received a patient who sustained a gunshot wound to the head. The patient is covered in blood and presents to the ED dead on arrival. The family comes into the ED crying and upset; they think that suicide may be a factor for consideration, and they want to see the patient's body. Which of the following is the best response by the nurse?

   A. Tell the family that you are sorry for their loss and that they can go see the patient once they are cleaned up so that they do not see the patient covered in blood.
   B. Let them see the patient after the nurse removes all the invasive lines that emergency medical personal placed so that it is not so traumatic for them.
   C. Prepare the family for how the patient looks and allow the family into the room.
   D. Cover the patient with a blanket, comfort the family, and give the clothes to the family in a sealed bag.

2. There was a severe motor vehicle accident, and the trauma team is currently treating the driver of one car and the passenger of the car that the driver hit. While assessing the driver, the driver begins to display belligerent behavior and the nurse notes a strong smell of alcohol on their breath. Which of the following actions is the proper way of addressing these findings?

   A. The nurse gets an order for a toxicology screen on the patient and collects the sample.
   B. The nurse documents the patient's behavior as "agitated" and notes the "smell of alcohol on their breath."
   C. The nurse personally does not feel any sympathy for the patient because this is a clear drinking-and-driving situation, so the nurse tells the patient, "Next time, call a cab."
   D. The nurse reorients the patient to the surroundings and treatment modalities and then tells them that they will provide them with information on an Alcoholics Anonymous program.

3. A patient is brought into the ED following an altercation in a bar. The patient was attacked by several people in the parking lot and the police have not been able to locate them. Which of the following is the most accurate statement regarding the emergency care of this patient?

   A. Emergency medical care should not be delayed to collect forensic data.
   B. Evidence must be collected as soon as the patient is in the ED.
   C. The patient's clothes are too soiled to be useful as forensic data.
   D. The police need to be present during resuscitation to ensure the data is secured.

4. Following a trauma, where would the forensic data/evidence collection occur?

   A. ED only
   B. Prehospital during transport
   C. ED, operating room, and ICU
   D. Only after the patient is stabilized and in intensive care

(*See answers next page.*)

1. C) Prepare the family for how the patient looks and allow the family into the room.

Preparing the family beforehand minimizes the shock of the situation and also prepares them to make the decision whether to actually see the patient or not at that time. The nurse should make the patient and the room as presentable as possible without tampering with possible evidence. The nurse should not wash the body or remove any invasive lines because they could contain forensic evidence. Comforting the family is a therapeutic nursing process; the clothes should not be packaged and sent with the family but should be kept for evidence.

2. A) The nurse gets an order for a toxicology screen on the patient and collects the sample.

The trauma nurse should get an order for a toxicology screen on the patient and collect the sample. The toxicology screen is an objective measure that would prove suspected assessment without passing judgment or inflicting incrimination. The behavior is documented correctly, but the nurse should not document alleged and subjective accusations such as *smell of alcohol on their breath*. Do not let personal judgment affect professionalism. Reorienting the patient, explaining treatment, and providing resources for a patient would be proper care. Making the assumption that the patient is an "alcoholic" is passing judgment and the ED is not the right time or place for making assumptions.

3. A) Emergency medical care should not be delayed to collect forensic data.

Emergency medical care should never be delayed to collect forensic data from a trauma patient. Patient care should come first. The goal is to collect evidence concurrent with the management of the patient. It does not necessarily need to be collected as soon as the patient arrives. Even if the clothing is soiled, it is still considered forensic evidence and should be packaged accordingly. The police do not need to remain in the resuscitation room in all cases.

4. C) ED, operating room, and ICU

The majority of forensic evidence collection typically occurs within the ED, but forensic evidence may continue to be found in the operating room and inpatient units as well. Data collection can occur concurrent with the care of the patient and does not have to occur only after stabilization and in the ICU.

5. A patient who has sustained a gunshot wound to the abdomen is brought in by emergency medical services (EMS). Which of the following is the best action by the trauma nurse?

   A. Do not damage the shirt when removing to prevent loss of forensic evidence.
   B. Cut around the bullet hole when cutting the patient's clothes off.
   C. Document the wound as being either an entrance or an exit wound.
   D. Circle the hole on the shirt with a marker.

(See answers next page.)

5. B) Cut around the bullet hole when cutting the patient's clothes off.
When removing the trauma victim's clothing, do not cut through the bullet holes or tears in the clothing. This preserves it for forensics. The shirt can be cut off but avoid cutting areas of potential evidence. Do not circle the hole or tear in the shirt because that may damage some of the residue, which may be forensic evidence. Do not document "entrance" or "exit" wounds.

End-of-Life Issues

19

Q What is it called when a person participates in making arrangements for end-of-life care?

A Advance planning

Advance planning refers to a person's preferences regarding care at the end of life. The healthcare clinician should follow this arrangement when the person is unable to make their own decisions or to communicate their wishes.

HINT

Living wills and advance directives are the legal documents of advance planning.

Q What is it called when you identify a person to make your healthcare decisions at a time when you are unable to make them yourself?

A Durable power of attorney for healthcare

Advance directives, determining a durable power of attorney for healthcare, and living wills are the patient's opportunity to inform healthcare clinicians of their preferences regarding critical illness and end of life. The Patient Self-Determination Act (PSDA) requires healthcare clinicians (primarily hospitals, nursing homes, and home health agencies) to give patients information about their rights to make advance directives under state law (Table 19.1).

Table 19.1 Advance directives

Durable power of attorney for healthcare	The person authorizes someone to make decisions on their behalf when incapacitated.
Living wills	Allows one to document their wishes concerning medical treatments at the end of life.

HINT

Living wills may include an individual's desire for analgesia, antibiotics, hydration, feeding, and the use of ventilators or cardiopulmonary resuscitation.

Q What is the best method for healthcare clinicians to use to share information with family members in an organized fashion?

A Family conferences

Family conferences allow for a scheduled time, away from the bedside, for healthcare clinicians to meet with the family. Family conferences are used to provide information about the patient, discuss the prognosis, and make joint decisions about treatments. Family members should be encouraged to be active participants in the family conference.

▶ HINT

Obtaining a consensus among healthcare clinicians is recommended before presenting treatment options and goals.

Q What is the frequent role of the nurse in the family conference and after family meetings with the physician?

A Translator of medical terminology

The nurse frequently assumes the role of the translator of medical jargon. Medical terminology is a language that is used by medical personnel. Physicians may be in a hurry when speaking with patients and family and are not always sensitive to the fact that the family may not understand the terminology. Explaining the information to the family in a different way can facilitate the communication.

▶ HINT

Nurses are advocates when taking on the role of communicator and medical translator.

Q What is the best practice for visitation of family with loved ones at the end of life?

A No restrictions

Family and patients need the time at the end of life to be together without restrictions. The ability to see, touch, and talk with the patient is reassuring to both the patient and the family members at the end of life. Not allowing the family to be there to say their goodbyes can complicate the grieving process.

▶ HINT

Patients do not usually want to experience the process of dying alone and benefit from the presence of others.

Q What does *DNR* stand for?

A Do not resuscitate

A DNR order can vary in its content, including requesting no resuscitative efforts to allowing limited efforts (medications or defibrillation only) if cardiac arrest occurs. A DNR does not mean "do not treat." The degree and amount of interventions initiated to "save" the patient should be determined separately from the decision to enact a DNR, which involves the decision of what to do if cardiac or respiratory arrest occurs.

▶ HINT

Another phrase being used to replace *DNR* is to *allow a natural death*.

Q When discussing withdrawal of specific life-supporting therapies, what is the assurance the family needs to have from the healthcare clinicians?

A Continued care

It is essential when working with patients and families that they understand withdrawal of specific life supports does not mean withdrawal of care. Palliative measures are to be performed while providing interventions with the goal of providing comfort and relief of pain during provided care.

▶ HINT

Patients and family should be treated with compassion and dignity during these times of decision.

Q After a decision is made to withhold or withdraw life-sustaining therapies, what type of care is provided for the patient?

A Comfort care

After the decision has been made to decrease the intensity of interventions, to withhold or withdraw life-sustaining therapies, and a DNR order is written, the focus shifts from saving the patient's life to providing comfort care to the patient. Comfort care may involve discontinuing any invasive diagnostic tests or therapeutic interventions, which do not contribute to comfort.

▶ HINT

Providing comfort care focuses heavily on relieving any pain or discomfort the patient may be experiencing with the use of analgesics, sedatives, and alternative methods (Box 19.1).

Box 19.1 Discomfort at the end of life

Discomfort
Pain
Breathing problems
Skin irritations
Digestive problems
Temperature sensitivities
Fatigue

Q What is the primary goal of hospice or palliative care?

A Relief of suffering

The primary goal of hospice and palliative care is to improve the quality of life for patients and family, through the relief of suffering during the end of life, and into the bereavement period for the family. Hospice care begins when decisions are made to move away from curative medical care to supportive care and a peaceful death, although palliative care can be initiated at the same time as curative interventions are being performed.

▶ HINT

Hospice is not the end of hope but a change in goals to maximize quality of life.

Q Honoring a patient's refusal of treatment uses which ethical principle?

A Autonomy

Autonomy is the patient's ability to make their own decisions regarding treatments and is legally and ethically acceptable.

HINT

In some situations, a patient may need to be evaluated to determine whether they are able to make their own decisions.

Q A patient at the end of life begins to make "gurgling" sounds or breathe noisily. What would be the best intervention to provide comfort to the patient at this time?

A Provide analgesia

When near death, patients frequently develop noisy breathing, and this is often called a *death rattle*. This gurgling sound or noisy breathing is a result of fluids collecting in the throat and by the throat muscles relaxing. Suctioning would cause discomfort and administering a diuretic is ineffective. Providing analgesia is the best intervention to provide comfort at the end of life.

HINT

Administration of oxygen does not necessarily improve dyspnea at end of life, may prolong life, and can actually increase discomfort.

Q A patient at the end of life expresses not wanting to eat. What would be the best response of the nurse?

A Do not force the patient to eat

Nausea, vomiting, constipation, and loss of appetite are common at the end of life. Encouraging eating by offering favorite foods in small amounts until the point at which the patient refuses to eat is acceptable. Do not force a person at end of life to eat. Going without food and/or water is generally not painful and losing one's appetite is a common and normal part of dying (Table 19.2).

Table 19.2 Interventions to provide comfort measures

Breathing issues	Raise the head of the bed. Use a vaporizer. Have a fan circulating air in the room.
Skin irritation	Gently apply alcohol-free lotion.
Face and mouth dryness	Apply lip balm. Apply a damp cloth over closed eyes. Offer ice chips if the person is conscious. Wipe the inside of the mouth with a damp cloth, cotton ball, or a specially treated swab.
Digestive problems	Limit intake. Provide anticholinergics. Provide antiemetics. Administer agents to decrease oral secretions.

(*continued*)

Table 19.2 Interventions to Provide Comfort Measures (*continued*)

Pain	Use the WHO ladder for pain management. Administer scheduled pain medications. Administer long-acting or slow-release opioids with short time to action for breakthrough pain.

WHO, World Health Organization.

HINT

Preparing the family for a patient's loss of appetite is important for acceptance.

Q If symptoms of pain and discomfort are intractable at the end of life and cannot be relieved despite appropriate interventions, what should be considered?

A Terminal sedation

Terminal sedation is used at the end of life when the patient is experiencing unbearable and unmanageable pain. The goal of end-of-life sedation is to obtund pain sufficient to relieve suffering, but not to hasten death.

HINT

Multidisciplinary care (palliative, psychosocial support, spiritual counseling) is to be tried first before terminal sedation.

Q What is the ethical principle that is commonly applied to the administration of opioids at the end of life even if the known risk of the opioids is respiratory depression?

A Principle of double effect

The principle of double effect distinguishes between consequences of intent and consequences that are unintended but foreseen. This principle is commonly applied to the administration of opioids at the end of life. The intent in administering opioids to a dying patient is to relieve pain and suffering, but opioids can depress breathing. The intent is pain management, but the unintended and foreseen effect is respiratory depression.

HINT

If the intent is for pain relief but respiratory depression occurs, this is both legally and ethically acceptable.

Q What is it called when a nurse knows the proper course of action to take, but family interpersonal constraints make it impossible to do so?

A Moral distress

Moral distress occurs when the nurse is unable to turn moral choices into moral actions, typically because of constraints from family or physicians. Nurses who identify that invasive procedures are only prolonging the inevitable may experience moral distress when the family continues to insist on all potential interventions.

▶ HINT

The American Association of Critical-Care Nurses (AACN) has developed the 4 As of moral distress: ask, affirm, assess, and act.

Q When a family states that they promise to be more attentive if their loved one survives this injury, what stage of grief are they experiencing?

A Bargaining

In the bargaining stage, the person is looking for ways to postpone the inevitable death. Most of the time, the bargaining of the family is for a change in a certain lifestyle that will prolong the life of a loved one (Box 19.2).

Box 19.2 Stages of grief

Denial
Anger
Bargaining
Depression
Acceptance

▶ HINT

The grief process is very individualized. Not all people go through all the stages of grief or within any particular order.

KNOWLEDGE CHECK: CHAPTER 19

1. An older adult patient is being treated after a motor vehicle/pedestrian trauma. The patient is lethargic, pale, and has a blood pressure of 90/62 mmHg. Intravenous fluids were initiated, and the physician was notified. The patient's daughter provides a do not resuscitate (DNR) form. The patient's hemoglobin comes back, and the result is 6.2 mg/dL. What does the nurse do next?

   A. The nurse understands that the patient has DNR status and provides comfort care only.

   B. The nurse notifies the physician of the critical lab result and obtains an order for two units of blood to be transfused.

   C. The nurse talks to the patient and tells the patient that they need a blood transfusion but that the nurse is not able to transfuse because of the DNR status.

   D. The nurse transfuses two units of packed red blood cells but tells the patient that they will not need any further procedures because of the DNR status.

2. Providing physical comfort measures to the patient at the end of life is an important part of palliative care. Which of the following would be the most appropriate intervention for the patient at the end of life?

   A. Provide supplemental oxygen.

   B. Place the patient in a lateral position.

   C. Apply lip balm to the lips when dry.

   D. Force the patient to eat to maintain strength.

3. A patient in the ICU is intubated and sedated. During the "sedation vacation," they remain unresponsive. The physician spoke to the family regarding the patient's poor prognosis. The spouse is clearly upset and states, "I wish I could talk to them just one more time, I need to tell them so many things." Which of the following responses would be the most appropriate in this situation?

   A. Encourage the spouse to talk to the patient even though the patient is unresponsive and sedated.

   B. The nurse encourages the spouse to talk to the patient, but informs the spouse that they most likely will not comprehend what is being said.

   C. "You are right, they won't be able to hear what you are saying. I'm terribly sorry for this poor prognosis."

   D. "It is highly unlikely that they can hear you. They don't even follow commands or react to pain when off sedation. There is no evidence to support that they will understand what you are saying to them, but you can try."

(*See answers next page.*)

1. B) The nurse notifies the physician of the critical lab result and obtains an order for two units of blood to be transfused.

A DNR order does not mean that healthcare clinicians do not treat the patient. Blood transfusions may stabilize the patient and provide relief from symptoms. The degree and the amount of interventions initiated to "save" the patient should be a separate decision from the DNR status. The DNR status tells healthcare clinicians what to do in case of cardiac or respiratory arrest. The nurse's next step is to discuss the treatment and obtain a blood transfusion consent form, but the first steps of notifying the physician and obtaining the order are initiated.

2. C) Apply lip balm to the lips when dry.

Dryness of the face and mouth can be a common discomfort near death and providing lip balm to the lips or wetting the mouth routinely with swabs may provide comfort. Providing supplemental oxygen may prolong life and make the patient more uncomfortable. Lateral positioning of the patient can decrease that "rattling" sound but will not reduce the fluids that are collecting in the back of the throat. When patients at end of life stop eating, it is recommended to not force the patient to eat.

3. A) Encourage the spouse to talk to the patient even though the patient is unresponsive and sedated.

Encourage the family to talk to the patient even though the patient is unresponsive and sedated. It is possible that even if a patient is unconscious, they may still be able to hear. It is also therapeutic for the spouse to talk to the patient so that a feeling of fulfilment can be achieved. Saying that "they won't be able to hear what you are saying" is incorrect and the nurse should always encourage communication even if the patient is unresponsive or sedated, it is never too late for the family to say how they feel. The last response is not a therapeutic response, there is no proven evidence that talking to the patient is unbeneficial.

4. Which of the following tests is required at the bedside to determine brain death before organ procurement can occur?

   A. Cerebral blood flow scan
   B. Meningeal testing
   C. Apnea test
   D. Babinski reflex

5. Which of the following should be corrected before brain death determination can occur?

   A. Metabolic alkalosis
   B. Tachycardia
   C. Hypothermia
   D. Apnea

(*See answers next page.*)

4. C) Apnea test

An apnea test is performed during brain death testing to determine the absence of the drive to breathe using a CO_2 challenge. A cerebral blood flow scan may be used in determining brain death but is not required and is not performed at the bedside. Meningeal testing is used if the patient is suspected of meningitis, not brain death. The Babinski reflex is not a component of brain death determination.

5. C) Hypothermia

Hypothermia mimics brain death and should be reversed before death is declared. Warming the patient externally and internally is recommended before brain death testing occurs. Metabolic acidosis is a greater concern than metabolic alkalosis in determining brain death. Apnea is actually a required criteria for brain death determination. Tachycardia is not tested for brain death determination.

Discharge Planning and Rehabilitation

20

DISCHARGE PLANNING

Q When does discharge planning begin in a trauma patient?

A On admission

Discharge planning begins on admission to the trauma center. Case management and social work can initially interview the patient or family regarding the home situation and potential care issues after discharge.

Q What is it called when a discharge occurs several days after the patient is determined to be ready for discharge?

A Delayed discharge

Delayed discharge is defined as patients who remain hospitalized beyond the time of being declared ready for discharge by the trauma team (Box 20.1).

Box 20.1 Causes of delayed discharge

- Delay in discharge paperwork
- Delayed consults by other specialties
- Delays in obtaining the discharge order
- Delays in arranging outpatient or home care
- Delayed pick up by families
- Uninsured patients

HINT

Discharge decisions should be a multidisciplinary process in which patient's appropriateness for discharge is determined.

Q What is a quality-of-care concern with delayed discharges?

A Infection

The longer the patient is hospitalized, the greater the risk of infection. These infections are hospital-acquired and are frequently related to invasive lines and catheters. Other quality-of-care concerns include development of pressure ulcers and increased risk of falls.

HINT

Delayed discharge and prolonged length of stay can also cause financial losses and use of resources.

Q What improves discharge and decreases length of stay?

A Multidisciplinary teamwork

Effective teamwork utilizing a multidisciplinary team can improve the discharge process. Coordinated care between healthcare clinicians includes rounding and reviewing the patient's ability for discharge daily. The team works together in both goal setting and treatment.

HINT

Multidisciplinary teams can include nursing, physicians, rehabilitation staff, respiratory therapy, social workers, and case managers.

Q What is a postdischarge intervention that can be used to decrease unplanned readmissions?

A Follow-up phone calls

Follow-up phone calls after discharge can be utilized to review the discharge instructions, ensure the patient has their medications and follow-up appointments, and answer any questions the patient or family may have regarding the care.

HINT

Preventing avoidable readmissions can improve quality of life in patients and families (Table 20.1).

Table 20.1 Transitions of care interventions

Predischarge	Postdischarge	Bridging Interventions
Patient education	Follow-up phone calls	Transition coaches
Discharge planning	Communication with ambulatory clinician	Patient-centered discharge instructions
Medication reconciliation	Home visits	Clinical continuity between inpatient and outpatient settings
Schedule follow-up appointments		

Q What is a complication that arises if a discharge occurs before the patient is medically ready for discharge?

A Unplanned readmission

A discharge that occurs before the patient is medically ready can result in an unplanned readmission. Discharging to an environment in which the level of care is not sufficient to meet the medical needs of the patient can also result in unplanned readmissions.

▶ HINT

Unplanned readmissions can poorly affect outcomes of the patient and increase financial losses of the trauma centers (Box 20.2).

Box 20.2 Factors that affect readmissions

Premature discharge
Inadequate support after discharge
Lack of follow up after discharge
Inaccurate medication reconciliation at discharge
Poor handoff during transitions of care
Complications (i.e., pressure ulcers, infections)
Discharged without prescriptions
Comorbidities
Leaving AMA

AMA, against medical advice.

Q What is the most common reason for delays in discharge to acute rehabilitation inpatient facilities?

A Lack of beds

Acute rehabilitation facilities may have limited bed availability, which can delay the discharge of trauma patients from the trauma center to an acute rehabilitation center. In addition, other delays include families making decisions on which facility to choose and transportation delays.

Q How does multidisciplinary rounding improve discharges and length of stay?

A Improved communication

Rounding with multidisciplinary team members allows for the review of the patient's status from the viewpoints of different healthcare clinicians. Performing these rounds together, in person, improves the communication and decision-making (Box 20.3).

Box 20.3 Methods to improve discharge times

Physicians write discharge orders during morning rounds
Residents write discharge orders early
Utilization of discharge nurses
Discharge lounges
Improved communication between trauma center and rehabilitation facility

▶ HINT

Rounding with the goal of coordinated discharge can improve the discharge time and appropriateness of discharge.

Q During discharge, the focus is on the patient's readiness for discharge. Who else should be assessed for readiness for discharge?

A The caretaker

The caretaker should be evaluated and assessed for their knowledge and ability to care for the patient after discharge. Providing the information and needed resources for the caregivers has been found to decrease the number of readmissions in 30 days.

▶ HINT

Availability and ability of the caregiver to provide appropriate level of care postdischarge plays into the location of the discharge.

Q After determining the patient is ready for discharge, what other step is required before discharge planning can be completed?

A Determination of location after discharge

Once the patient is determined to be ready for discharge, the most appropriate location for the discharge needs to be determined. This is based on the medical needs of the patient, need or ability to participate in rehabilitation, and caregiver's ability to provide the level of care (Box 20.4).

Box 20.4 Location of discharge involvement

Physician
Family members and patient
Case manager
Social worker
Physical therapist
Occupational therapist
Insurer

Q What is a major determinant used to decide on placement between an acute inpatient rehabilitation facility and skilled nursing facility (SNF)?

A The ability of the patient to participate in rehabilitation

There are multiple factors that are reviewed to determine placement of a trauma patient at discharge (Box 20.5). When a patient requires rehabilitation, the ability of the patient to be able to participate in the rehabilitation is a major factor used to determine whether the patient is a candidate for an acute rehabilitation facility versus SNF.

Box 20.5 Determinants of patient location after discharge

Cognitive status
Activity level
Functional status
Therapy tolerance and motivation
Comorbidities and medical stability
Mental and emotional states
Caregiver presence and capability
Availability of home-care services
Medical diagnosis
Finances and insurance

HINT

Acute inpatient rehabilitation requires the patient to have the ability to participate in active and intensive rehabilitation.

Q Which facility is more likely to accept patients with complex wounds or ventilator dependent?

A Long-term acute care (LTAC) facilities

LTAC facilities are able to manage patients who have complex wounds, ventilator dependence, and multiorgan involvement. They provide closer monitoring and ability to provide complex procedures and interventions.

HINT

Average length of stay in an LTAC is typically greater than 24 days (Table 20.2).

Table 20.2 Types of care facilities

Type of Facility	Patient Requirements
Inpatient acute rehabilitation	Patient must be able to participate in the multidisciplinary rehabilitation.
LTAC	Patient requires closer monitoring and greater skilled nursing care.
SNF	Patient must require rehabilitation but it is needed less frequently or requires less patient participation.
Extended care	Patient requires assistance with ADL.
Home-based services	Patient may have varying levels of need and support provided in-house.

ADL, activities of daily living; LTAC, long-term acute care; SNF, skilled nursing facility.

Q What is it called when the patient's medication is verified during transitions of care?

A Medication reconciliation

Performing an accurate medication reconciliation is important to prevent medication errors once the patient is discharged from the trauma center. The discharge medication list is reviewed with the patient and primary caregiver.

HINT

During medication reconciliation, the nurse has the opportunity to ensure the patient understands their medications.

Q What is a method used during patient education to ensure the patient or primary caregiver understands the instruction?

A Teach-back method

Teach back is a method used during patient education to ensure the patient understands the instructions. This technique has the nurse ask the patient to explain the recently taught concept in their own words.

HINT

Teach-back technique allows the nurse to correct any misunderstanding in real time.

REHABILITATION

Q When does acute rehabilitation begin following a major trauma?

A On admission

Rehabilitation should begin early in the acute care facility following a trauma. This should occur as soon as the trauma patient is stable enough to tolerate rehabilitation. Typically, acute care rehabilitation includes physical therapy (PT), occupational therapy (OT), and speech pathology therapy. Early mobility has been found to improve outcomes.

HINT

Even early range-of-motion (ROM) exercise is a form of PT in patients unable to participate in activity.

Q What is the ultimate goal for rehabilitation?

A Reintegration

Trauma rehabilitation extends beyond the care provided in the rehabilitation facility to reintegration of the patient to the home and community. The primary purpose of rehabilitation is to enable the patient to function at the highest possible level after their injury. Rehabilitation is often the longest and hardest part of the trauma journey.

HINT

Neuropsychological sequelae are a recognized component of recovery from a traumatic event.

Q What is a functional outcome tool that can be used in rehabilitation?

A Functional Independence Measure (FIM)

FIM can be used to evaluate a patient's functional ability. It is an 18-item ordinal tool designed to evaluate disability. Other tools include Glasgow Outcome Scale (GOS) and Barthel Index for activities of daily living (ADL). Functional assessment tools are used to determine the effectiveness of rehabilitation.

HINT

Goal of rehabilitation is to obtain and maintain optimal level of functioning.

Q Following a traumatic brain injury (TBI), rehabilitation may include physical rehabilitation. What is another focus of TBI patients in rehabilitation?

A Cognitive and behavioral modification

Following moderate to severe TBI, it is recommended that comprehensive rehabilitation services be provided to improve function and quality of life after injury. This comprehensive rehabilitation includes cognitive and behavioral modification in TBI patients (Box 20.6).

Box 20.6 Common problems addressed during inpatient rehabilitation

Memory
Language and speech
Judgment and problem-solving
Physical concerns
Impulsiveness
Mood changes
Sensory issues

HINT

TBI in older adult patients requires aggressive rehabilitation due to the vulnerability of this population.

Q What type of physician specializes in rehabilitation medicine?

A Physiatrist

A physiatrist's specialty is rehabilitation medicine. The physiatrist evaluates the patient in the inpatient rehabilitation center to determine needs tailored to the individual patient. This includes medications and therapies (Box 20.7).

Box 20.7 Members of a rehabilitation team

Rehabilitation nurse
Physiatrist or neurologist
Psychologist/neuropsychologist
Physical therapist
Occupational therapist
Speech–language pathologist
Recreation therapist
Social worker/case manager
Nutritionist/dietician
Primary caretaker
Prosthetist
Recreation therapist

Q Which of the rehabilitation therapists primarily works with the upper extremities to improve function and ability to perform ADL?

A Occupational therapist

The occupational therapist's focus in rehabilitation is the upper extremities and ability to perform ADL. PT focuses on the lower extremities and patient's gait and ambulation. Rehabilitation nurses manage all aspects of the patient's care and prevention of complications.

HINT

Balance and prevention of falls are also areas of focus for PT.

Q What is the intervention in which a device is used to assist the patient to complete a task?

A Use of assistive technology

Assistive technology refers to devices that are used to assist or to make a task easier or safer. These include mobility aids such as walkers, bathroom-assist devices such as raised toilets, and electronic and computerized devices such as voice-activated computers (Table 20.3). *Adaptive methods* refer to therapists changing the way a task is done to make it easier or safer.

Table 20.3 Assistive devices

Mobility devices	Canes Walkers Crutches Wheelchairs
Bathroom and self-care aids	Raised toilet seats Grab bars
Prosthetics	Prosthesis Orthoses (braces)
Environmental modifications	Ramps

HINT

Mobility devices that are not properly fitted or used correctly can increase falls and injuries.

Q The brain has the ability to "rewire" or grow new pathways in the recovery phase. What is this called?

A Neuroplasticity

Neuroplasticity is the ability of the brain to change and adjust following an injury. The brain has the ability to reorganize pathways and create new connections and pathways. This includes functional plasticity, which is the ability to adapt uninjured areas to pick up the function of the injured brain tissue, and structural plasticity, which is the ability of the brain to actually grow new connections and neurons.

HINT

Rehabilitation can focus on neuroplasticity to improve patient's functional outcomes.

Q What population is a higher risk for complications and poorer outcomes in rehabilitation?

A Geriatric

Geriatric patients haveincreased disability with similar injuries when compared to a younger population. Musculoskeletal injuries, in particular, affect mobility and ability of the patients to be able to live independently.

HINT

Geriatric patients have many comorbidities and greater risk for complications.

KNOWLEDGE CHECK: CHAPTER 20

1. What is a postdischarge intervention that can be used to decrease unplanned readmissions?

   A. Patient satisfaction survey for the patient to complete after discharge
   B. Follow-up phone call after discharge
   C. Neuropsychological evaluation after discharge
   D. Assistance with insurance after discharge

2. What is a major determinant used to decide on placement between an acute inpatient rehabilitation facility and skilled nursing facility (SNF)?

   A. Physician's order for placement
   B. Patient's choice between acute rehabilitation and SNF
   C. Ability of patient to participate in rehabilitation
   D. Ventilator-dependent patients would require SNF

3. Which of the following is most important in preventing a medication error following a transition of care?

   A. Nurse to review home medication list
   B. Physician to perform reconciliation of medication list
   C. Patients should continue on all their previous home meds
   D. The nurse should discharge patient on all current medications

4. Which of the rehabilitation therapists primarily works with the upper extremities to improve function and ability to perform activities of daily living (ADL)?

   A. Physical therapist
   B. Speech therapy
   C. Physiatrist
   D. Occupational therapist

5. When does rehabilitation start after a traumatic injury?

   A. During the acute in-house rehabilitation
   B. Immediately before discharge
   C. At the time of transfer to a progressive care unit
   D. At the time of admission to the hospital

(See answers next page.)

1. B) Follow-up phone call after discharge

Follow-up phone calls after discharge can be utilized to review the discharge instructions, ensure the patient has their medications and follow-up appointments, and answer any questions the patient or family may have regarding the care. This can help prevent unplanned readmissions. Patient satisfaction surveys can be used to improve process and future care of patients but does not prevent readmissions. Not all patients require neuropsychological evaluations. Assistance with insurance does not prevent readmissions.

2. C) Ability of patient to participate in rehabilitation

There are multiple factors that are reviewed to determine placement of a trauma patient at discharge. When a patient requires rehabilitation, the ability of the patient to be able to participate in the rehabilitation is a major factor used to determine whether the patient is a candidate for an acute rehabilitation facility versus an SNF. Physicians are involved with placing orders and patients have input but if the patient is evaluated and not determined to be able to participate in the rehabilitation process at the level required, the patient will not be accepted. Ventilated patients would be placed in a long-term acute care facility not an SNF.

3. B) Physician to perform reconciliation of medication list

Performing an accurate medication reconciliation is important to prevent medication errors once the patient is discharged from the trauma center. The discharge medication list is reviewed with the patient and primary caregiver. If nursing just reviews the medication list without action, this will not prevent medication errors. Certain medications the patient took before they came to the hospital may need to be discontinued or changed. Medications prescribed in the hospital may not need to be continued at home.

4. D) Occupational therapist

The occupational therapist's focus in rehabilitation is the upper extremities and ability to perform ADL. The physical therapistst focuses on the lower extremities and patient's gait and ambulation. Speech therapists work with the patient's swallow and speech. A physiatrist's specialty is in rehabilitation medicine. The physiatrist evaluates the patient in the inpatient rehabilitation center to determine needs tailored to the individual patient.

5. D) At the time of admission to the hospital

Rehabilitation begins at the time of admission with actions such as recognizing and treating complications. The longer the time between injury and rehabilitation, the less likely the patient will be able to rehabilitate fully. Rehabilitation interventions should be initiated in the ICU before transfer to the progressive care unit or discharge to an acute care in-house rehabilitation center.

PART VI

Professional Issues: Trauma Quality Management

Trauma Quality Management

21

Q What is a database of information regarding traumatically injured persons and hospitals receiving injured persons called?

A Trauma registry

A trauma registry is a database in which information regarding the person involved in a traumatic injury and hospitals that care for the trauma patient are collected; the data are used to evaluate and improve the quality of patient management. The trauma registry can also be used to improve trauma prevention, education, research, and outcomes.

HINT

When participating with a trauma registry, data are submitted regarding all admissions, readmissions, interfacility transfers, and deaths involving trauma.

Q What are programs in the hospital that monitor services and initiate measurable changes in care to improve outcomes?

A Quality improvement (QI) or performance improvement (PI) programs

QI programs monitor and detect problems, effectively initiate change in trauma care services, and offer sustainable means to implement improvement initiatives. QI or PI programs focus on creating systems to prevent errors from happening. There is less focus on blame and reactive stances (Table 21.1).

Table 21.1 Example of error types

Rule-based mistakes	Deviation from accepted guidelines or protocols
Knowledge-based mistakes	Errors made from lack of knowledge by the clinician, either from inexperience or a new situation
Errors of execution	Correct decision is made, but the actual execution is incorrect
Diagnostic errors	Incorrect identification of an injury so management is incorrect

HINT

PI shifts the focus more on human performance, whereas QI focuses on the interaction of the system and the human component.

Q When analyzing the trauma program, it is noted that there are delays in obtaining chest radiographs. The trauma coordinator reviewed the times at which x-rays were taken and compared them to the hospital's set goals. What is this is called?

A Gap analysis

Gap analysis is part of the assessment process; it is the comparison of the actual outcome to a predetermined or identified goal. Gap analysis is used to determine whether the care provided is what the institute wants to deliver (Box 21.1).

Box 21.1 Process of quality improvement or performance improvement

Consider desired outcomes or performance.

Identify gaps between desired and actual performance.

Identify root causes.

Select interventions to close the gap.

Measure changes in performance.

Q Who should be involved in QI for trauma patients?

A Members of multiple disciplines

Trauma care is multidisciplinary, extending across multiple departments and involving a wide range of hospital staff as well as various physical locations within the hospital. Everyone involved with the trauma patient may be a part of the QI or PI process. There should be a dedicated leader of the QI team who has the authority to recommend and make improvements.

HINT

Multiple disciplines are necessary for the achievement of optimal patient outcomes, and all should participate in QI.

Q What is essential for a PI to be successful?

A Action

Following analysis, a corrective strategy or action plan is essential to effectively change a suboptimal performance or process. Just analyzing a situation and discussing the issues will not make the change occur; only implementation of an action plan can change the situation.

HINT

Program improvement should be continuous. The trauma program should continually perform analyses and institute action plans to improve patient care (Table 21.2).

Table 21.2 Examples of action plans

Guidelines, pathways, and protocols	Development of new practices Implementation
Targeted education	In-service training Posters Seminars Rounds
Peer review	Morbidity and mortality conferences
Action targeted on specific clinicians	Further education Disciplinary action Restriction of privileges
Enhancement of resources	Additional personnel Communication Facility improvement

Q What does the phrase *closing the loop* mean in QI programs?

A Measuring corrective actions

The program should measure what is achieved by the corrective strategies to confirm that they have accomplished the intended effects. Confirmation of the impact of the action plan is the closure needed to ensure an improvement was made.

Documentation of the gap analysis, action plan, and loop closure is the final step in PI.

Q What is the name of the formal peer-review process for reviewing deaths and complications on a regular basis?

A Mortality and morbidity (M & M) conference

M & M conferences are held to review all trauma deaths and complications. This is a formal peer-review process that has been used as a foundation for medical quality-improvement programs. These conferences should be seen as not just a discussion of deaths and adverse events, but also as an opportunity to improve (Box 21.2).

Box 21.2 Examples of performance improvement

Morbidity and mortality conferences
Trauma PI committee
Preventable death panel review
Case review
Rounds

PI, performance improvement.

HINT

Deaths are typically determined to be either nonpreventable, potentially preventable, or preventable.

Q A trauma patient using a face mask for supplemental oxygen is brought into the ED with a Glasgow Coma Scale (GCS) score of 6. The patient continues to deteriorate and goes into respiratory arrest. The physician is unable to obtain an airway and the patient expires. How would this death be classified?

A Preventable

A standard of care is to obtain an airway on a patient with a significantly depressed level of consciousness. This patient was admitted with a GCS of 6. An airway was not obtained until after the respiratory arrest.

HINT

An example of a preventable death is one resulting from airway obstruction or isolated splenic injuries (Table 21.3).

Table 21.3 Definitions

Preventable death	Injuries considered survivable Typically involves obvious deviation from standards of care
Potentially preventable death	Injuries severe, but survivable Death could potentially have been prevented if certain steps had been taken Some deviations from standards of care
Nonpreventable death	Injuries not survivable, even with optimal management

HINT

Even if a death is considered nonpreventable, the process should still be reviewed for potential improvement.

Q What are preidentified variables that are routinely tracked to identify whether acceptable standards of care are being met?

A Audit filters

Audit filters can identify issues that may lead to adverse events, complications, and death. These frequently are used to identify "near misses" even if no complication occurred and the patient had a good outcome (Box 21.3).

Box 21.3 Key time variables in trauma

Estimated time of injury
Time until arrival at the scene by prehospital personnel
Time of arrival at the hospital
Time until transfusion
Time of general surgical evaluation
Time until disposition to operating room, ICU, or floor

HINT

The trauma QI committee should review cases found by the audit filters (Boxes 21.4 and 21.5).

Box 21.4 Examples of prehospital trauma audit filters

Field scene time more than 20 minutes
Missing EMS report or significant information
Appropriateness of triage and facility selection
Airway management

EMS, emergency medical services.

Box 21.5 Examples of ED trauma audit filters

Abdominal injury with hypotension without laparotomy within 1 hour of arrival
Subdural hematoma without a craniotomy within 4 hours of arrival
Open fracture without debridement within 8 hours of arrival
Absence of hourly vital sign checks or neurological assessment on multisystem trauma patients
GCS <12 without a head CT scan within 2 hours
Unplanned return to OR within 48 hours

GCS, Glasgow Coma Scale; OR, operating room.

Q What is an injury called that is caused by medical management rather than the underlying disease and that prolongs hospitalization, produces a disability at discharge, or both?

A Adverse event

The terms *complication* and *adverse event* are sometimes used interchangeably, but a complication can occur even without suboptimal care because of an underlying disease. An error or adverse event can be considered a failure to follow an acceptable standard of care. An error that does not result in a bad outcome is considered a "near miss." A sentinel event is a severe adverse event with bad outcomes that prompts an immediate review with an action plan. Complications should be tracked for rates that are considered higher than normal (Box 21.6).

Box 21.6 Potential complications to audit

CAUTI
CLABSI
Wound dehiscence
Aspiration pneumonia
Sepsis
Surgical site infections
Skin breakdown
Compartment syndrome

CAUTI, catheter-associated urinary tract infection; CLABSI, central-line associated bloodstream infection.

▶ HINT

An adverse event results in a complication, but not all complications result from an adverse event. Not all adverse events are sentinel events.

Q What is the investigation called when a sentinel event occurs?

A Root cause analysis (RCA)

When a particularly bad outcome occurs with an adverse event, a separate QI process called an *RCA* must occur. An RCA is a process used to identify the etiology of an unanticipated outcome. The individuals involved in the RCA should come from multiple disciplines. RCA is a one-time investigation into a particular event.

▶ HINT

An RCA is not an ongoing collection and analysis, but rather a one-time event in which a particular case is investigated.

KNOWLEDGE CHECK: CHAPTER 21

1. Which of the following is the emphasis of quality management in trauma?
   - **A.** Reviews only the mortality.
   - **B.** Involves multidisciplinary teams.
   - **C.** Focuses on individual errors.
   - **D.** Involves reviewing cases without any corrective action.

2. Which of the following is considered the most significant barrier to a quality-improvement program?
   - **A.** Identify the problem, but fail to correct it
   - **B.** Difficulty in determining preventable from nonpreventable deaths
   - **C.** Inability to identify the problem
   - **D.** Lack of adherence to protocols

3. Which of the following is the primary goal of morbidity and mortality conferences?
   - **A.** Determine whether the trauma surgeon is meeting acceptable statistics.
   - **B.** Identify opportunities for improvement.
   - **C.** Identify all the nonpreventable deaths.
   - **D.** Track sentinel events.

4. Which of the following is considered the step that is used to "close the loop" of a problem identified in the care of patients in the trauma facility?
   - **A.** Identify the problem.
   - **B.** Develop reasonable corrective action plans.
   - **C.** Implement the plans.
   - **D.** Evaluate whether the action had the intended consequences.

5. An identified variable that is routinely tracked to identify whether predetermined standards are being met is called:
   - **A.** Scorecards
   - **B.** Outcome scores
   - **C.** Audit filters
   - **D.** Closed loop

(*See answers next page.*)

1. B) Involves multidisciplinary teams.

Quality improvement is a method of evaluation and improving processes of patient care that emphasizes a multidisciplinary approach to problem-solving that focuses on the system. Improving quality of the system includes implementing corrective actions where and when needed. The goal of quality-improvement programs is to shift the focus away from individual errors to system-wide errors. Quality improvement does not focus only on mortality as do morbidity and mortality conferences.

2. A) Identify the problem, but fail to correct it

A common problem with the quality-improvement program in trauma centers is that problems may be identified but are not corrected. The lack of adherence to a developed protocol is considered a quality-improvement problem that should be addressed but is not as significant a barrier as inability to close the loop. Most of the time, the problem can be identified and a decision can be reached on preventable versus nonpreventable deaths.

3. B) Identify opportunities for improvement.

The primary goal of morbidity and mortality conferences is to identify opportunities for improvement in outcomes. The deaths are reviewed to determine preventable (not non-preventable) deaths and to identify the problems to be able make changes to improve outcomes. Quality improvement is not intended to identify personnel issues as much as to look at systemic problems. Sentinel events are tracked but are not the primary focus for morbidity and mortality conferences.

4. D) Evaluate whether the action had the intended consequences.

Quality improvement involves identifying problems, developing reasonable corrective action plans, following through on implementing these plans, and evaluating whether the corrective action has had its intended consequences, which is the "closing the loop" component of the quality-improvement plan. Just implementing an action does not necessarily mean the action had the intended outcomes.

5. C) Audit filters

Audit filters are identified variables that are routinely tracked to determine whether predetermined acceptable standards are being met. Adverse events or complications are examples of audit filters, which may be tracked in trauma systems. Audits should identify "near misses" in patient care that do not result in a poor outcome but might indicate a patient care process that can be improved.

Research

Q What type of research directly involves the use of human subjects to verify clinical effectiveness?

A Clinical research

Clinical research is an investigation of human subjects intended to determine clinical or pharmacological effects and outcomes of a product, drug, or clinical practice. Clinical research is used to increase knowledge and understanding of products, drugs, or processes in diagnosis, prognosis, treatment, and cure of disease processes. Patient-oriented research examines mechanisms of disease processes and the effects of drugs or therapies on disease processes.

HINT

All aspects of clinical research are important to patient outcomes.

Q Transferring of the laboratory research knowledge to the bedside or clinical research is called what?

A Translational research

Translational research is the transferring of knowledge across the research and practice continuum. Translational research involves two steps: One is research in laboratory or preclinical areas and two is the development of human trials. This is to improve the trajectory from preclinical to clinical practice.

HINT

Translational research also involves moving research studies toward best practice.

Q When developing a research question, the PICOT format is commonly used. What does the *P* in PICOT stand for?

A Population

The PICOT (population, intervention, comparison, outcome, time) format is a helpful approach used to develop a research question. *P* stands for population, which is the sample of subjects to be studied. One of the first steps in research is developing a research question. It should be clear, concise, and provide direction to the research project. PICOT will help with the development of a clear question (Table 22.1).

Table 22.1 PICOT

P = Population	Refers to the population to be studied.
I = Intervention	Refers to the treatment that will be provided to the subjects.
C = Comparison	Defines the reference group that will be compared to the study group (intervention group).
O = Outcome	Refers to measurements of outcomes that will be used in the study.
T = Time	Refers to the duration of data collection.

HINT

Populations can be "ideal" for best outcomes or more likely to encounter patients with comorbidities.

Q What is it called when scientific data from research is translated to patient care?

A Evidence-based medicine (EBM)

EBM is the integration of best research evidence with clinical expertise and patient values. EBM is the conscientious and judicious use of clinical research and current best practice to make decisions about care and assist patients to make well-informed decisions about their care. EBM is used to develop national guidelines and pathways. These guidelines are developed with different levels of recommendations based on the strength of the research findings.

HINT

The three components of EBM include integration of best research evidence, clinical expertise, and patient values.

Q What should be carried out early when developing a research question?

A Literature review

A review of existing studies should be carried out early in the research process to determine whether the question was already studied or the problem identified. When reviewing the research that pertains to a formulated question, determine whether the setting is similar, whether the research method selected is consistent with the stated research question, and whether it follows a logical order and steps are clearly defined.

HINT

If the study was a sample study, did the sample represent the group to be studied?

Q What type of research, qualitative versus quantitative, uses the cause or correlation between variables through testing of hypothesis?

A Quantitative

Quantitative research seeks to understand the causel or correlation between variables through testing of a hypothesis. Qualitative research seeks to understand situations within real-world context through use of interviews and observation (Tables 22.2, 22.3, and 22.4).

Table 22.2 Differences between qualitative and quantitative research

Qualitative	Quantitative
Experimental	Discovery
Random assignment	Exploration
Causal/correlational relationships	Understand phenomenon
Random sample	Purpose sample of group
Large study	Focus groups
Control groups	Typically small study
Clinical research	Interviews
Prospective or retrospective	Surveys
Inductive process	Field observation
Involves interactions between researcher and subject	Deductive process
	Numeric findings

Table 22.3 Quantitative methods

Descriptive research	Methodology that describes phenomena as they exist
Correlational research	Methodology in which variables are not manipulated
Quasi-experimental	Methodology that manipulates some independent variables but cannot assign subjects to experimental or control groups
Experimental research	Methodology that randomly assigns subjects to two groups and compares their outcomes

Table 22.4 Qualitative methods

Phenomenology	Methodology in which researcher carries out individual interviews, records them and then analyzes the data for congruent themes
Grounded theory	Methodology in which the researcher carries out individual interviews and draws conclusions from those interviews
Ethnographic studies	Methodology in which researcher observes the subjects to collect data and data analysis is related to observations of behavioral patterns

HINT

Examples of quantitative research includes descriptive research, correlational research, quasi-experimental research, or experimental research.

Q A study reviewed past medical charts to identify the most common presentation of the disease process. What is the type of research using this method of data collection?

A Retrospective

Retrospective studies look backward and review situations that have already occurred. This method typically uses chart reviews of large sample populations. Prospective studies look at subjects in real life and have more control over confounding factors. Prospective studies typically use control and experimental groups. Case-control studies are more often retrospective while cohort studies are more likely prospective studies (Table 22.5). Frequently used to identify risk factors and disease outcomes.

Table 22.5 Case control versus cohort studies

Case-Control Study	Cohort Study
Smaller numbers are required	Requires large numbers
Outcome measured before exposure	Outcome measured after exposure
Quicker results	Takes longer to complete
Prone to selection bias	Prone to attrition bias
	Expensive
	Longitudinal over time

▶ HINT

Biases are more common in retrospective than prospective studies.

Q When studying tools/instruments used in the medical field, both reliability and validity are used to determine effectiveness of the tool. What does reliability measure?

A Consistency

Reliability means there is a consistency in the results of the tool when used under the same conditions. Reliability may be tested using different times, different observers, and different sections of the test itself. Validity is the degree to which a method accurately measures what it intends to measure (Table 22.6).

Table 22.6 Validity testing

Construct validity	Method is consistent with current theories and knowledge.
Content validity	Method includes all aspects of what is being studied.
Criterion validity	Method is consistent with another tool that has been determined to be valid.

▶ HINT

Inter-rater reliability indicates the reliability of the tool when utilized by different observers.

Q Which of the following measures the probability of a positive test result when assessing accuracy of the test, sensitivity or specificity?

A Sensitivity

Sensitivity refers to the probability of a positive test, whereas *specificity* refers to the probability of a negative test. Sensitivity and specificity are used to describe the accuracy of a test that reports the presence or absence of a condition. If the goal of the test is to identify everyone who has a condition, the number of false negatives needs to be low. If the goal is to accurately identify people who do not have the condition, the number of false positives should be low, requiring high specificity.

HINT

False positives are the measurement of specificity and false negatives are the measurement of sensitivity.

Q What is the purpose of the Institutional Review Board (IRB) in research?

A Protect rights of subjects

The IRB functions to protect the rights and welfare of the participants in research studies.

Q When enrolling a subject into a research study, what is used to ensure the subject is aware of their rights?

A Informed consent

When enrolling someone as a participant in a study, informed consent must be obtained in advance. Informed consent obtained prior to a study allows the participant to make independent decisions about the risk and benefits of participation (Box 22.1).

Box 22.1 Components of informed consent

Statement study involves research.

Review risks/benefits.

Discuss alternative treatments.

Review confidentiality.

State one's rights as a research subject.

Affirm that participation is voluntary.

Outline early study termination.

Indicate costs associated with involvement.

KNOWLEDGE CHECK: CHAPTER 22

1. Which of the following statements best describes clinical research?
   - **A.** Investigation of human subjects intended to determine clinical or pharmacological outcomes
   - **B.** Transferring of knowledge across the research and practice continuum
   - **C.** Always involves use of investigational and control groups
   - **D.** Involves pharmacological study research but does not include product research

2. Which of the following are the two steps identified in translational research?
   - **A.** Obtain consent and educate patients.
   - **B.** Do research in lab and develop human trials.
   - **C.** Examine effects of medications and identify safe dosing.
   - **D.** Identify best practices and develop guidelines.

3. When developing a research question, PICOT format is commonly used. What does the *C* in *PICOT* stand for?
   - **A.** Communication
   - **B.** Collaboration
   - **C.** Comparison
   - **D.** Complications

4. The nurses working on their clinical ladder are developing a research project. They are trying to set up the criteria for the control group and interventional group. Using the PICOT format, which step are they working on?
   - **A.** P—Population
   - **B.** I—Intervention
   - **C.** C—Comparison
   - **D.** O—Outcome

5. Which of the following is used to develop national guidelines and pathways?
   - **A.** Transitional research
   - **B.** Qualitative research
   - **C.** Quantitative research
   - **D.** Evidence-based medicine (EBM)

(*See answers next page.*)

1. A) Investigation of human subjects intended to determine clinical or pharmacological outcomes

Clinical research is best described as an investigation of human subjects intended to determine clinical or pharmacological outcomes. Transferring knowledge across the research and practice continuum is translational research. Use of investigation and control groups is a part of clinical research. Clinical research can involve both pharmacological study research and product research.

2. B) Do research in lab and develop human trials.

Translational research transfers knowledge across the research and practice continuum. Translational research involves two steps: research in laboratory or preclinical areas and the development of human trials. The goal is to move the clinical trials toward best practice and guideline development, but that is not the two-step process of translational research. Obrtaining consent and patient education may occur in clinical trials but is not a part of the process for translational research. Medication safety and efficacy trials are defined as stage II and III clinical trials.

3. C) Comparison

PICOT format is a helpful approach to the development of a clear, research question. The *P* refers to the population to be studied. *I* stands for the intervention to be performed. The *C* refers to the comparison of the study group to the interventional group. The *O* refers to outcome and *T* referes to the time or duration of data collection.

4. C) Comparison

The *C* is the comparison of the study group to the interventional group. The nurses are at this step in the development of their PICOT questions. The *P* is the population to be studied. The *I* is the development of the intervention to be performed. The *O* is the outcome to be monitored. The *T* is the time or duration of data collection.

5. D) Evidence-based medicine (EBM)

EBM is the conscientious and judicious use of clinical research and current best practice to make decisions about care and assist patients in making well-informed decisions about their care. EBM is used to develop national guidelines and pathways. EBM may utilize both qualitative and quantitative research. Translational research involves the transfer of knowledge across the research and practice continuum.

Staff Safety and Critical Incident Stress Management

Q What is the key to preventing violence in a hospital setting?

A Recognizing the potential escalation of violence

The key to preventing violence in the hospital setting includes early recognition of potentially violent patients, family members, or situations. Other interventions that may reduce the risk of violence include controlling environmental factors that provoke violent behaviors; a show of force; and, in some situations, chemical or physical restraints.

HINT

Situations that may induce patient violence include stress of the unknown regarding a diagnosis or procedure (Box 23.1).

Box 23.1 Potential situations that trigger violence in the ED

Small space
Long waiting times
Limited visitation
Patients in pain
ED is accessible 24 hours a day
Continuation of trauma

Q What is the best physical position the nurse should take when confronting an angry person who may become violent?

A Do not face the person directly

When interacting with an angry person who is likely to escalate to violence, stand at a slight angle. Never stand directly facing the person and do not turn your back to the person. Stand close enough to have a conversation, but not too close so you remain out of reach.

HINT

This stance is less provocative and intimidating to the person and provides a narrower target, which reduces exposure.

Q What is the best response of the nurse when a family member begins to complain about the long wait for admission?

A Allow a degree of complaining

Sometimes complaining or venting is a way to express one's frustration and concerns. Allowing some degree of expression of emotion can diffuse the situation. Avoid arguing or defending the actions of the healthcare clinicians or yourself. Remain calm and maintain control of your emotions.

HINT

After a degree of patient venting, calmly and firmly set limitations.

Q What would be an appropriate response of an ED nurse if a patient in the ED suddenly pulls out a gun?

A Protect yourself

Apply the concepts of time, distance, and shielding. Avoid exposure to threat, put distance between yourself and the threat, and put protective barriers or equipment between yourself and the threat.

HINT

In most situations, it is best not to fight back or attempt to remove the patient's weapon.

Q What is the risk to ED personnel when caring for patients exposed to chemical or biological agents?

A Secondary contamination

Secondary contamination of healthcare clinicians can occur with improper or incomplete decontamination of exposed patients, exposure to a toxic substance carried on the patient's clothing or hair, and risk of exposure to the exhalaled fumes of chemical toxins in closed spaces. Ensure appropriate procedures are being followed during decontamination to limit exposure to healthcare clinicians.

HINT

Healthcare clinicians can become contaminated themselves as well as becoming spreaders of disease.

Q What is the best way for healthcare clinicians to protect themselves from exposure to chemical or biological agents during the decontamination process?

A Wear appropriate personal protective equipment (PPE)

PPE should be specific to the potential exposure, and appropriate gowning and use of these PPE devices can lower the risk of exposure. Staff training for disasters should include correct donning and removal of PPE following exposure.

HINT

Different biologics and chemicals may require different PPE. If the substance is unknown, the staff should wear the maximal protective devices until the substance is determined (Box 23.2).

Box 23.2 Personal protective equipment for unknown substances

Powered air-purifying respirator
Chemical-resistant protective garment
Head covering
Double-layered protective gloves
Chemical-resistant protective boots

Q Who has the priority for prophylactic antibiotics or chemical antidotes during mass exposures or contaminations?

A First responders and healthcare clinicians

First responders and healthcare clinicians place themselves at high risk when responding to or treating patients who have been exposed to infectious disease, chemicals, or biological warfare. Healthcare clinicians should be trained to protect themselves from exposure and should be the highest priority for receiving prophylactic antibiotics or chemical antidotes, if available.

HINT

Safety for self should always be the highest priority for healthcare clinicians.

Q What is a physical or psychological event or threat to the well-being and safety of an individual called?

A Critical incident

A critical incident can be any event (e.g., shooting, death, natural disaster) that causes a distressing or emotional response to a physical or psychological event. This response can cause the person to be unable to function during or after the event. It overwhelms their usual coping mechanism. The critical incident can cause a profound change in the person's psychological functioning.

HINT

Those affected may include any emergency or public safety personnel (responders) involved in the traumatic event.

Q When a person experiences a significant traumatic event or disaster, what is the most common initial reaction?

A Shock

Shock and denial are the two most common initial reactions when someone experiences a significant traumatic event or disaster. This shock phase can last days to weeks and is characterized by confusion; disorganization; and an inability to perform simple, daily tasks. Denial takes the form of the person refusing to believe the event is happening or has happened.

HINT

Trained medical responders may not experience the shock phase.

Q Following the initial phase of shock, what is a common emotional response a person may feel?

A Anger

The phase following the initial shock is commonly called the *impact phase.* It involves strong emotions such as anger, anxiety, crying, and outrage. The experience of helplessness and depression can follow the shock phase.

HINT

Self-doubt and self-blame can contribute to some of the strong emotions experienced following a traumatic event.

Q Does everyone move through each stage of loss to the recovery phase following a critical event?

A No

Without proper counseling and being able to work through the traumatic event, people may get stuck in the impact stage. They commonly cycle from depression to anger. These people experience high levels of tension and stress.

HINT

Posttraumatic stress disorder (PTSD) and drug or alcohol addictions are a complication that can occur without proper recovery and rehabilitation.

Q What is the purpose of critical incident stress management (CISM)?

A To lower the impact of trauma on the involved person

CISM should be initiated in any situation that could potentially create distress for those involved in the event. The purpose is to mitigate the impact of the trauma. It involves participation in a structured group that uses storytelling combined with sharing practical information to normalize the group's reaction (Box 23.3).

Box 23.3 Goals of critical incident stress management

Mitigation of the impact of the traumatic event
Facilitation of the normal recovery process
Restoration of adaptive functions in psychologically healthy people
Identification of group members who may benefit from additional support

▶ HINT

Counselors professionally trained in CISM should lead the interventions.

Q What is the recommended immediate intervention following a critical or traumatic event called?

A Defusing

Defusing occurs immediately after the event and is a formal three-step process. This is typically the first intervention that occurs immediately after the event and provides one-to-one support. So soon after a traumatic event, many people are not ready for debriefing. Defusing can be run by anyone experienced in counseling or support groups. Another name for this intervention is *immediate small-group support (ISGS)*.

▶ HINT

If defusing cannot occur within 12 hours, then the intervention of debriefing should be used.

Q What is the supportive intervention technique that is a formal process initiated after the critical incident?

A Debriefing

Critical incident stress debriefing (CISD) is a formal eight-step process that is recommended within days to 2 weeks after a critical event. This method becomes less effective the longer it occurs after the event. This intervention is intended for a small group of people who have encountered the same powerful traumatic event. It involves a supportive, crisis-focused discussion of the critical event.

▶ HINT

CISD is not a substitute for psychotherapy for people in need of follow-up counseling and is not a stand-alone intervention.

Q When should a CISD occur?

A When a group shows signs of distress

Typically, CISD is used when the personnel from a particular homogenous group are demonstrating signs of distress caused by strong emotional reactions to the event. It aims at restoring group cohesion and performance.

▶ HINT

The distress may impair the ability of the personnel to function.

Q What is the primary factor that makes up the group involved in the debriefing?

A Homogeneity

The group should be small enough for participation in discussions and should be homogenous. Group members should have about the same level of exposure to the event. An example is ED personnel who witnessed a hostage situation in the ED (Box 23.4). Even though other nurses in another area may have experienced fear and psychological trauma, it was at a different level than those in the ED.

Box 23.4 Common situations requiring debriefing

Death in the line of duty
Emergency worker or peer suicide
Tragic deaths of children
Disasters (natural and man-made)
Bombings
Terrorist attacks
Shootings
Pandemics

HINT

There may be several groups participating in the debriefing following a critical incident. These group members are paired according to their role and level of involvement (Box 23.5).

Box 23.5 Group requirements

Group contains a homogenous mixture of members.
Involvement in the event is complete.
Members have the same level of exposure to the event.
All members are psychologically ready.
Members are not overly fatigued or distraught.

Q Is a debriefing designed to involve the cognitive or the affective response of the group members?

A Both

The process of debriefing is designed to take a person from the cognitive aspect to the affective aspect and then back to the cognitive. The participants are encouraged to participate in the group, but participation is voluntary.

HINT

Emotional content can occur anywhere within the process.

Q During a CISD, following the introduction, what is the first phase of the debriefing?

A Facts phase

The group members are asked to talk very briefly about what happened in the critical event. All are given the opportunity to speak if they wish. This format is used to get the members talking. It is easier to talk about the actual traumatic event than to discuss with others the impact the event had on one's own life.

HINT

The facts phase is the beginning, but it is not the real focus; it should remain very short.

Q Which phase is the transition from the cognitive to the affective aspect?

A Thoughts phase

When the group members are asked about their thoughts of the critical event, this moves the participants from the fact phase, or cognitive domain, into the beginning of the affective domain. The facilitator starts by inquiring about their thoughts, as these are easier to deal with than the deeper pain they may be experiencing.

HINT

The question asked around the room is: "What was your first thought when you began thinking?"

Q Which phase is considered to be the most crucial phase in the CISD intervention?

A Reaction phase

The reaction phase is the most crucial phase because it focuses on the impact of the event on the group members. This change of focus may become difficult for the group members. Different emotions may be exhibited, including anger, sadness, fear, or confusion. Members are allowed to talk about the impact until the group no longer brings up new issues or concerns.

HINT

The question at this phase is: "What is the very worst thing about this event for you personally?"

Q What phase begins to move the group back to the cognitive domain?

A Symptoms phase

The symptoms phase begins to delve into what symptoms or changes the members have been experiencing since the traumatic event. This opens the way for the leaders to begin to teach.

HINT

The question asked at this phase is: "What behavioral, cognitive, or emotional symptoms have you been experiencing since the event?"

Q Following a mass shooting, the ED nurse tells you they have been experiencing excessive fatigue and an inability to sleep. What could these symptoms represent?

A Distress from the critical incident

Critical incidents produce common symptoms in people involved in a traumatic event (Box 23.6). Symptoms of distress are also commonly experienced by first responders and healthcare professionals involved in the traumatic event.

Box 23.6 Symptoms of critical incidents

Restlessness
Irritability
Excessive fatigue
Sleep disturbances
Anxiety
Startle reactions
Depression
Moodiness
Muscle tremors
Difficulty concentrating
Nightmares
Vomiting
Diarrhea
Suspicion

HINT

Healthcare clinicians have been found to be at risk of developing PTSD.

Q What phase of CISD allows the group members to begin to realize that their symptoms are normal for the situation they have experienced?

A Teaching phase

The teaching phase is used to provide explanations for why the members are experiencing certain symptoms or aftereffects from the traumatic event. It is also a phase used to introduce stress management and interventions that may be used to allow the person to cope with their emotions. The final phases include summarizing the discussions and some social interaction to assist in anchoring the group members together (Box 23.7).

Box 23.7 Phases of critical incident stress debriefing

Introduction
Facts
Thoughts
Reactions
Symptoms
Teaching
Reentry
Follow-up

▶ HINT

Specific topics that may be pertinent to the members of the group may also be discussed at this time. If members were involved in a plane crash, for example, future travel may be discussed.

Q What is the primary rule when people are sharing their thoughts or feelings about the critical event?

A Do not criticize others

The sharing of thoughts and feelings about the critical event or disaster should always remain positive and supportive. No one should criticize someone else during this sharing process; group members should use active listening. Everyone's feelings should be shared and accepted. Everyone should also know that what is said is absolutely confidential.

▶ HINT

Everyone in the group needs to feel they can contribute to the group discussion and be accepted.

Q How does CISM assist with the prevention of PTSD?

A It allows a person to work through the crisis

Not all people who have been through a major trauma develop PTSD. It has been shown that when a person is able to work through the crisis surrounding the event, the incidence of PTSD is significantly lower.

KNOWLEDGE CHECK: CHAPTER 23

1. When the trauma nurse meets the family of a patient for the first time, the nurse introduces the healthcare team and each individual member. The nurse also describes what the patient looks like and the current situation in a calm manner, allowing the family to process the information and encouraging them to express their feelings, ask questions, and visit the patient. This nurse is best exemplifying which of the following?

   A. Therapeutic communication
   B. Crisis intervention strategies
   C. Stress intervention strategies
   D. Concepts of psychosocial needs

2. Crisis intervention is frequently part of nursing care for the trauma patient. Denial is an important part of the grieving process. The nurse should handle denial by:

   A. Redirecting to the truth
   B. Confronting the feeling of denial
   C. Allowing denial and avoiding being honest with the patient
   D. Using reflection to face thoughts of denial

3. Which of the following is the best definition of workplace violence?

   A. Physical abuse that does not include verbal abuse
   B. An act of physical violence only
   C. An act of aggression directed toward persons at work or on duty
   D. An act of theft only

4. When a trauma patient is brought into the ED in police custody, which of the following is the best nursing action when caring for the patient?

   A. The patient can be allowed to go to the restroom alone as long as a healthcare worker remains outside the restroom.
   B. For safety purposes, do not allow the patient to be handcuffed or restrained in any manner.
   C. Ask the police officers to leave the room during assessment for the patient's privacy.
   D. Do not allow the patient to distract the nurse during assessment or while performing interventions.

5. Which of the following is the best management of workplace violence?

   A. Crisis management classes for healthcare clinicians
   B. Prevention of workplace violence
   C. Performing deescalating techniques when violence occurs
   D. Providing force to restrain the violent patient

(See answers next page.)

1. B) Crisis intervention strategies
The nurse is exemplifying crisis intervention strategies for the family of the trauma patient. Therapeutic communication is part of crisis intervention, but the whole picture involves more than communication; it also incorporates facilitation of care. A crisis is a sudden, unexpected threat to life, whereas stress is the actual arousal of the body in response to a situation; therefore, the strategies are geared differently. Stress interventions are not harmonious with crisis interventions. The nurse is incorporating concepts of psychosocial needs by informing the family, but compassion and maintenance of hope develop with the rapport and delivery of care.

2. D) Using reflection to face thoughts of denial
Reflective verbalized content can confront the patient's thought process in a nonthreatening way. The nurse should allow the defense of denial, which may be needed at that time. The nurse should not confront the patient and should always be honest.

3. C) An act of aggression directed toward persons at work or on duty
Workplace violence is an act of aggression directed toward persons at work or on duty and ranges from offensive language to homicide. Violence reported by hospitals includes assault and battery, hostage situations, homicide, kidnapping, armed robbery, theft, vandalism, and bomb threats. Violence can range from verbal abuse all the way to homicide.

4. D) Do not allow the patient to distract the nurse during assessment or while performing interventions.
The trauma nurse should use extreme caution when working with a patient in police custody. To avoid personal injury, the trauma nurse should not let the person in custody distract or manipulate them during the course of an assessment or treatment. Allow police officers to remain in the room during assessment and treatment when patients are in custody to maintain the safety of healthcare clinicians. The trauma nurse should never leave a patient in custody unattended, even with bathroom privileges.

5. B) Prevention of workplace violence
Prevention of violence is the best management. The training of hospital employees needs to include how to recognize potential violence, defuse the violence, and deal with the aftermath of the violence. Deescalating techniques are recommended but are used more to prevent violence than when it actually occurs. When working with an aggressive patient, use the least amount of physical force necessary, remain focused and centered, and attempt to redirect the patient's behavior. Crisis management is taught, but the best way to manage violence is to prevent it.

Disaster Management

24

Q What is a low-probability but high-impact event that causes a large number of people to become ill or injured?

A Disaster

Disasters are low-probability events, but if they do occur, they can have a high impact on the hospital and the community. These events cause a significant, short-term increase in demand for emergency services.

HINT

During the time of a disaster, hospitals frequently have to initiate a plan to free up resources and physical space.

Q Disasters can be grouped into two main categories: natural and man-made. How would a major train crash be classified?

A Man-made

Man-made disasters include transportation incidents, terrorist bombings, and biological or chemical attacks (Box 24.1). Natural disasters include weather-related events (hurricanes, tornados, and earthquakes) and disease outbreaks (Box 24.2).

Box 24.1 Examples of man-made disasters

Terrorism
Riots
Strikes
Bombs
Hostage situations
Transportation incidents
Structural collapses
Explosions
Fires
Chemical (toxic wastes)
Biological (sanitation)

Box 24.2 Examples of natural disasters

Hurricanes
Tornados
Earthquakes
Landslides
Tsunamis
Blizzards
Dust storms
Floods
Volcanic eruptions
Communicable disease epidemics

HINT

Chemical emergencies can be unintentional, such as a spill, or intentional, as in a terrorist attack (Box 24.3).

Box 24.3 Categories of terrorist threats

Chemical
Biological
Radiological
Nuclear
Explosive

Q What do hospitals need to have in place if they receive warning of an impending disaster?

A An evacuation plan

All hospitals need to develop an evacuation plan, and staff need to be aware of the plan and prepared through in-service training. If there is a warning of an impending disaster (e.g., hurricane) and the patients would be safer in a different facility, then evacuation needs to occur in an orderly and timely fashion.

HINT

If the hospital is able to evacuate the majority of its patients, then fewer patients are in harm's way and fewer casualties will occur.

Q What is a step in preventing a disaster in your hospital?

A Recognize the hazard

Disasters can happen at any time, and awareness of surroundings and people can assist with identifying potential hazards such as unusual behavior, unexplained liquids or smells, and suspicious packages. Know to whom to report this suspicious activity or behavior within your facility.

HINT

An example of an unusual behavior that should be flagged as suspicious and reported is a visitor found in a restricted area that is well marked.

Q What is the first step in disaster management when preparing for a disaster?

A Mitigation

In preparing for disasters, the hospitals, counties, and regions perform a hazards vulnerability analysis. This step involves determining the hazards for which a hospital is at risk so that actions can be taken ahead of time to minimize the risks. This is performed annually. Hospitals need to focus their preparation on the most likely or potentially serious hazard. It is not recommended that a plan be developed for every potential disaster.

HINT

When performing a hazards vulnerability analysis, hospitals need to review both natural disasters (such as hurricanes) and man-made disasters (such as a plane crash).

Q What stage of disaster management is the hospital performing when in the process of stockpiling enough antibiotics for 5 days?

A Preparation

Preparation is the stage during which the hospital takes steps to prepare for the disaster (Box 24.4). These steps may include stockpiling certain medications for a defined number of days. This is done in response to the potential lack of access to critical medications during a disaster. Another example is developing mutual-aid agreements and contracts with other healthcare facilities to take patients during the time of a disaster.

Box 24.4 Common insufficiencies found in disasters

Available beds
Ventilators
Isolation rooms
Medications
Staff

HINT

The development of a disaster plan and the education of staff are part of the preparation for disaster management.

HINT

Some staff may have a difficult time getting to the hospital because of the actual disaster.

Q What does the National Incidence Management System (NIMS) establish in the hospitals?

A The Incident Command System (ICS)

The NIMS outlines the ICS, which defines the organizational structure for response. The ICS contains five functional areas: command, operations, planning, finance or administration, and logistics.

HINT

The hospital ICS may be used in any unusual situation and is not reserved for a disaster only.

Q If a disaster is called and a nurse of the hospital involved is off duty, what is the best action of the nurse?

A Do nothing until called

When a critical incidence command is set up for a hospital emergency or disaster, if more staff are required to handle the disaster, the staff will be notified by a prearranged communication system. It is recommended that off-duty staff wait for the call and not call in or just show up at the hospital.

HINT

Some staff may be needed during the incident and immediately following the incident. Call sheets should be developed and maintained before any unseen disaster.

Q The command center structure in the hospital includes a person with the title "public information officer." What role does this person have during a disaster?

A Works with the media

The command infrastructure needs to have a process in place for, or a person who is in charge of, patient care, media, safety, logistics of critical supplies, and staff or family support. These roles and processes should be well defined before the incident.

HINT

Only the designated public information officer should be talking with the media during a critical incident or a disaster.

Q During a disaster, what is important to maintain with the community?

A Communication

Hospitals may need to work closely with the police and fire departments, power companies, utility companies, and water department during the disaster. Communication and alternative communication routes should be established during preparation to prevent a loss in obtaining or providing critical information regarding the disaster. Phone lines and cellular towers may be out, causing a loss of phone communication during an emergency. The alternative may be using walkie talkies or radios (Box 24.5).

Box 24.5 Issues that occur with poor communication

Patients transported to inappropriate facilities
Hospital becoming overwhelmed with too many patients
Lack of sufficient alert before patients arrive
Inappropriate allocation of resources in the community

▶ HINT

Healthcare clinicians working in the hospital during the disaster require real-time and up-to-date information about what is happening.

Q During the disaster, a triage unit is set up in front of the hospital. If a patient is considered likely to be salvageable but requires immediate intervention, what color would be assigned to the patient?

A Red

During triage of patients in mass casualty events, colors are placed on each victim depending on the patient's level of acuity. Red is used for patient injuries that are considered to be life-threatening but salvageable. These patients require immediate intervention for survival and are the priority during mass casualty events (Box 24.6).

Box 24.6 Disaster triage

Black: Deceased or likely to die from injuries despite treatment
Red: Likely salvageable with immediate intervention
Yellow: Requires medical care, but unlikely to die without immediate interventions
Green: Walking wounded, but likely to survive even if medical treatment is not provided

▶ HINT

Most victims end up in the nearest hospital whether the hospital has the appropriate capabilities or not. Do not assume the patient was appropriately triaged in the field or properly decontaminated.

Q What is the most common route of arrival to hospitals following a mass casualty event?

A Private transportation

The most common route for patients to arrive at the ED following a disaster or mass casualty event is by private transportation. Mass casualty victims arrive by private car, taxis, buses, and police vehicles. If able, victims may walk to the nearest ED. These are called the *walking wounded*.

▶ HINT

The most seriously injured patients often arrive in the ED first, followed by the walking wounded.

Q When a hospital has reached the maximum number of patients, exceeding the hospital's medical infrastructure, what is this called?

A Surge capacity

Surge capacity refers to the ability to manage increased patient care volume that otherwise would severely challenge or exceed the existing medical infrastructure. Surge capacity may involve physical space, medical personnel, necessary equipment, or medications and supplies. *Surge capability* is the ability to manage patients requiring unusual or very specialized medical evaluation and intervention, often for uncommon medical conditions.

HINT

A large number of people may present to the ED at the same time following a mass casualty event, causing an initial surge to maximize capacity to handle the wounded.

Q After the disaster, the recovery stage occurs. What is a primary action required during this phase?

A Evaluation

During the recovery stage after a disaster, the primary action is to evaluate the status of the hospital and the community and to determine what needs to be done now to restore them to their previous status. Interventions include restoring the physical building if damaged during the disaster, replenishing stocks of supplies and medications, assessing bed status, and disposing of garbage and other waste.

HINT

Recovery is basically restoring the institution back to its previous status.

Q What is considered a standard of care that must be maintained even in circumstances of disaster and mass casualties?

A Maintaining airway and breathing

During the periods of uncontrolled, increased volumes of patients that can occur during a disaster or a mass casualty event, certain standards of care may be abandoned, but a few are critical standards that should be present always. These include maintaining airway, breathing, and circulation (ABCs), maximizing patient and staff safety, and maintaining or establishing infection-control measures. Elective procedures, routine care, and complete documentation may not always be upheld when responding to a disaster or mass casualty event.

HINT

In an emergency, the goal is to save lives. This works on the principle of the greatest good for the greatest number. This is called *sufficiency-of-care mode*.

Q What is the mechanism that may be used in a disaster to allow healthcare students or healthcare volunteers to work under guidance in the hospital?

A Emergency response competencies

These are competencies that can be used during a disaster to credential a person to be able to work under guidance during a disaster when more staff is needed to care for the increased volumes of patients. Emergency medical services (EMS) are another good source of nurse and physician extenders. The National Disaster Medical System has teams of volunteers from around the country. Volunteers should not be self-assigned or self-directed but should be working under direct guidance of employed healthcare clinicians.

HINT

Delegation of some care may be given to technicians or support staff or involve family of the patients during these times of crisis.

Q What is a primary method used in an emergency situation to free up beds for victims from the mass casualty?

A Discharge noncritical patients

Victims of the emergency situation or disaster may be at a higher level of acuity than current patients. Depending on the number of victims and resources, hospitals typically expand beyond capacity and require more beds to care for the victims. Discharging patients who are noncritical is an important step in increasing the hospital's capacity to care for the influx of patients.

HINT

Other options include cancelling elective surgeries, transferring patients to other hospitals that are not a part of the emergency, and using extra space to place more beds.

Q What does The Joint Commission require hospitals to perform regarding disaster management?

A Disaster drills

The Joint Commission requires hospitals to have an emergency management plan and to test the plan with practice drills. Disaster drills are needed to evaluate the plan and make appropriate changes, but they may not actually address the educational needs of the staff.

HINT

Education and competency of emergency nurses in a disaster is a recommendation for each hospital.

Q What do patients suspected of exposure to chemical or biological agents require before entry into the hospital's ED?

A Decontamination

Patients suspected of exposure to chemical or biological agents require decontamination before entry into the hospital. EMS may do field decontamination, but often some of the people exposed walk into the ED without field decontamination. If the patients are not decontaminated appropriately and enter the ED, it can be shut down for operation.

HINT

Hospitals must be prepared to lock down to prevent contaminated people from entering the ED before decontamination in extreme cases.

KNOWLEDGE CHECK: CHAPTER 24

1. A community-based disaster has just occurred. A tornado has caused mass destruction, resulting in 220 people being injured; 50 of these injuries are life-threatening, and 95 are casualties. This situation can be best described as:

   A. Multiple patient incident
   B. Multiple casualty incident
   C. Mass casualty incident
   D. Single hospital response team

2. Which of the following are categorized as the most toxic of all chemical agents, with a mechanism of action that inhibits acetylcholinesterase and that is spread through inhalation or contact?

   A. Nerve agents
   B. Vesicants
   C. Pulmonary agents
   D. Blood agents

3. A patient was exposed to tabun, a type of nerve agent, and is now experiencing rhinorrhea, salivation, and seizures. What is the appropriate antidote for this patient?

   A. Dimercaprol
   B. Sodium nitrate
   C. Atropine
   D. Nothing; there is no antidote

4. An ED has seen five patients in the past week with fevers higher than 101°F, productive cough with associated chest pain, and purulent sputum. These patients all had evidence of bronchopneumonia on chest x-rays. Because of this pattern, the physician follows up with the previously collected sputum samples and reviews the gram-negative rods results. Which of the following would best describe the concern of these presentations?

   A. They present symptom clusters.
   B. They are indicative of infectious agent involvement.
   C. These symptoms are indicative of the plague.
   D. They are symptoms of normal flu.

5. Which of the following provides hospitals with a chain of command, organizational charts, and checklists, and facilitates communication among other facilities in disaster situations?

   A. Hospital Emergency Incident Command System
   B. Emergency Medical Treatment and Labor Association
   C. Emergency Disaster Command Station
   D. Hospital Emergency Medical Disaster System

(See answers next page.)

1. B) Multiple casualty incident

This is considered a multiple casualty incident because there are greater than 10 but fewer than 100 casualties. A multiple patient incident is categorized as fewer than 10 casualties, and a mass casualty incident results in greater than 100 casualties and involves responses from multiple hospitals.

2. A) Nerve agents

Nerve agents are the most toxic of all chemical agents and affect the cardiovascular, respiratory, gastrointestinal, musculoskeletal, and central nervous systems, with inhibition of acetylcholinesterase as the main mechanism of action. Vesicants are also known as *blister agents* and are contracted by inhalation or topical exposure, damaging the cardiovascular and central nervous systems. Pulmonary agents are contracted by inhalation and primarily affect the respiratory system. Blood agents interfere with oxygenation and are inhaled or ingested.

3. C) Atropine

Atropine and 2-PAM Cl are the only antidotes for nerve agents such as tabun, sarin, or VX (venemous agent X). Dimercaprol is the antidote for lewisite, which is a type of vesicant. Hydroxocobalamin, amyl nitrate, sodium thiosulfate, and sodium nitrate are antidotes for blood agents such as cyanide. There are no antidotes for pulmonary agents. These patients should receive aggressive airway/breathing management.

4. A) They present symptom clusters.

Symptom clusters suggest that there could be a possibility of infectious agent exposure with mass exposure. Infectious agents can cause individual infections but not necessarily multiple injuries.

5. A) Hospital Emergency Incident Command System

This is the role of the Hospital Emergency Incident Command System (HEICS). The Emergency Medical Treatment and Labor Act (EMTALA) is a federal law that requires the stabilization and treatment of anyone who comes to an ED, regardless of insurance status or ability to pay. Emergency Disaster Command Station and Hospital Emergency Medical Disaster System are not actual terms in disaster management.

Trauma Team Well-Being and Team Dynamics

25

Q What is the purpose of the trauma team?

A Successful resuscitation

The trauma team is a group of medical staff with varying backgrounds and levels of expertise. The trauma team is greater than the sum of its parts. These healthcare clinicians collaborate to provide high-quality care. Trauma teams work under high stress with patients whose health concerns may be very complex. These teams are called to assemble suddenly at unpredictable times.

HINT

Teamwork and leadership are critical to a trauma team.

Q What must exist between the trauma team members to make an effective team?

A Trust and respect

Team members must have mutual respect and trust to function effectively as a team. Individual members must be knowledgeable, skillful, and competent in managing trauma resuscitations. The team members must have complementary skills.

Q What is key to each team member when performing coordinated care during a resuscitation?

A Understanding of their role

There are many key attributes the trauma team members require for more coordinated, successful resuscitation (Box 25.1), but the primary attribute is role delineation. Each member of the team should have a clear understanding of their role during the resuscitation. Training and practice sessions improve the dynamics of the team.

Box 25.1 Key attributes of trauma team members

- Clear understanding of roles
- Demonstration of trust and respect of other team members
- Flexibility
- Resilience
- Effective communication
- Accountability
- Commitment
- Competency

(continued)

Box 25.1 Key attributes of trauma team members (*continued*)

Consistency of performance
Striving for excellence
Interpersonal empathy
Adaptability
Flexibility to changing situations

HINT

Communication is another key attribute that helps to ensure clear and accurate information is exchanged regarding the patient to improve outcomes.

Q Which is more important in teamwork, the performance of the team or individual achievements?

A Team performance

The goal of the team is optimal team performance, not individual achievements. Team orientation is about the group performance as a whole, with less emphasis on individual achievement. This may be a barrier in some teams. due to the culture of rewarding individual performance.

HINT

The goal of the team is team performance, not individual achievements.

Q What is a common cause of fatal errors in trauma care?

A Miscommunication

Miscommunication among the trauma team members can lead to fatal errors. Communication is a skill that needs to be learned and practiced. It remains one of the most challenging aspects of working with trauma teams.

Q Which role on a trauma team is responsible for directing the other team members?

A Team leader

The team leader controls, manages, and directs the trauma resuscitation. The team leader should ensure that each team member is performing their assigned role effectively (Box 25.2). The team leader will assign tasks and roles to the other members of the team. When team leaders become more involved in performing procedures than in managing the resuscitation, the team becomes less effective. Team leaders must be willing to intercede when other team members are not performing up to acceptable standards.

Box 25.2 Examples of trauma team roles

Team leader
Airway specialist
Airway assistant
Physician assessment
Physician procedures
Trauma surgeon
Anesthesiologist
Circulating nurse
Monitoring nurse
Scribe
Radiographer technician
Respiratory therapist
Laboratory technicians
Pharmacists

HINT

Typically, the team leader is an ED or trauma physician with the highest level of trauma knowledge and skills.

Q Who is responsible for determining the definitive treatment plan of the trauma patient during resuscitation?

A Team leader

The team leader (Box 25.3) must rapidly assess the situation, listen to emergency medical services (EMS), evaluate the patient, and make decisions on required diagnostics and treatment. Once decisions are made, the leader needs to make sure the team is aware of the evolving situation and the required interventions.

Box 25.3 Trauma team leader's responsibilities

Is knowledgeable in trauma and resuscitation
Ensures effective communication
Knows the team's strengths and weaknesses
Fosters teamwork
Delegates tasks
Assists with strengthening team member's skills
Grooms others for leadership roles
Acknowledges team members when they are performing well
Holds team members accountable for their actions
Knows their own limitations

HINT

A key attribute for the team leader as well as for team members is the ability to anticipate or predict the trauma patient's course based on mechanism of injury.

Q When EMS arrives with the trauma patient, what is the most important task between the EMS crew and the trauma team?

A Handoff

The trauma team, especially the team leader, should listen to the EMS crew to receive information regarding mechanism of injury and prehospital assessment. Some of the information is obtained prior to patient arrival, which allows for preparation and briefing of the team members.

HINT

A handoff is the transfer of patient information from one healthcare clinician to another. Listen to the handoff before beginning to work on the patient.

Q When using the acronym *ISBAR* while providing the handoff, what does the *A* stand for?

A Assessment

ISBAR (identify, situation, background, assessment, recommendation; Box 25.4) is a format that can be used when providing a report or handoff to the next team. Acronyms used by healthcare clinicians during handoffs can improve clarity and completeness of the information. This is a structured approach used to avoid missing important information for the care of the patient.

Box 25.4 ISBAR handoff

I	Identify
S	Situation
B	Background
A	Assessment
R	Recommendation

Q When the team leader requests an action or procedure be done, what is the process used to confirm completion of the procedure?

A Closed-loop communication

Once the team leader requests a procedure or action be performed, the team member should acknowledge the request and confirm once it is completed. Closed-loop communication allows the team leader to know that their requests have been heard and allows for any clarification by the team members. Team members should call out any important changes.

HINT

Team leaders should state the name of the team member when requesting an action or procedure be performed. This decreases the risk that it will not be done.

Q What is a key factor in a trauma team to ensure safety and prevent errors?

A Speaking up

When a team member is concerned or believes that an error is about to be committed by another team member,it is essential that the person speaks up. This ability to speak up without repercussions creates an environment of safety. There are many ways to handle the situation. It usually begins with questioning and discussions, but when it progresses to the point of patient safety, a team member should demand that the individual stop so the situation can be reevaluated before further interventions are made.

HINT

The key is patient safety. Challenge assumptions during the resuscitation.

Q What is it called when the team members are acutely aware of the patient's changing state?

A Situation awareness

Situation awareness is the continual assessment and awareness of the patient's status and physiological changes. The team leader and members are continuously updated with these repetitive assessments. The ability to adapt to the changes found in the assessments and anticipate the other team members' needs contributes to a successful team.

HINT

The team leader needs to continually monitor the team's ongoing performance.

Q What is a barrier to effective teamwork in a trauma resuscitation?

A Strong egos

Teamwork requires shared decision-making and listening to others on the team. Team dynamics are crucial to the quality of care that is provided by the team. Processes need to be in place to overcome barriers to effective teamwork (Box 25.5). The culture of the trauma center is also important in developing effective processes. The trauma center's culture involves knowledge, beliefs, customs, and habits.

Box 25.5 Barriers to effective teamwork

Lack of trust
Strong egos
Stress
Sleep deprivation and fatigue
Poor staffing
Pandemics
Lack of role delineation
Failure to hold members accountable
Poor delegation of tasks

(continued)

Box 25.5 Barriers to effective teamwork (*continued*)

Reluctance to speak up and question decisions
Failure to prioritize task demands
Lack of experienced team members
Environmental factors
Loud environment
Lack of needed protective gear

HINT

Culture creates sustainability.

Q When a conflict does occur among the trauma team members, what needs to occur?

A Conflict resolution

Conflicts among team members will happen; it is inevitable. The ability to resolve the conflict allows for the learning and growth of the team. Teams must be able to allow both support and confrontation among the team members. Without confrontation, issues may be glossed over and can lead to impaired team performance. Without the ability to challenge each other, the team runs the risk of "group thinking," which leads to errors and bad outcomes.

Q What environmental factor can interfere with a resuscitation?

A Noise level

High noise levels can interfere with verbal communication and feedback during a resuscitation. Noisy environments can cause the healthcare clinicians to become louder in relaying findings or interventions. The high noise level can lead to missed communication and missed clinical events and creates team dysfunction.

HINT

The noise level within the resuscitation room can interfere with the ability to hear critical alarms.

Q What is an educational technique that is recommended in training trauma teams to anticipate the course of the patient's resuscitation?

A Simulation

Simulation or role-playing with case scenarios is a great training method for trauma teams to learn to effectively listen to the EMS crew and other clinicians during a handoff. Simulations involve formulating a plan, assigning roles, and practicing the resuscitation. Cross-training the team members to learn each other's roles will increase flexibility when unforeseen situations arise. Training should also include team building and effective teamwork.

HINT

Each training session should have specific and well-defined goals and specific tasks to be targeted.

KNOWLEDGE CHECK: CHAPTER 25

1. What is the primary goal of the trauma team?

   A. Collaboration with sharing of knowledge
   B. Providing a skill set to the patient
   C. Successful resuscitation
   D. Supportive group at trauma center

2. Which of the following is a required characteristic of a successful team?

   A. Trust
   B. Knowledge
   C. Skill
   D. Competency

3. A trauma is alerted and the trauma team assembles, awaiting the arrival of the patient. Each member of the trauma team gets into position and begins prepping for certain functions during the resuscitation. What is this called?

   A. Teamwork
   B. Respect
   C. Role delineation
   D. Flexibility

4. Which of the following attributes of the trauma team during a resuscitation most likely contributes to successful resuscitation?

   A. Resilience
   B. Accountability
   C. Commitment
   D. Communication

5. During a trauma resuscitation, the nurse on the team is moving around and performing multiple tasks that are outside of the identified roles and tasks of the trauma nurse. Which of the following best describes this barrier to successful resuscitation?

   A. Role delineation
   B. Individual achievements
   C. Team orientation
   D. Communication

(*See answers next page.*)

1. C) Successful resuscitation

The purpose of a trauma team is to successfully resuscitate the trauma patient. The trauma team is composed of a group of medical staff with varying backgrounds and levels of expertise, but the primary purpose is not sharing knowledge or providing a skill set. It is important for the team to work well together, but it is not considered a support group.

2. A) Trust

A team requires trust and respect to function effectively as a team. Individual characteristics of the team members include knowledge, skill, and competency.

3. C) Role delineation

There are many key attributes the trauma team members require for more coordinated, successful resuscitation, but the primary attribute is role delineation. Each member of the team should have a clear understanding of their role during the resuscitation. *Teamwork* refers to the actual dynamics of the team. Respect, trust, and flexibility are required for teamwork but are not specifically associated with preparation of each role before patient arrival.

4. D) Communication

To improve outcomes, communication is the key team attribute for ensuring clear and accurate information regarding the patient during a resuscitation. Resiliency, accountability, and commitment are all attributes of the trauma team, but the attribute most likely to affect outcomes and ensure successful resuscitation is effective communication during the resuscitation.

5. B) Individual achievements

The goal of the team is optimal team performance, not individual achievements. This may be a barrier in some teams due to the culture of rewarding individual performance. Team orientation is about group performance as a whole, with less emphasis on individual achievement. Role delineation and communication are not barriers but are required characteristics of the trauma team for improved outcomes.

Education and Outreach

26

Q What type of education involves continuing education for trauma nurses?

A Intramural education

Intramural education involves continuing education for trauma nurses and is a required metric at all levels of trauma centers. This includes real-time debriefing following a trauma case.

HINT

Advanced trauma life support is an example of intramural education.

Q Who is the recipient of extramural trauma education?

A The community

Extramural education involves education in the community for trauma prevention. Injury prevention is a principal area of community outreach that can affect trauma outcomes. The goal of community outreach programs (Box 26.1) is to prevent as many injuries as possible through education and safety. Data and quality improvement (QI) drive the community education. An example of a trauma outreach program is driver education for people charged with driving while intoxicated.

Box 26.1 Examples of community outreach programs

- Young adult driver safety
- Older adult driver safety
- Fall prevention
- Stop the Bleed
- Car seat safety
- Pedestrian safety
- Emergency preparedness
- Suicide prevention training
- Naloxone (Narcan) training for overdoses

HINT

Injury prevention should be specific to the community.

Q Besides intramural and extramural education, trauma education also focuses on what other group?

A Prehospital healthcare clinicians

Trauma centers should provide trauma education to prehospital personnel. This includes trauma prevention, stabilization of trauma patients, and pre-alerting trauma centers. Trauma centers should establish a relationship with emergency medical services (EMS) agencies and become involved with QI.

HINT

EMS education and including EMS personnel in QI projects builds teamwork between EMS and trauma centers.

Q What is the national awareness campaign to encourage bystanders to help in a bleeding emergency?

A Stop the Bleed

Stop the Bleed is a national awareness campaign that encourages bystanders to become trained, equipped, and empowered to help in a bleeding emergency. Uncontrolled bleeding is the number one cause of preventable death from trauma. Laypeople at the scene can close the gap between bleeding to death and controlling bleeding until EMS arrives.

HINT

Someone who is severely bleeding can bleed to death in as little as 5 minutes.

Q Who is encouraged to stop the bleeding from a trauma in the field?

A Anyone

The "first person at the scene" bystander is encouraged to initiate the process of controlling the blood loss. It does not require a medical background to learn how to stop the bleeding. The Stop the Bleed campaign encourages the initiation of application of pressure or tourniquets prior to arrival of first responders.

HINT

Bystanders are at the scene before EMS arrives and can save lives by stopping the bleeding of traumatic injuries.

Q In the Stop the Bleed campaign, what is taught as the first step to stop bleeding?

A Locate the site of the bleeding

The first step to stopping the bleed is finding the location of the bleed. The campaign teaches to cut the clothing at the site to be able to see the wound. It teaches the differences between serious and nonserious bleeding. Alerting or calling 911 is encouraged prior to intervening.

HINT

With serious bleeding, one is taught to apply a tourniquet 2 to 3 inches above the wound.

Q What is one taught to look for to identify a serious bleed in the Stop the Bleed campaign?

A Blood squirting

Laypeople are taught that serious bleeding can be identified by blood continuously flowing, blood squirting, or blood pooling on the surface under the patient. They are taught that if the bleeding is nonserious, they should apply direct pressure to control blood loss until bleeding stops.

HINT

If bleeding does not stop with direct pressure, it is recommended that the layperson should call 911.

Q When should a layperson stop holding direct pressure on a bleeding wound?

A If they are in danger

If the bystander is holding pressure to stop the bleeding, they should continue to hold the pressure until the bleeding has stopped, medical personnel have arrived, or the bystander has been put in danger.

HINT

An important point to teach is that the bystander should ensure their own safety first before assisting the victim.

Q In the Stop the Bleed campaign, what is taught with regard to placing a tourniquet near a joint?

A Avoid placing a turniquet on the joint

When applying a tourniquet, teach the participants to avoid placing it on a joint. Teach them to place it above the joint if necessary.

HINT

The class also teaches the areas that are not amenable to using a tourniquet (e.g., neck wounds).

Q When teaching car seat safety, where is the safest place in the car?

A In the middle of the back seat

Car seat safety is a common outreach program taught by trauma nurses. Teaching the safest location for a car seat is important to lower risk of injuries in automobile crashes. It is recommended that children from birth to age 2 to 4 years ride in rear-facing car seats. The back seat is safer than the front seat for children. Airbag deployment with the car seat in the front seat can cause serious or fatal injury to the child.

HINT

The best way to protect a child from injury in a car crash is restraint in the right car seat in the right way.

Q What is commonly used to determine the type of car seat, harness, or seat belt that is appropriate for the child?

A Height and weight

Some of the recommendations for car seats are age related, but the majority of recommendations are based on the child's height and weight. This is used when the child has advanced from rear-facing to front-facing car seats, from car seats to booster seats, and from five-point harnesses to car seat belts.

HINT

Properly fitted car seats are based on weight and height of the child and are important to improve efficacy of protection from injury.

KNOWLEDGE CHECK: CHAPTER 26

1. Which of the following describes continuing education for trauma nurses?
   A. Extramural education
   B. Intramural education
   C. Principle of adult learning
   D. Inservice training

2. Which of the following would be a type of intramural trauma education?
   A. Debriefing following trauma resuscitation
   B. Holding a community fair for trauma prevention
   C. Providing education at a high school on trauma prevention
   D. Presenting to a local representative to initiate change in legislation

3. Which of the following is the primary goal of education in the community?
   A. Inform the public which hospital to go to if they experience a trauma.
   B. Increase public awareness of legislation regarding trauma.
   C. Prevent as many injuries as possible through education and safety.
   D. Lower risk of admissions to the trauma center.

4. Which of the following statements is accurate regarding the trauma center's interactions with emergency medical services (EMS)?
   A. Trauma centers should be involved with quality improvement in prehospital emergency care.
   B. EMS will transport to the nearest hospital regardless of the trauma designation.
   C. Trauma centers do not have a role in EMS education due to conflict of interest.
   D. EMS systems are separate from trauma centers and typically are not involved in the other's education or quality.

5. What is the name of the national awareness campaign to encourage bystanders to help in a bleeding emergency?
   A. Hold Pressure, Save a Life
   B. BEST: Bleeding Established Safe Techniques
   C. Bleed Prevention
   D. Stop the Bleed

(*See answers next page.*)

1. B) Intramural education

Intramural education involves continuing education for trauma nurses and is a required metric at all levels of trauma centers. Adult learning may be the principle through which the education is taught, but it does not describe the required education. *Inservice training* is a form of education but is not the term used to describe required education for trauma nurses. Extramural education is education provided to the community.

2. A) Debriefing following trauma resuscitation

Debriefing following a trauma resuscitation is an example of intramural trauma education, or education for the trauma nurse. A community fair and a high school presentation are examples of extramural education, or education to the community regarding trauma.

3. C) Prevent as many injuries as possible through education and safety.

Injury prevention is a principal area of community outreach that can affect trauma outcomes. The goal of community outreach programs is to prevent as many injuries as possible through education and safety. Trauma center designation education is primarily for emergency medical services, not the community. Lowering the number of admissions to a trauma center may be a consequence of the education but is not the primary goal. Public awareness of trauma legislation is not the primary purpose of community education.

4. A) Trauma centers should be involved with quality improvement in prehospital emergency care.

Trauma centers should provide trauma education to prehospital personnel. This includes trauma prevention, stabilization of trauma patients, and pre-alerting trauma centers. Trauma centers should establish a relationship with the EMS agencies and become involved with quality improvement.

5. D) Stop the Bleed

Stop the Bleed is a national awareness campaign to encourage bystanders to become trained, equipped, and empowered to help in a bleeding emergency. Uncontrolled bleeding is the number one cause of preventable death from trauma. Laypeople at the scene can close the gap between bleeding to death by controlling bleeding until emergency medical services arrive.

Ethical Issues

Q What is the term for a situation in which two or more unattractive courses of action are possible, but none of them is an overwhelmingly rational choice?

A Ethical dilemma

Ethical dilemmas exist when two or more unattractive courses of action are possible but none is the overwhelmingly rational choice; both are equally compelling alternatives and a moral argument can be made for and against each alternative.

HINT

Ethical dilemmas are increasing in number and intensity in hospitals.

Q What type of crisis does acting against one's conscience cause?

A Moral distress

To act against one's own conscience causes feelings of shame or guilt and violates one's sense of wholeness and integrity. Moral distress is caused when the ethically appropriate action is known but cannot be acted upon.

HINT

Nurses frequently resort to their own personal values and receive guidance from other nursing peers when formulating their ethical beliefs (Box 27.1).

Box 27.1 Development of an ethical belief system

Parents' values and influence
Family's values and influence
Religious beliefs
Cultural traditions
Past experiences

Q What is the ethical dilemma of withholding intravenous (IV) fluids from a patient at the end of life called?

A Removal of life-sustaining therapies

End-of-life issues and removal of life-sustaining therapies (nutrition, hydration, and ventilation) frequently can become ethical issues in the hospital (Box 27.2).

Box 27.2 Ethical issues in the hospital

Futility issues
"Do not resuscitate" issues
"Slow codes"
Removal of life-sustaining therapies
Euthanasia
Physician-assisted suicides
Scarce resources
Organ donors/recipients
Protection of children's rights

HINT

Frequently, ethical dilemmas are a result of contradictory beliefs, competing duties, conflicting principles, and a lack of clear clinical or legal guidelines.

Q What role should emotions play in making ethical decisions?

A None

Many decisions made in the ICU have an ethical component. Decisions need to be made based on a learned skill, not just an emotional response. Ethical decision-making should use a systematic process, and ethical principles provide direction. Without this guidance, decisions are made based on emotions, intuitions, or fixed policies.

HINT

Everyone is unique and influenced by their own personal, cultural, and religious values.

Q When an ethical dilemma is presented to the ethics committee, what is the first step in the process?

A Data collection

Data collection includes the gathering of medical facts, including the prognosis, alternatives, and assessment of patient and family knowledge. Social facts are also collected, including the patient's living environment, family and significant others, economic concerns, and current or previously stated wishes (Box 27.3).

Box 27.3 Steps in making ethical decisions

Collect data: Gather medical facts, including prognosis, alternatives, and assessment of patient/family knowledge; social facts are also collected, including the patient's living environment, family and significant others, economic concerns, and current or previously stated wishes.

Identify the conflict: Look at the values and determine where they conflict or agree, determine who is involved in the conflict; state the ethical position of the families, patients, and healthcare clinicians.

(*continued*)

Box 27.3 Steps in making ethical decisions (*continued*)

Define the goals of therapy: Is the goal prolongation of life, relief of pain, or maximum recovery?

Identify the ethical principles: List the ethical principles that may be used in the situation and rank them to identify the primary principle; ethical principles may conflict.

Review alternative courses of action: Compare the alternatives with the goals; predict possible consequences of the alternatives and prioritize acceptable alternatives.

Choose the course of action: This is the action that confronts the fewest ethical principles.

Develop and implement plan of action: This requires the input of the healthcare clinicians and decision makers.

Evaluate the plan: After the action is implemented, evaluate whether the plan effectively met the ethical principles and initial goals.

HINT

The ethics committee uses a process similar to the nursing process, which begins with an assessment.

Q What is the ethical principle that is based on the greatest good for the greatest number of people called?

A Utilitarianism

Utilitarianism is also called *situation ethics*. This principle defines *good* as happiness or pleasure. It is based on two principles: the greatest good for the greatest number and the end justifies the means. When using this principle, the situation determines whether the act is right or wrong.

HINT

Believers in utilitarianism do not believe in absolute rules but believe that rules can change according to the situation.

Q What is the ethical principle that is based on moral rules and unchanging principles called?

A Deontology

Deontology, in its purest form, focuses on the act, rather than the consequences of the act. Morality is defined by the act, not its outcome. The main principles are human life has value, one is to always tell the truth, and—above all—do no harm.

HINT

Deontology standards do not change no matter the situation, location, time, or people involved.

Q When a hospital or country is experiencing scarcity of a resource, what ethical principle is used to determine allocation of the resource?

A Justice

Justice incorporates ideas of fairness and equality. Most decisions relating to the allocation of scarce resources involve the use of this principle. Every patient needs to be treated similarly, avoiding discrimination on the basis of age, sex, perceived social worth, financial ability, or cultural/ethnic background.

▶ HINT

The determination of which person on an organ transplant list will receive a donor organ is based on the principle of justice.

Q Which ethical principle is commonly used when justifying the removal of life support for a patient in the ICU?

A Beneficence

Beneficence refers to healthcare's responsibility to benefit the patient, usually through acts of kindness, compassion, and mercy. This principle weighs the balance between benefit and harm and asks which action maximizes the benefit and minimizes the harm. The principle of beneficence is used to analyze futile care and withdrawal of life support.

▶ HINT

Although the principle of nonmaleficence is "to do no harm," the definition of *harm* becomes crucial when applying this principle.

Q Who is the healthcare decision maker in the ethical principle of autonomy?

A The patient

Autonomy is the right to self-government (Box 27.4). This is the freedom to make choices that affect one's life. In the hospital setting, it refers to the belief that a competent patient has the right to make their own decisions about care and should be able to refuse therapy. This justifies our duty to obtain informed consent and to be truthful and encourages the use of advance directives. Conflict occurs when the decision is in conflict with the beliefs of healthcare clinicians or even family members. *Veracity* is the requirement to provide patients and decision makers with all the information needed to make an autonomous decision.

Box 27.4 Components of autonomy

The autonomous person is respected.
The autonomous person must be able to determine personal goals.
The autonomous person has the capacity to decide on a plan of action.
The autonomous person has the freedom to act on those choices.

▶ HINT

Autonomy is used to justify the use of a family member as a primary decision maker if the patient is unable to make decisions at that time; the right of autonomy is recognized by the legal system.

Q What is it called when healthcare professionals have the duty to benefit the patient, which outweighs the right of personal choice?

A Paternalism

The principle of paternalism maintains that the benefits provided outweigh the consideration of autonomy, the patient's condition severely limits their ability to choose autonomously, and the intended action may be universally justified in similarly relevant circumstances. Physicians may implement this belief by providing only partial information to the patient based on their own beliefs and personal preferences.

HINT

When parents withhold the care of a child, but the physicians believe that the intervention is in the child's best interests, then the hospital may take on the decision-making for the child. When this occurs, the decision is based on the ethical principle of paternalism.

Q At the end of life, terminal sedation is based on which ethical principle?

A Principle of double effect (PDE)

PDE states that an act must be morally good or indifferent, and a bad effect must not be the means by which one achieves a good effect. The intention must be to achieve the good effect, with the bad effect occurring as an unintended side effect only. The good effect must be at least equal to the bad effect.

HINT

PDE is used to justify the administration of medication to relieve pain even though this may lead to the unintended, although foreseen, consequence of hastening death by causing respiratory depression.

Q What is the ethical dilemma in which physicians and their consultants, consistent with the available medical literature, conclude that further treatment cannot, within a reasonable probability, cure, ameliorate, improve, or restore the quality of life that would be satisfactory to the patient?

A Futile care

In each situation, futile care may be hard to define. The survival rates or mortality rates of a certain disease process or situation is commonly used to assist with the definition of futility of care (Box 27.5).

Box 27.5 Criteria used to assess futility

Severity of illness
Chronic health conditions
Life expectancy
Quality of life
Expected long-term outcomes
Social support
Duration of therapy
Cost of treatment

HINT

An example of futile care may be an emergency thoracotomy for a blunt chest trauma or an irreversible coma or vegetative state.

Q What is the document that identifies a person who will have the power to make medical decisions in the event that the patient is unable to do so?

A Durable power of attorney for healthcare

A durable power of attorney for healthcare is a legal document that identifies someone who will have the power to make medical treatment decisions in the event that the patient is unable to do so. This power of attorney is initiated at a time when the patient loses the capacity to participate in the decision-making process (Box 27.6). This is part of one's advance directives, which may also include a living will.

Box 27.6 Barriers to initiating advance directives

Reluctance to talk about death
Belief that it is not needed at this time of life
Patient waiting for physician to initiate the conversation
Difficulty completing the forms
Ignorance of the option
Witness requirements that hinder completion in the hospital setting
Healthcare professionals possibly not knowledgeable about the process

HINT

A dilemma may appear to exist when a patient has a living will that says they do not want to be intubated, but healthcare clinicians have already intubated the patient.

Q Which ethical principle is used to support physician-assisted suicide?

A Autonomy

Physician-assisted suicide involves a medical professional providing a patient the means to end their own life. The supporting ethical principle for this is autonomy, whereas the conflicting principle for this is nonmaleficence.

HINT

It is well accepted that a patient may refuse treatment even if healthcare professionals believe the treatment is in the patient's best interests. This is withholding treatment and is not considered assisted suicide.

ADVOCACY

Q When do nurses become advocates for their patients?

A On a daily basis

Advocacy of nurses for their patients is a part of the daily practice of nurses in the clinical area. Advocacy is an important part of nursing and is a significant component of trust between the patient and the nurse. Advocacy means to act on someone's behalf.

HINT

Advocacy can also become a career in itself for a nurse.

Q What is the role of the nurse when advocating between the physician and the patient?

A Mediator

The advocacy role in nursing (Box 27.7) can be defined as being a mediator between the physician and the patient. This occurs often when the physician's recommendations are at odds with the patient's or family's concerns or beliefs. Nurses are the ones who spend the most time with patients and families and become knowledgeable about their beliefs, culture, and concerns.

Box 27.7 Nurse advocate roles/actions

Act as mediator.
Act as patient representative.
Ensure patients know their rights.
Defend the rights of patients.
Protect patient interests.
Protect the patient.
Provide information for decision-making.
Support and respect patient and family decisions.
Provide support for ethical decision-making.
Ensure continuity of care.
Educate about treatment options.
Provide resources.
Keep the team informed.
Coach better health decisions.
Ensure safety.
Allocate resources.
Facilitate access to healthcare.
Prevent racial disparities in care.
Facilitate advanced care planning.

HINT

When the nurse plays the mediator role and informs other healthcare clinicians of the patient's concerns or beliefs, this improves patient outcomes and compliance.

Q What is a significant advocacy role of nurses for patients in the trauma center?

A Education

Nurses are patient educators. Assisting the patient and family to understand processes and procedures will allow more informed decisions about their care. Some healthcare decisions are very difficult to make by the patient's loved ones, and the nurse can be an advocate by providing information for decision-making.

HINT

End-of-life decisions are some of the most difficult decisions families have to make, and nurses are in the position to facilitate these decisions.

Q Would nursing advocacy for the patient more likely involve empathy or sympathy?

A Empathy

Empathy is a component of nursing advocacy. It includes understanding the patient and their condition, feeling close to the patient, and showing compassion for the patient and family members. Understanding the patient's expectations can improve the relationship between the nurse and the patient.

HINT

Put yourself in the patient's shoes to help understand what the patient needs.

Q Compassion occurs as a response to what human situation?

A Suffering

Compassion occurs in response to another person's suffering when one is affected by the suffering and pain of another. Nurse advocacy seeks solutions to alleviate others' pain and suffering.

HINT

With advocacy, the nurse seeks solutions to alleviate suffering.

Q What is a common barrier to compassion and advocacy in nursing?

A Burnout

Burnout refers to a state of mental, physical, and emotional exhaustion and is commonly caused by excessive working hours and workload. Burnout leads to disengagement and detachment. Burnout is a barrier to being compassionate and advocating for patients (Box 27.8).

Box 27.8 Barriers to advocacy

Burnout
Lack of competency
Lack of dedication
Moral distress
High-stress situations and work environments
Poor communication skills
Lack of knowledge
Lack of confidence
Complacency

▶ HINT

Patients tend to see nurses with good communication skills as being their best advocates.

Q What is an essential skill for being a nurse advocate at the bedside?
A Communication

The ability of the nurse to implement good communication skills with the patient, family, physician, and other healthcare clinicians is essential to act as an advocate for the patient. In the role of mediator, the nurse needs to be able to identify issues and develop solutions. This requires the ability to listen and communicate (Box 27.9).

Box 27.9 Skills needed for advocating in nursing

Communication skills
Leadership ability
Negotiating skills
Ability to make decisions
Empathy
Active listening

▶ HINT

Nurses are frequently in the position to "translate" medical jargon for physicians.

Q What is an example of a difficult situation in which the nurse should be an advocate but that advocacy has the potential to cause difficulty with a superior?
A Challenging decisions of physicians

Nurses may be in positions in which they need to question or challenge a physician's decision. This can be a difficult situation due to occupational hierarchy, and thus nurses may not raise their concerns regarding the patient's care. This type of situation is detrimental to patient care and outcomes. Nurses require confidence and good communication skills to advocate for the patient to a physician. By challenging, speaking up, or escalating the concern when a potential error is identified, nurses may prevent errors and poor outcomes from occurring. This is the role of nursing advocacy.

HINT

See something, say something.

Q What type of patient requires all reasonable steps be taken to protect the patient from harm?

A A vulnerable patient

All reasonable steps should be taken to prevent harm to vulnerable populations, including those who cannot make their own decisions, do not have support systems, or are at risk for abuse, neglect, or harm.

HINT

Nurses are in great positions to act as advocates for vulnerable populations.

KNOWLEDGE CHECK: CHAPTER 27

1. What is the term used to describe a situation in which a person acts against their own conscience or moral beliefs?

   A. Empathy
   B. Moral distress
   C. Beneficence
   D. Moral agent

2. An older adult patient is in the ICU on a ventilator following a multisystem trauma. The physician has discussed a do-not-resuscitate (DNR) order with the family. The patient's spouse states that the patient would not want to live like this, but the patient's adult son is adamant that everything possible should be done and will not discuss a DNR order. Which of the following would be the most appropriate intervention by the nurse?

   A. Tell the spouse that the son is right and that the spouse should support this decision.
   B. Ask the physician to make the decision relating to a DNR order.
   C. Refer the situation to the ethics committee if the disagreement cannot be resolved.
   D. Continue treatment until the family can make a decision together.

3. Which of the following ethical principles considers the balance between benefit and harm, in which an action maximizes the benefit and minimizes the harm?

   A. Paternalism
   B. Autonomy
   C. Nonmaleficence
   D. Beneficence

4. Which of the following ethical principles is commonly used for acts of kindness and mercy?

   A. Beneficence
   B. Nonmaleficence
   C. Veracity
   D. Fidelity

5. Which of the following best describes the withholding of intravenous (IV) fluids in a patient at the end of life?

   A. It is unnecessary at this point.
   B. It is considered withholding of life support.
   C. It is considered euthanasia and is unethical.
   D. It is frequently done due to scarce resources.

(*See answers next page.*)

1. B) Moral distress

Moral distress is caused when the ethically appropriate action is known but cannot be acted upon. To act against one's own conscience causes feelings of shame or guilt and violates one's sense of wholeness and integrity. Empathy is the capacity to understand or feel what another person is experiencing. Beneficence is an ethical principle used in ethical dilemmas. A moral agent is a person who is able to make moral choices based upon the notion of right and wrong.

2. C) Refer the situation to the ethics committee if the disagreement cannot be resolved.

Ethics committees should be consulted when an ethical dilemma is not readily resolved. Common causes and scenarios for ethical dilemmas include contradictory beliefs, competing duties, conflicting principles, and lack of clear clinical or legal guidelines. The physician can make a recommendation but cannot make the decision for the family. The nurse should not support one family member's opinion but should facilitate decision-making among the family members.

3. D) Beneficence

The ethical principal of beneficence considers the balance between benefit and harm, in which an action maximizes the benefit and minimizes the harm. This is the principle frequently used to analyze futile care and withdrawal of life support. Autonomy means *self-governing* and is the freedom to make choices that affect one's life. Nonmaleficence is an ethical principle that requires that actions do not inflict harm. Paternalism is based on the belief that healthcare professionals have the duty to benefit the patient.

4. A) Beneficence

The ethical principle of beneficence considers the responsibility of healthcare clinicians to benefit the patient, usually through acts of kindness, compassion, and mercy. Nonmaleficence is an ethical principle that requires that actions not inflict harm. The definition of *harm* becomes crucial when applying this principle and includes deliberate harm, risk of harm, and harm that occurs during beneficial acts. Veracity is the requirement to provide patients and decision makers with all of the information needed to make an autonomous decision. Fidelity relates to the concept of faithfulness and the practice of keeping promises. It includes the loyalty that exists in a nurse–patient relationship.

5. B) It is considered withholding of life support.

Stopping or withholding hydration (IV fluids) and nutrition and removing endotracheal tubes are considered to be removal of life-sustaining therapies at end of life. These commonly occur and can be necessary. It is not euthanasia and is not performed due to scarcity of resources.

PART VII

Practice Test

Trauma Certified Registered Nurse Practice Test

28

1. A patient was struck by a baseball bat on the right side of the head, sustaining a coup–contrecoup injury. Which of the following injuries is most likely associated with this mechanism?

   A. Intraventricular hemorrhage (IVH)
   B. Epidural hematoma (EDH)
   C. Hydrocephalus
   D. Retinal hemorrhages

2. A patient involved in a motor vehicle crash was hit head on and sustained a traumatic brain injury (TBI) when their head impacted the windshield. Which of the following terms refers to this mechanism of injury?

   A. Indirect injury
   B. Acceleration
   C. Deceleration
   D. Coup–contrecoup

3. A patient is a college football player who has sustained several minor traumatic brain injuries (TBIs) during football games. The patient has been demonstrating signs of difficulty concentrating and issues with memory. Which of the following is the most likely cause of the patient's symptoms?

   A. Chronic subdural hematoma
   B. Hydrocephalus
   C. Chronic traumatic encephalopathy
   D. Temporal mesial atrophy

4. A pediatric patient was brought into the ED unresponsive and has been determined to have experienced violent shaking by the patient's father. Which of the following is a more common complication of shaken baby syndrome?

   A. Retinal hemorrhages
   B. Cerebral contusions
   C. Cerebellar hematomas
   D. Locked-in syndrome

5. Which artery is most commonly involved in producing an epidural hematoma (EDH) following traumatic brain injury?

A. Carotid
B. Middle meningeal
C. Vertebral
D. Middle cerebral

6. Which of the following labs is used to improve the accuracy of identifying cerebrospinal fluid (CSF) in nasal drainage after a basilar skull fracture?

A. D-dimer
B. Immunoglobulin G (IgG) levels
C. Hemoglobin (Hgb) level
D. Beta-2 transferrin

7. Which of the following best describes the traumatic brain injury known as *diffuse axonal injury (DAI)*?

A. Sudden deceleration injury with head impacting windshield
B. Result of the tearing of the middle meningeal artery
C. Presence of interstitial cerebral edema
D. Rotational mechanism causing a shearing of the neuronal axons

8. Traumatic injury to the brain tissue with development of a contusion is associated with focal edema surrounding the contusion. Which of the following is the type of cerebral edema caused by direct tissue injury?

A. Vasogenic
B. Cytotoxic
C. Vasospasm
D. Basal

9. A patient develops bilateral periorbital ecchymosis after a traumatic brain injury (TBI). What is this patient's injury?

A. Depressed skull fracture
B. Cervical fracture
C. Basilar skull fracture
D. Rhinorrhea

10. Following admission to the ED, a traumatic brain injury (TBI) patient has the following findings:

Blood pressure (BP): 105/64 mmHg

Heart rate (HR): 110 beats/min

Respiratory rate (RR): 20 breaths/min

Oxygen saturation (SaO_2): 95%

Which of these findings is most concerning for the patient?

A. HR = 110 beats/min
B. BP = 105/64 mmHg
C. RR = 20 breaths/min
D. SaO_2 = 95%

11. Which of the following signs of neurological deterioration is the most sensitive and early sign of increased intracranial pressure (ICP)?

A. Change in level of consciousness
B. Dilated, nonreactive pupils
C. Increased systolic pressure with widened pulse pressure
D. Bradycardia

12. Which of the following statements is most accurate regarding a minor traumatic brain injury (TBI)?

A. A minor TBI will have a Glasgow Soma Scale (GCS) score of 9 to 12.
B. An initial loss of consciousness is required to call the injury a concussion.
C. Minor TBI may have transient neurological abnormalities for weeks to months after injury.
D. GCS scores are very accurate in determining the severity of TBIs.

13. Following a motor vehicle crash, the patient had a rapid deterioration in consciousness in the ED. A stat noncontrast CT scan was obtained, which found an epidural hematoma with a shift. Which of the following pupil changes would the nurse expect to find if the patient develops uncal herniation?

A. Dilated ipsilateral nonreactive pupil
B. Bilateral dilated nonreactive pupils
C. Dilated contralateral nonreactive pupil
D. Bilateral pinpoint pupils

14. A traumatic brain injury (TBI) patient in the ICU has an intracranial pressure (ICP) monitor, and the ICP has been 25 to 30 mmHg. Hyperosmolar therapy with mannitol (Osmitrol) is being administered every 4 hours. The following labs are obtained: Na+ = 148, K+ = 3.8, and serum osmolality = 325 mOsm/L. Which of the following would be the most correct statement regarding this patient?

- **A.** Increase the frequency of mannitol (Osmitrol) infusions to lower the ICP.
- **B.** Hold the next dose of mannitol (Osmitrol) until serum osmolality is less than 320 mOsm/L.
- **C.** Avoid administering 3% normal saline at this time due to the patient's hypernatremia.
- **D.** Administer steroids to help lower the patient's ICP.

15. A multisystem trauma patient has injuries including traumatic brain injury (TBI) and femur fractures. The patient is in pain and requires opioids to manage the pain. Which of the following should be monitored closely in this patient to prevent secondary neurological injuries?

- **A.** Pupillary changes
- **B.** Constipation
- **C.** Serum sodium levels
- **D.** Blood pressure

16. Which of the following long-term complications is most commonly associated with basilar skull fractures?

- **A.** Loss of smell
- **B.** Loss of hearing
- **C.** Paresis of the contralateral side
- **D.** Nasal congestion

17. Following a traumatic brain injury, the patient had no recollection of events for 12 hours after the trauma, even though they were conscious in the hospital and answering questions. Which of the following terms is best used to refer to this type of amnesia?

- **A.** Retrograde
- **B.** Posttraumatic
- **C.** Transient global
- **D.** Antegrade

18. A patient in the ICU following a traumatic brain injury (TBI) requires an intracranial pressure (ICP) monitor due to level of consciousness. The patient's mean arterial pressure (MAP) is 70 mmHg, and their ICP is 20 mmHg. Which of the following is the correct calculated cerebral perfusion pressure (CPP) in mmHg?

- **A.** 10
- **B.** 140
- **C.** 50
- **D.** 70

19. During monitoring of a traumatic brain injury (TBI) patient's intracranial pressure (ICP), it was noted that the ICP remained greater than 30 mmHg despite hyperosmolar therapy. Which of the following actions could be performed to lower the patient's ICP at this time?

    A. Administering high-dose steroids
    B. Hyperventilating to partial pressure of carbon dioxide between 30 and 35 mm Hg
    C. Maintaining systolic blood pressure greater than 200 mmHg
    D. Continuing to administer hyperosmolar therapy; no other action is necessary

20. Which of the following would be the most appropriate intervention in a patient with a basilar skull fracture?

    A. Placing the endotracheal tube nasally
    B. Packing the nose if rhinorrhea is present
    C. Using bilevel positive airway pressure if the patient requires supplemental oxygen
    D. Placing the gastric tube orally

21. The patient has experienced a mild traumatic brain injury. Following the injury, the patient is complaining of ocular pain, tearing, redness, blurred vision, and a headache. Which of the following is most likely the cause for the presenting symptoms?

    A. Subconjunctival hemorrhage
    B. Corneal abrasion
    C. Choroidal hemorrhage
    D. Retinal necrosis

22. Which of the following is the most likely method for treating a parotid duct injury?

    A. Tube cannulation for 3 to 6 months
    B. Removal of the duct
    C. Bypass procedure
    D. Self-limiting condition; does not require intervention

23. A patient presents to the ED with corneal abrasion. The nurse is explaining to the orienting new nurse the treatment of this type of injury. Which of the following is a correct statement regarding the treatment for a corneal abrasion injury?

    A. A light semi-pressure dressing is applied to the eye.
    B. The dressing is taped from the forehead to the ear.
    C. Oral antibiotics are administered for 14 days.
    D. A firm-pressure dressing is applied to the eye.

24. Which of the following types of chemical burn to the eye has the ability to penetrate deeper tissue and cause damage to the intraocular structures, leading to glaucoma and cataracts?

    A. Acid
    B. Base
    C. Neutral
    D. Corrosive

25. What is considered the gold standard for diagnosing facial fractures/injuries?

A. Plain films
B. Angiography
C. CT
D. Oral contrast studies

26. For which of the following traumatic eye injuries would the nurse avoid checking eye motility?

A. Open-globe injury
B. Hyphema
C. Chemical burns to the eye
D. Orbital fracture

27. A patient has an orbital blowout fracture. This injury has caused entrapment of the ocular muscles, and extraocular eye movements are restrained. The nurse explains the procedure that will be performed to determine the presence and severity of the entrapment. Which of the following is the correct process for this injury?

A. Oral antibiotics and nasal decongestants
B. Needle decompression of the ocular muscle
C. Reconstruction of orbital floor and medial wall with mesh, synthetic orbital plates, or bone grafting
D. Forceps used to grab the rectus muscle and rotate the globe in all directions

28. A patient presents the ED reporting increased eye pain. The patient reports that fragments of sawdust entered their eye last week. On examination, there is an enlarged gray area on the corneal surface. What is this reflective of?

A. Conjunctivitis
B. Corneal infection
C. Conjunctival infection
D. Corneal abrasion

29. A patient comes into the ED after an altercation in which they sustained a blow to the face. The patient's profile shows a compressed nose, and the frontal view appears to be widened and flattened. What type of injury did this patient most likely sustain?

A. Nasal fracture
B. Ethmoid fracture
C. Telecanthus injury
D. Naso-orbital-ethmoid injury

30. The nurse is assessing a patient with orbital ecchymosis and edema. The trauma nurse is having the patient follow the nurse's pen as the nurse moves it across the full range of horizontal and vertical eye movements. The patient is having difficulty with extraocular movements. What type of fracture is most likely associated with this presentation?

A. Zygomatic fracture
B. Orbital blowout fracture
C. LeFort I fracture
D. Orbital rim fracture

31. Which of the following is recommended after the recognition of fractured ribs one through three following a blunt trauma to the chest?

 A. Arteriogram
 B. Barium swallow
 C. CT coronary angiogram
 D. Bronchoscopy

32. Orbital fractures can be associated with ocular injuries. Which of the following terms refers to the pooling of blood within the anterior chamber of the eye?

 A. Vitreous hemorrhage
 B. Hyphema
 C. Optic nerve injury
 D. Opacification of the globe

33. A flail chest associated with sternal fracture is commonly associated with which of the following life-threatening thoracic injuries?

 A. Aortic dissection
 B. Diaphragm rupture
 C. Splenic laceration
 D. Liver laceration

34. Following a sudden deceleration mechanism of injury, the patient sustains an aortic transection. What is the most common location of the aortic transection following a trauma?

 A. Aortic arch
 B. Ascending aorta
 C. Level of the isthmus
 D. Level of the diaphragm

35. Which of the following is commonly found in a delayed presentation of bronchial injury above the level of the carina?

 A. Persistent pneumothorax
 B. Hemothorax
 C. Cuff leak on endotracheal tube
 D. Decreased lung compliance

36. Following a high-speed motor vehicle crash, the patient is suspected of having an aortic transection. Which of the following chest x-ray findings would be the most indicative of this injury?

 A. Kerley B lines
 B. Widened mediastinum
 C. Presence of hemothorax
 D. Enlarged cardiac silhouette

37. Which diagnostic study is recommended to diagnose a bronchial injury following blunt trauma to the chest?

A. Chest x-ray
B. Bronchoscopy
C. Sputum culture
D. Tracheal pressure

38. Which of the following is the most accurate statement regarding diaphragm injuries?

A. They cause immediate loss of diaphragm movement.
B. They result in immediate stomach herniation into the thoracic cavity.
C. Their most common mechanism is penetrating trauma.
D. The left side is more commonly injured.

39. Which of the following arteries is most commonly involved in the development of a hemothorax?

A. Aorta
B. Subclavian artery
C. Circumflex coronary artery
D. Internal mammary artery

40. Which of the following radiographic diagnostic studies is most specific to identifying diaphragm injury after trauma?

A. Ultrasonography
B. Anteroposterior chest x-ray
C. CT
D. Lateral chest x-ray

41. Following a significant blunt chest injury, the patient is noted to be hypotensive and tachycardic. Which of the following types of shock is the best explanation for hypotension following cardiac contusions?

A. Hemorrhagic
B. Distributive
C. Cardiogenic
D. Neurogenic

42. A patient with which of the following would be considered a candidate for an emergency thoracotomy following chest trauma?

A. Tension pneumothorax
B. 1,500-mL chest tube output after insertion
C. Blunt trauma to the chest in cardiac arrest
D. Sternal fracture

43. Which of the following abdominal organs is more likely to be injured in blunt trauma to the abdomen?

A. Sigmoid colon
B. Stomach
C. Spleen
D. Jejunum

44. Which of the following is most likely the symptom of delayed diaphragmatic rupture?

A. Hemorrhage
B. Shortness of breath
C. Pulseless electrical activity
D. Elevated lipase and amylase levels

45. Following a blunt trauma, the presence of air in the abdomen is identified. Which of the following is the most likely cause?

A. Stomach laceration
B. Liver laceration
C. Aortic transection
D. Ruptured spleen

46. The physician tells the patient that they have a minor pancreatic injury from their motor vehicle crash today. After the physician leaves, the patient asks the nurse, "What happens now? Do I need surgery? How is this going to be fixed?" The best response would be:

A. "We most likely will have to take you to the operating room to remove the pancreas."
B. "We most likely will have to take you to the operating room to aggressively debride the pancreas."
C. "We have to make sure you are up-to-date on all your vaccinations."
D. "We might have to place a temporary drain in the area of the pancreas."

47. A patient is diagnosed with thoracic aortic dissection following a high-speed motor vehicle collision. The patient is hypertensive and tachycardic. Which of the following would the nurse expect the ED physician to order?

A. Esmolol (Brevibloc)
B. Sodium nitroprusside (Nipride)
C. Fluid bolus
D. Diltiazem (Cardizem)

48. A driver in a motor vehicle collision sustains injuries from the seat belt. Which of the following would be the most likely to be injured?

A. Spleen
B. Liver
C. Pancreas
D. Bladder

49. Following a blunt injury to the abdomen with diaphragm injury, which of the following would most likely be an early sign of herniated bowel?

   A. Shortness of breath
   B. Bloody diarrhea
   C. Vomiting blood
   D. Constipation

50. The nurse is precepting a new ICU nurse in the trauma unit. The patient they are caring for is diagnosed with abdominal compartment syndrome, and the orientee is preparing to perform bladder pressure readings. Which of the following statements by the orientee would require correction by the preceptor?

   A. "An indwelling bladder catheter needs to be inserted using sterile technique."
   B. "The transducer needs to be leveled to the symphysis pubis."
   C. "Two hundred mL of dextrose should be instilled into the bladder before a pressure reading is obtained."
   D. "The physician needs to be notified for pressure readings greater than 20 mmHg."

51. A 14-year-old patient was performing tricks on their bicycle when they fell over the handlebars. They are complaining of midepigastric abdominal pain. Which of the following is indicative of a pancreatic injury?

   A. Elevated platelets
   B. Leukocytosis
   C. Low serum lactate level
   D. Elevated serum amylase level

52. A patient sustained a liver laceration 10 days before that has been repaired. They also underwent a splenectomy. The nurse has stabilized the patient and now is preparing the patient for transfer to the trauma telemetry unit. While reviewing the labs, the nurse notes that the complete blood count (CBC) results are:

   Red blood cells (RBCs): 5.1

   White blood cells (WBCs): 10

   Hemoglobin (Hgb): 9.4

   Hematocrit (Hct): 37

   Platelets: 519

   On which of the following medications should the patient be placed before transfer?

   A. Enoxaparin sodium (Lovenox)
   B. Pegfilgrastim (Neulasta)
   C. Aspirin
   D. Folic acid

53. The nurse is assessing a crying pediatric patient complaining of "belly" pain who has marked abdominal distention. The trauma nurse should expect which test to be performed initially?

A. CT of the abdomen
B. Focused assessment sonography for trauma (FAST)
C. Peritoneal lavage
D. Kidney, ureter, and bladder (KUB) x-ray

54. What is the mechanism of injury that commonly causes fetal death in a house fire?

A. Maternal burns
B. Decreased fetal circulation
C. Carbon monoxide poisoning
D. Maternal hypervolemia

55. Which of the following is the most appropriate positioning of a pregnant trauma patient?

A. Reverse Trendelenburg
B. Prone
C. Supine
D. Tilt to left side

56. Which of the following is the most accurate statement regarding the care of a pregnant trauma patient?

A. Vasopressors improve fetal perfusion.
B. The supine position is recommended.
C. Thoracostomy tube placement is higher than in nonpregnant trauma patients.
D. Airway management is the same as in nonpregnant trauma patients.

57. A 5-year-old child was hit in the right lateral chest with a baseball bat. The radiographic results reveal no rib fractures, but the patient is crying and saying that their chest hurts. The nurse should still be assessing the patient for a possible:

A. Cardiac injury
B. Liver injury
C. Renal injury
D. Lung contusion

58. A patient presented with a splenic injury and is now complaining of abdominal pain in the left upper quadrant. The pain is referring to the neck. What is this referred pain called?

A. Positive Saegesser's sign
B. Positive Kehr's sign
C. Positive cervicalgia sign
D. Positive Kernig's sign

59. A pregnant trauma patient is being evaluated in the ED. The patient is tachypneic and tachycardic. Which of the following is an expected finding on the patient's arterial blood gas due to normal physiological changes in pregnancy?

A. Compensated respiratory alkalosis
B. Hypoxia
C. Compensated metabolic acidosis
D. Hypercarbia

60. What is the fifth vital sign in a pregnant trauma patient?

A. Pain
B. Fetal heart tones
C. Pulse oximetry
D. Capnography

61. A patient at 28 weeks' gestation comes to the ED following a minor trauma. The patient begins to complain of a headache, blurred vision, and epistaxis. Which complication should the nurse be suspicious of?

A. Preeclampsia
B. Eclampsia
C. Hypervolemia
D. HELLP syndrome

62. A patient at 32 weeks' gestation comes to the ED with a stab wound to the abdomen. The patient requires multiple blood transfusions and is blood type O negative. What distinct laboratory test is indicated to deliver proper treatment for this patient?

A. Kleihauer–Betke (KB) test
B. Beta human chorionic gonadotropin (HCG) level
C. Prothrombin time (PT) and partial thromboplastin time (PTT) level
D. Hemoglobin and hematocrit levels

63. Which of the following terms is best used when referring to ligament injuries that cause the pelvis to spread wider?

A. Straddle injury
B. Open-book pelvic fracture
C. Vertical shear
D. Subtrochanteric fracture

64. Fat emboli are usually caused by long-bone fractures and pelvic fractures. The patient typically has respiratory compromise, including tachypnea and hypoxia. Which of the following are the pulmonary signs of fat emboli?

A. Productive cough with coarse crackles
B. Dry cough with scattered rhonchi
C. Productive cough with diminished breath sounds
D. Dry cough with inspiratory wheezes

65. Of the five "Ps" in the neurovascular assessment, which of the following is the most vital part of the assessment of a patient with compartment syndrome?

A. Pain
B. Pressure
C. Pulselessness
D. Paralysis

66. An increased blood flow to a previously ischemic muscle resulting in the washout of lipid-soluble intracellular metabolites causes which of the following complications of compartment syndrome?

A. Inadequate decompression
B. Reperfusion injury
C. Volkmann's ischemic contractures
D. Hypoperfusion

67. A patient who suffers a pelvic fracture may require the application of a pelvic binder to reduce bleeding, limit movement, and stabilize the fracture. What is the proper placement of a pelvic binder?

A. At the level of the greater trochanters
B. Over the iliac crest
C. Above the level of the greater trochanters
D. Over the abdomen

68. A patient with a fat embolism typically develops pulmonary interstitial edema. This places the patient at a high risk for:

A. Pneumonia
B. Chronic obstructive pulmonary disease (COPD)
C. Sepsis
D. Acute respiratory distress syndrome (ARDS)

69. Which of the following cutaneous findings is a sign of fat emboli?

A. Hives
B. Petechiae
C. Purpura
D. Rash

70. A nurse is precepting a new hire to the trauma ED. The team receives a patient with signs of compartment syndrome. The experienced nurse questions the new orientee about the care for this patient. Which of the following statements from the orientee would reveal an opportunity for further education about compartment syndrome and the management of care?

A. "We need to elevate the extremity."
B. "We need to remove any constrictive clothing."
C. "The physician should remove constrictive casts."
D. "The extremity should be in a neutral position."

71. The trauma nurse in the ED receives an amputated extremity from the paramedics for a patient who was in a motorcycle collision. What is the proper way to handle an amputated extremity in the ED?

A. Wash with hypertonic solution.
B. Wrap in penicillin-moistened sterile gauze.
C. Use iodine on the severed injury.
D. Place extremity directly on ice or dry ice.

72. There are three major classifications for amputation injuries. Which of the following is the injury that can best be described as a result of forceful stretching and tearing away from tissue?

A. Guillotine
B. Avulsion
C. Crush
D. Cut

73. A 65-year-old patient comes to the ED with a severed finger from a knife incident while cooking. Blood pressure is 92/60 mmHg, heart rate is 98 beats per minute, respiratory rate is 22 breaths per minute, and oxygen saturation is 96% on 2 L via nasal cannula. The bleeding has stopped, and a moist dressing is placed on the site. The amputated extremity was kept cool on ice prehospital. Which of the following is the most accurate statement?

A. A finger is not a functional requirement and need not be reimplanted.
B. Fingers are good candidates for reimplantation.
C. Hands are more commonly reimplanted than a finger.
D. Finger reimplants have a high failure rate because of loss of tissue.

74. A patient suffered a guillotine-style bilateral hand amputation from a factory injury involving heavy machinery. The patient is a strong candidate for reimplantation because of the functional need of the extremity. Which of the following is typically considered an indication for reimplantation because of the function of the extremity?

A. Nondominant hand
B. Thumb
C. Fifth digit of hand
D. Sites distal to proximal interphalangeal

75. A burn patient is being resuscitated according to the Parkland formula and is determined to require 14,000 mL of fluid resuscitation within 24 hours. How much fluid should be administered in the first 8 hours?

A. 7,000 mL
B. 3,500 mL
C. 14,000 mL
D. 4,666 mL

76. A patient was struck by lightning. The patient was stabilized and has been in the ICU for 24 hours. Fluid resuscitation remains in progress, and strict input and output monitoring has been ordered. The nurse notes dark, pigmented urine. Which of the following would apply to this situation?

A. Keep the urine output at 75 to 100 mL/hr.
B. Keep the urine output to at least 30 mL/hr.
C. Keep the urine output at 100 to 150 mL/hr.
D. Keep the urine output at 150 to 200 mL/hr.

77. The management of a partial amputation differs somewhat from a complete amputation. The proper treatment for a partial amputation includes all but which of the following?

A. Splint the attached part.
B. Apply saline-moistened sterile dressing.
C. Place the amputated portion on ice.
D. Perform pulse oximetry on distal extremity.

78. A patient was struck by a car while riding their bike. One foot has been severed from the leg. They are brought into the ED with their foot preserved by paramedics. However, the patient is bleeding profusely, the posterior tibial artery has been severely damaged, and there is significant tissue loss. Which of the following is the most accurate statement?

A. Lower extremities are considered essential and are reimplanted in the majority of patients.
B. Significant tissue loss due to vascular injury may prevent the reimplantation of the lower extremity.
C. Loss of sensation to the reimplanted foot does not affect the ability to ambulate.
D. Limb length discrepancies should not affect the decision to reimplant the lower extremity.

79. The nurse received a patient postreimplantation of the thumb. The digit's color becomes bluish and cool to touch and has brisk capillary refill. The nurse notifies the surgeon. What would the trauma nurse expect the surgeon to order?

A. Lowering of the extremity
B. Medicinal leech therapy
C. Surgical revascularization
D. Antiplatelet medication

80. A patient presents with cyanide poisoning after being exposed to burning plastics in a house fire. The patient is confused and dizzy and is complaining of a headache. The patient's respiratory rate is 32 breaths per minute, pulse oximetry is 94% on a non-rebreather face mask, and heart rate is 121 beats per minute. Which of the following is the most appropriate intervention in this patient?

A. Initiate bilevel positive airway pressure.
B. Intubate and place on high levels of positive end-expiratory pressure.
C. Administer sodium nitrate.
D. Administer sulfur nitrate.

81. The initial treatment for a patient who experienced an electrical burn should ensure adequate ventilation and intravenous fluid administration. What will the nurse anticipate?

A. Maintaining fluid intake at "to keep open" rate to prevent overload
B. Administering 2-L fluid bolus followed by an infusion of 100 mL/hr for 24 hours
C. Administering fluid to maintain a urine output of 75 to 100 mL/hr
D. Administering fluid at a rate of 4 mL/kg/body surface for 24 hours

82. An electrical burn patient has been stabilized and transferred to the ICU for further monitoring. The patient is lethargic but hemodynamically stable. After 6 hours, the patient is more alert, remains hemodynamically stable, and has clear, amber urine. The nurse decreases the intravenous fluid administration as ordered. How much urine output should be maintained for this patient?

A. 1.5 to 2 mL/kg/hr
B. 30 mL/hr
C. 0.5 to 1 mL/kg/hr
D. 50 mL/hr

83. In instances of burn trauma, infants and young children are recommended to receive 4 mL of intravenous solution multiplied by their body weight in kilograms multiplied by the percentage of the total body surface area burned. An 18-month-old has been burned by a pot of boiling water. The infant weighs 10 kg and has burned 18% of the body surface area. How should the fluid resuscitation be administered?

A. 360 mL of lactated Ringer's followed by 360 mL of 5% dextrose normal saline
B. 720 mL of lactated Ringer's along with 5% dextrose at 45 mL/hr
C. 360 mL of normal saline followed by 360 mL of 5% dextrose
D. 720 mL of normal saline along with 720 mL of 5% dextrose normal saline

84. Which of the following is a recommended measure that the nurse can take to aid in temperature regulation in a burn patient?

A. Applying ice to burn sites
B. Applying cool dressing to the burn
C. Increasing the room temperature to 86°F
D. Applying topical lidocaine to the burn

85. Which of the following mechanisms of injury would result in an inhalation injury below the level of the glottis?

A. Direct thermal injury
B. Chemical exposure
C. Superheated air
D. Steam inhalation

86. Patients with surface burns involving phenol contamination should be treated with attention to other capacities that can be affected by this substance. Which of the following levels should be evaluated?

A. Serum calcium
B. Blood urea nitrogen
C. Myoglobin
D. Serum bicarbonate

87. The ICU is precepting a new orientee to the burn unit. The preceptor asks the orientee to tell her about some complications commonly experienced by burn patients. Which of the following answers would be the most accurate?

A. Hypokalemia
B. Pulmonary edema
C. Hyperthermia
D. Hypernatremia

88. A 3-year-old patient comes to the ED with burn injuries to bilateral feet. When obtaining the history, the nurse discovers that the patient obtained these burns when getting into a bathtub that was filling up with hot water. What would be the recommendation to the parents regarding this situation?

A. The water heater at home should be set below 120°F.
B. The water temperature should be tested before the child gets into the bathtub.
C. A thermometer should be placed in the bathtub.
D. Safety mechanisms should be placed on the hot water tap in the bathtub.

89. Following a burn, alteration in capillary permeability occurs. All of the following are appropriate nursing interventions for this patient except:

A. Administer lactated Ringer's or normal saline boluses.
B. Position the patient in reverse Trendelenburg position.
C. Administer blood transfusions.
D. Position the patient with the legs elevated.

90. An electrical injury was sustained by a 14-year-old patient at home through an electric socket, which is an alternating-current electrical injury. Which of the following statements is true regarding this type of injury?

A. A direct-current injury causes tetany.
B. An alternating-current injury is more dangerous than a direct-current injury.
C. A direct-current injury is the most dangerous injury.
D. An alternating current passes in one direction straight through the body.

91. Which statement best describes why a patient reconstructs a traumatic event and tells it repetitively to multiple people?

A. This is a step toward acceptance.
B. The patient is dealing with anger about the event.
C. The patient is wanting sympathy.
D. This allows the patient to tell their version of the story.

92. The goals of resuscitation for a burn patient are to stabilize vital signs, to maintain urine output greater than 0.5 to 1 mL/kg/hr, and to have the patient maintain proper mentation. Which of the following is the best statement regarding the use of intravenous fluids in burn resuscitation?

A. Intravenous fluids should be warmed before administration.
B. Colloid solutions should be used in the initial treatment process.
C. Intravenous fluids should be administered in a central line.
D. Intravenous fluids should be limited to prevent volume overload.

93. There is a point during a prolonged hospitalization stay when the family begins to "pitch in" on the patient's care. Which of the following is the best example of the "pitching in" stage?

A. The family member demonstrates fear of touching the tubing.
B. The family member suctions the patient.
C. The family member performs bathing and skin care only.
D. The family member brings treats for the nurses.

94. A patient has a blood pressure (BP) of 88/64 mmHg, a heart rate (HR) of 126 beats per minute, and a respiratory rate (RR) of 36 breaths per minute in the field following a motor vehicle crash. The paramedics make the decision to transport this patient to a level 1 trauma center. Which of the following criteria is used to make this determination?

A. Mechanism of injury
B. Physiologic considerations
C. Anatomical considerations
D. Special considerations

95. Transfer agreements with other facilities outline treatment and transfer protocols that can accurately address and treat special trauma conditions. Which of the following would not be an appropriate trauma condition to use for a transfer agreement?

A. Burns
B. Amputations
C. Fractures
D. Brain injuries

96. Which of the following statements is most accurate regarding patients with brain death?

A. Patients with brain death can continue to exhibit pupillary reaction to light.
B. Spontaneous motor movement can occur in patients with brain death.
C. The nurse should initiate the conversation of organ procurement with the family.
D. An electroencephalogram can be obtained to determine brain death instead of a bedside evaluation.

97. The family member of a trauma patient makes the following comment to the nurse: "I noticed the heart rate went down to 96 when it once was 113. Is this okay?" Which of the following best describes the need of the family member?

A. Learning
B. Information
C. Vigilance
D. Hope

98. The spouse of a trauma patient is pacing around the room; the nurse enters to speak with them about starting tube feedings. The spouse immediately becomes frustrated and responds, "I don't know what to do, I don't know whether I want them to have a feeding tube, I can't make any decisions right now." What does this best exemplify?

A. Stages of grief
B. Ineffective coping
C. Crisis intervention
D. Stress response

99. Which of the following injuries would indicate the need to limit fluid resuscitation prehospital?

A. Open femur fracture
B. Obvious pelvic fracture
C. Blunt abdominal injury from seat belt
D. Penetrating injury to abdomen

100. Which of the following is required to meet Emergency Medical Treatment and Active Labor Act guidelines when a patient seeks medical assistance?

A. Medical screening examination
B. Surgery to stabilize the patient
C. Obtaining all radiographic studies required for diagnostics before transfer
D. Case management initiation of transitions after acute care

101. How would the nurse best explain the primary difference between occupational therapy (OT) and physical therapy (PT) to the family of a trauma patient?

A. PT is more important during the rehabilitation process.
B. OT and PT work as a team to improve the patient's outcomes.
C. There is no difference between OT and PT clinically.
D. PT primarily works with the legs and OT primarily works with the arms.

102. Which of the following is a common complication that occurs in patients with brain death?

A. Syndrome of inappropriate antidiuretic hormone (SIADH)
B. Cerebral salt-wasting syndrome (CSWS)
C. Diabetes insipidus (DI)
D. Cushing's syndrome

103. What is the overall goal of the Trauma Quality Improvement Program (TQIP)?

A. To collect accurate data from trauma facilities
B. To identify improvement processes
C. To identify medical staff who are making errors
D. To establish benchmark comparisons of trauma centers

104. While reading a research study, the nurse notes that control and experimental groups were used for the study with a hypothesis. Which of the following would best describe the research study?

A. Qualitative
B. Quantitative
C. Retrospective
D. Case study

105. What intervention can be most helpful in supporting staff following a mass casualty event?

A. Involve staff in stress support groups.
B. Use the critical incident stress management (CISM) team.
C. Consult a mental health professional.
D. Involve peer support groups.

106. What is the priority of care for large numbers of contaminated people presenting to the ED with traumatic wounds?

A. Obtaining airways and ventilation
B. Applying pressure bandages to bleeding extremities
C. Performing decontamination strategies before providing care
D. Obtaining two large-bore peripheral intravenous catheters

107. Which of the following best describes the primary goal of rehabilitation following a major trauma?

A. To regain independence and maximal recovery
B. To return to the preinjury level of functioning
C. To return to a productive life
D. To increase the length of life

108. What is the data-collection system that is composed of uniform data elements that describe the injury events, demographics, prehospital information, diagnosis, care, and outcomes of injured patients?

A. National Trauma Data Bank
B. Trauma Registry
C. Action Registry
D. Impact Registry

109. Which of the following research methods will have more biases?

A. Retrospective
B. Prospective
C. Quasi-experimental
D. Experimental

110. During a trauma resuscitation, the physician ordered the massive blood transfusion protocol. The nurse acknowledged the request and informed the team when it had been ordered. What type of communication is this?

A. Repetitive
B. Closed-loop
C. One-way
D. Two-way

111. When the emergency medical services (EMS) crew arrives with a trauma patient, what is the most important task between the EMS crew and the trauma team?

A. Handoff
B. Securing an airway
C. Establishing relationship among teams
D. Positive reinforcement to EMS team

112. Which of the following best describes plans to care for high volumes of patients in an unexpected event?

A. Crisis planning
B. Disaster planning
C. Community planning
D. Hurricane relief center

113. Which of the following statements is an accurate statement about ethical dilemmas?

A. Ethical dilemmas occur because families are not knowledgeable in medical aspects of care.
B. The egos of healthcare clinicians are the cause of ethical dilemmas.
C. Ethical dilemmas exist when two or more unattractive courses are possible but neither is the overwhelmingly rational choice.
D. End-of-life situations are the only ones in the hospital that can cause an ethical dilemma.

114. Which of the following influences the nurse's ethical beliefs?

A. Nothing; ethical beliefs cannot be influenced.
B. The nurse has their own set of beliefs and does not rely on others.
C. The nurse may receive guidance from and be influenced by peers.
D. The nurse is influenced by physicians because they are the decision makers.

115. A patient's neurological assessment reveals bilateral nonreactive pupil dilation, decreased level of consciousness, and a Cheyne-Stokes breathing pattern. The nurse suspects which type of herniation?

A. Uncal
B. Subfalcine
C. Central
D. Tonsillar

116. The nurse is caring for a spinal cord patient. A halo vest is being used to stabilize the injury. What is the most important task to be completed when caring for a patient using a halo vest?

A. Ensure the weights are hanging freely at all times.
B. Ensure that the wrench is taped to the vest.
C. Cut patient hair around the pin sites.
D. Ensure that the liner is applied before the vest.

117. During a resuscitation, the trauma nurse recognizes that the dosage the physician ordered was incorrect. Which of the following would be the best action of the nurse?

A. Continue performing their role in the resuscitation.
B. Distract the team and get the correct dosage to the medication nurse.
C. Stop the resuscitation immediately.
D. Say something to the physician before the drug is administered.

118. A nurse caring for an older adult patient with a very poor prognosis finds that the aggressiveness of the care being provided is against their belief system. Which of the following best describes the nurse's feelings?

A. Moral distress
B. Posttraumatic stress disorder
C. Depression
D. Grief

119. An ethical dilemma regarding removal of life support was brought to the ethics committee. What is the initial step of the process to assist with the dilemma?

A. Collect data.
B. Identify the conflict.
C. Define goals of the outcomes.
D. Identify the ethical principles.

120. A fracture of the anterior vertebrae usually occurs with hyperflexion and axial compression injuries. This injury can also have associated posterior dislocation. This type of fracture is called:

A. Simple
B. Compression
C. Anterior body
D. Burst

121. Which of the following mechanisms of injury would most likely increase the risk of a diffuse axonal injury (DAI)?

A. Penetrating injury
B. Flexion injury
C. Direct blow to the head
D. Rollover vehicle crash

122. A patient presents with an odontoid type II fracture without cord involvement. Which of the following would the trauma nurse anticipate for intervention?

A. Soft-collar application
B. C4–C5 surgical fusion
C. Halo immobilization
D. Traction with weights

123. Which type of incomplete cord syndrome is most commonly a result of hyperextension injuries?

A. Central cord
B. Anterior cord
C. Posterior cord
D. Brown–Sequard

124. Which of the following is the most accurate statement regarding urethral injury?

A. Blunt mechanism of injury most commonly results in anterior urethral injury.
B. Chance of injury is greater in males because the urethra is longer and fixed by a ligament.
C. Urethral injuries are most commonly caused by penetrating trauma.
D. Diagnostic evaluation of the urethra following trauma is best performed with a cystogram.

125. Following a motor vehicle collision (MVC), a passenger who was wearing a seat belt is diagnosed with a bladder rupture. Which of the following would be the most common site of rupture?

A. Anterior portion of bladder
B. Posterior portion of bladder
C. Extraperitoneal bladder
D. Intraperitoneal bladder

126. What is the best way to refer to an avulsion injury of the renal artery?

A. Pedicle injury
B. Extraperitoneal injury
C. Greenstick injury
D. Renal artery dissection

127. Which of the following is the best diagnostic study to evaluate for the presence of a suspected spinal cord injury without radiological abnormalities (SCIWORA)?

A. Angiography
B. Myelography
C. MRI
D. CT

128. Which of the following is the most common mechanism of injury for urethral trauma?

A. Gunshot wound
B. Penetrating trauma
C. Straddle injuries
D. Perineal impalement

129. The patient presents with blood at the meatus following blunt mechanism to the lower abdomen. What would you expect the physician to order to evaluate for associated injuries?

A. CT chest scan
B. Kidney, ureter, and bladder (KUB) x-ray
C. Pelvic x-rays
D. Femur x-rays

130. Which of the following diagnostic examinations is recommended to identify extraperitoneal bladder injuries following pelvic fractures?

A. Intravenous pyelogram (IVP)
B. Cystogram
C. Urethrogram
D. Kidney, ureter, and bladder (KUB) x-ray

131. Which of the following is the gold standard for diagnosing and grading kidney injuries?

A. Kidney, ureter, and bladder (KUB) x-ray
B. CT scan
C. Abdominal ultrasound
D. Cystogram

132. Which of the following is a cardinal sign of kidney and bladder injuries?

A. Microscopic hematuria
B. Pain on urination
C. Anuria
D. Gross hematuria

133. A patient presents in the ED following a motorcycle collision. Upon assessment, it is noted that the patient has blood at the meatus. Which of the following orders would the trauma nurse be most likely expect at this time?

A. Insert Foley catheter.
B. Obtain MRI of abdomen.
C. Prepare patient for suprapubic catheter.
D. Obtain retrograde urethrogram.

134. Which of the following injuries is most likely to require the early placement of a suprapubic catheter to improve healing?

A. Posterior urethral injury
B. Intraperitoneal bladder rupture
C. Extraperitoneal bladder rupture
D. Kidney injury

135. A patient with a body mass index of 39 kg/m^2 presents with shortness of breath following a motor vehicle collision (MVC). Which of the following is the most common contributing factor to increased work of breathing in patients with obesity?

A. Elevated diaphragm
B. Hypercapnia
C. Chronic hypoxia
D. Pneumothorax

136. Which of the following is a more commonly associated pulmonary complication in patients with obesity?

A. Aspiration pneumonia
B. Obstructive sleep apnea
C. Acute respiratory distress syndrome
D. Pulmonary contusions

137. Following a blunt abdominal trauma, the physician orders an intravenous pyelogram (IVP). Which of the following is the physician suspecting?

A. Ureteral injury
B. Urethral injury
C. Duodenum rupture
D. Scrotal injury

138. Which of the following interventions is most likely to be expected if the patient presents with a large segment of ureteral damage?

A. Bed rest for 7 to 10 days
B. Transureteroureterostomy
C. Ureteral stent placement
D. Immediate placement of suprapubic catheter

139. A patient is determined to have a body mass index (BMI) of 38 kg/m^2. What is the BMI classification of the patient?

A. Overweight
B. Class I obesity
C. Class II obesity
D. Class III obesity

140. Which of the following statements regarding mechanism of injury in bariatric patients is the most accurate?

A. Seat belts are often worn correctly, reducing injuries in motor vehicle collisions in patients with obesity.
B. Patients with obesity more commonly sustain facial fractures.
C. A fall is the least common mechanism of injury for patients with obesity.
D. Abdominal stab wounds are typically less serious in patients with obesity.

141. Which of the following is the most accurate statement regarding evidence collection in trauma patients?

A. The patient's belongings can be given to the family because most of the evidence is on the patient's body.
B. Evidence should be preserved and collected for all trauma patients.
C. Only intentional injuries require evidence collection for trauma patients.
D. Evidence should be collected from victims, not from perpetrators.

142. What type of spinal cord injury is more commonly seen in pediatric patients than in adult patients?

A. Anterior cord syndrome
B. Brown–Sequard cord syndrome
C. Spinal cord injuries without radiographic abnormalities
D. Central cord syndrome

143. Blood cultures are positive for gram-negative bacteria in a trauma patient in the ICU. What is the best term for this finding?

A. Bacteremia
B. Septicemia
C. Fungemia
D. Septic shock

144. While managing a trauma patient in septic shock in the ICU, the nurse knows the recommended mean arterial pressure (MAP) is which of the following?

A. Greater than 90 mmHg
B. Less than 80 mmHg
C. Greater than 65 mmHg
D. Less than 60 mmHg

145. Which of the following patients would be at the highest risk for developing a fungal infection in the blood?

A. A pediatric patient with traumatic brain injury
B. A patient experiencing a second episode of infection after being on antibiotics
C. An abdominal trauma patient with bowel rupture
D. A geriatric trauma patient with multiple orthopedic injuries

146. In sepsis, due to the overwhelming inflammatory response, the patient begins to release immature white blood cells (WBCs). What are the immature WBCs called?

A. Bands
B. Megakaryocytes
C. Kupffer cells
D. Monoclonal cells

147. A bullet is found in the clothing of a trauma patient during resuscitation. What is the best instrument to use to handle the bullet?

A. Metal forceps
B. Gloved hands
C. Tweezers
D. Rubber-tipped forceps

148. After a multisystem trauma, the patient develops tachycardia, high fever, and increased respiratory rates. Which of the following would be suspected?

A. Hypovolemia
B. Sepsis
C. Pulmonary embolism
D. Pulmonary contusions

149. Which of the following is a common and severe complication of septic shock?

A. Increased intracranial pressure (ICP)
B. Abdominal compartment syndrome
C. Acute respiratory distress syndrome (ARDS)
D. Cardiogenic shock

150. Which of the following is a cardiac effect of sepsis?

A. Hypertrophied cardiomyopathy
B. Decreased ejection fraction
C. Decreased cardiac output
D. Mitral valve insufficiency

151. Catheter-associated urinary tract infections (CAUTIs) are associated with higher rates of morbidy and mortality. Which of the following would be an indication for a urinary catheter to be used in a trauma patient?

A. Urinary incontinence
B. Accurate intake and output in a critically ill patient
C. Diuretic therapy being administered to an awake patient
D. A postsurgical patient

152. Which of the following laboratory values can be used to determine when antibiotics can be discontinued?

A. Prolactin
B. Calcium levels
C. C-reactive protein
D. Procalcitonin level

153. Which of the following protocols, when implemented, can decrease mortality in a hemorrhagic shock trauma patient?

A. Utilization of a 4:1 (packed red blood cell [PRBC]:fresh frozen plasma [FFP]) ratio
B. Delayed resuscitation protocol
C. Initiation of massive transfusion protocol
D. Use of artificial intelligence for determining blood loss

154. Which of the following complications is most commonly associated with large-volume crystalloid resuscitation?

A. Hypokalemia
B. Hypophosphatemia
C. Third-spacing
D. Hypernatremia

155. A male trauma patient is demonstrating signs of severe hemorrhagic shock and will require massive blood transfusions. Which of the following would be acceptable to administer with type and crossmatch for this patient?

A. O positive
B. AB negative
C. B negative
D. A negative

156. When identifying the biomechanics of a traumatic injury, *force* is defined as mass multiplied by what?

A. Size of impact surface
B. Rate of acceleration
C. Body weight
D. Kinetics

157. Which of the following nursing interventions has been found to lower the incidence of ventilator-associated pneumonia (VAP)?

A. Use of saline lavages prior to suctioning
B. Intubation with antibiotic impregnated endotracheal tube
C. Oral decontamination
D. Routine suctioning every 2 hours

158. A patient presents in hemorrhagic shock following a penetrating trauma to the chest. The massive transfusion protocol (MTP) was initiated. Which of the following blood transfusion reactions would be the most common concern?

A. Transfusion-associated circulatory overload
B. Febrile nonhemolytic transfusion reactions
C. Transfusion-related sepsis
D. Transfusion-related hypokalemia

159. When would it be appropriate to use laboratory results to make decisions regarding blood product transfusions?

A. During the resuscitation to direct the transfusions
B. Before resuscitation to determine the amount of transfusion required
C. After major bleeding is controlled
D. Never; labs are not recommended to guide resuscitation

160. Which of the following is considered to be the first step in trauma prevention?

A. Identification of patterns of injury
B. Development of prevention programs
C. Prediction of potential severity of injury
D. Identification of risks for trauma

161. Following a high-profile trauma, the trauma nurses involved were provided with real-time debriefing. What is the best term for this intervention?

A. Extramural trauma education
B. Intramural trauma education
C. Trauma outreach
D. Quality improvement

162. A person drinks alcohol at a party and then becomes involved in a motor vehicle collision on the way home. What is identified as the risk factor for this injury?

A. Environmental factors
B. Agent involved in injury
C. Human factor
D. Social factors

163. The trauma center is focusing on a community that is noted to have a younger population, with a large number of children in grade school or junior high school. Which of the following would be the most appropriate community outreach program to be initiated in this community?

A. Fall prevention
B. Prevention of head injuries with helmets
C. Car seat safety
D. Driver's education

164. Which of the following is the most life-threatening symptom of anaphylaxis and anaphylactoid reactions?

A. Hypotension
B. Loss of consciousness
C. Urticaria
D. Angioedema

165. Which of the following triggers is more likely associated with an immunoglobulin E (IgE) mediated anaphylaxis reaction?

A. Insect stings
B. Use of contrast media
C. Use of angiotensin-converting enzyme (ACE) inhibitors
D. Use of nonsteroidal anti-inflammatory drugs (NSAIDs)

166. In severe anaphylactic shock, which of the following is the first-line drug to manage complications?

A. Calcium channel blockers
B. Corticosteroids
C. Antihypertensives
D. Epinephrine

167. When dealing with trauma outreach programs, how is the focus of the outreach program determined?

A. It is established by emergency medical services.
B. It is determined by the local government.
C. It is based on the preferences of the trauma center.
D. It is based on data analysis of trauma in the community.

168. Following discharge, a trauma patient is having difficulties with postdischarge emotions regarding the trauma. As part of outreach, the trauma center frequently offers what type of program for this kind of patient?

A. Clinic follow-up appointments
B. Psychiatric support
C. Trauma support group
D. Education outreach on trauma prevention

169. Which of the following is most responsible for angioedema present in both hypersensitivity reactions of anaphylaxis and anaphylactoid reactions?

A. Release of catecholamines with the stress response
B. Stimulation of tumor necrosis factor (TNF)
C. Mast cells releasing chemical mediators
D. Triggering of the renin–angiotensin system (RAS)

170. A patient presents to the ED with urticaria, chest tightness, and wheezing. Which of the following would be the highest priority of care for the patient?

A. Blood pressure management
B. Airway protection
C. Isolation of the patient
D. Transferring of the patient to higher level of care

171. What is the primary cause of cardiogenic shock?

A. Myocardial ischemia
B. Myocardial contusion
C. Pulmonary embolism
D. Cardiac tamponade

172. A trauma patient requiring a diagnostic contrast study states that they are allergic to contrast agents. What is the best next action?

A. Proceed without contrast agent.
B. Do not perform the diagnostic procedure.
C. Pretreat with corticosteroids and antihistamines.
D. Take the patient to interventional radiology.

173. Although inotropic agents, such as dobutamine (Dobutrex), can increase myocardial contractility in cardiogenic shock, adverse effects may occur. Which of the following is the most significant adverse effect of inotropic agents in cardiogenic shock?

A. Tachycardia
B. Increased myocardial demand
C. Arrhythmias
D. Hypotension

174. Which of the following is the most prominent finding in cardiogenic shock?

A. Tachycardia
B. Low cardiac index
C. Tachypnea
D. Fever

175. Which of the following compensatory mechanisms is activated during hypovolemic shock to improve circulating blood volume?

A. Thyroid stimulating hormone (TSH)
B. Sympathetic nervous system (SNS)
C. Brain natriuretic peptide (BNP)
D. Renin–angiotensin system (RAS)

Trauma Certified Registered Nurse Practice Test Answers

29

1. **B) Epidural hematoma (EDH)**
   EDH is the injury most commonly associated with a coup–contrecoup mechanism. Under the point of impact, the middle meningeal artery is frequently torn, and rapid development of EDH occurs. IVH and hydrocephalus are not commonly associated with coup–contrecoup injury, and retinal hemorrhages are more commonly seen with shaken baby syndrome.

2. **C) Deceleration**
   Deceleration occurs when a moving head hits a stationary object, such as a windshield. This is also called a *direct injury*. An indirect injury is a TBI without direct impact to the head. Acceleration occurs when a moving object impacts a stationary head. *Coup–contrecoup* refers to a bilateral injury, typically from a lateral impact.

3. **C) Chronic traumatic encephalopathy**
   Chronic traumatic encephalopathy is a result of multiple TBIs, which cause changes in concentration and memory, chronic headaches, and mood changes. TBI does not cause hydrocephalus or temporal mesial atrophy. Chronic subdural hematomas are more likely to occur in the older adult population.

4. **A) Retinal hemorrhages**
   Shaken baby syndrome is also called *abusive head trauma*. The violent shaking of the infant causes bilateral subdural hematomas, retinal hemorrhages, and cerebral edema. Cerebral contusion is not a common complication unless the head impacts an object. Cerebellar hematomas and locked-in syndrome are typically due to strokes and are not associated with shaken baby syndrome.

5. **B) Middle meningeal**
   The middle meningeal artery is most commonly lacerated in blunt trauma to the head, causing the development of an EDH. The carotid artery and vertebral artery are more commonly involved with dissections following trauma but do not produce EDH. The middle cerebral artery is not typically injured with trauma but is involved in strokes.

6. **D) Beta-2 transferrin**
   Beta-2 transferrin is a variant of transferrin and is used as an endogenous marker for CSF in bodily fluids, including nasal drainage. It is the most specific test for CSF. D-dimer is used to assist with identifying venous clots such as venous thromboembolism. IgG and Hgb levels are not indicated to identify the presence of CSF in body fluids.

7. **D) Rotational mechanism causing a shearing of the neuronal axons**
DAI is the "shearing" of the axons commonly associated with rotational mechanism of injury. The head impacting a stationary object, such as a windshield, is a direct injury due to deceleration. Tearing of the middle meningeal artery causes epidural hematomas. Neither are considered DAI. Presence of interstitial cerebral edema is called *vasogenic edema;* it is not a traumatic DAI.

8. **A) Vasogenic**
Vasogenic edema is interstitial edema caused by direct tissue injury. Cytotoxic cerebral edema is intracellular edema and is caused by hypoxic and anoxic brain injuries, not direct tissue injury. Vasospasm and basal cerebral edema are not terms that refer to cerebral edema.

9. **C) Basilar skull fracture**
Basilar skull fractures present with bilateral periorbital ecchymosis, called *raccoon eyes,* or bruising on the mastoid process, called *Battle's sign.* Rhinorrhea is another sign of a basilar skull fracture, not the initial injury itself. Depressed skull fracture and cervical fracture are associated with TBI but do not produce bilateral periorbital ecchymosis.

10. **B) BP = 105/64 mmHg**
Hypotension and hypoxia are the two most important determinants of neurological outcomes following TBI. A BP of 105/64 mmHg is borderline hypotension and can cause hypoperfusion to the brain. An HR of 110 beats per minute indicates tachycardia but does not have as significant an effect on the brain. An RR of 20 breaths per minute with an SaO_2 of 95% is normal and does not indicate hypoxia. Typically, supplemental oxygen is not administered unless the SaO_2 is less than 94%.

11. **A) Change in level of consciousness**
A change in level of consciousness (alertness and/or orientation) is the most sensitive sign of an increased ICP. Dilated, nonreactive pupils; bradycardia; and increased systolic pressure with widened pulse pressure can all indicate an increased ICP and possible herniation, but they are not considered early signs.

12. **C) Minor TBI may have transient neurological abnormalities for weeks to months after injury.**
Minor TBI may involve postinjury neurological abnormalities that typically resolve over weeks to months. A GCS score of 9 to 12 would be classified as a moderate TBI. Minor concussion would have a GCS score of 13 to 15. TBI, even minor, does not require a loss of consciousness. GCS scores are used but are not always accurate in defining the severity of a TBI.

13. **A) Dilated ipsilateral nonreactive pupil**
Uncal herniation is a lateral displacement and herniation of brain tissue caused by a unilateral expanding mass. The pupil affected by the herniation is the ipsilateral pupil. It will dilate and become nonreactive. Bilateral dilated and nonreactive pupils can indicate a downward herniation. Pinpoint pupils typically involve the brain stem.

14. B) Hold the next dose of mannitol (Osmitrol) until serum osmolality is less than 320 mOsm/L.

When administering mannitol (Osmitrol), close monitoring of the serum osmolality is recommended, and mannitol (Osmitrol) should be held if the serum osmolality is greater than 320 mOsm/L. This patient's osmolality is 325 mOsm/L. Mannitol (Osmitrol) is administered every 4 to 6 hours; it is not recommended to increase the dose due to serum osmolality. Administering 3% saline would potentially help lower the ICP and would not be held unless serum Na+ is greater than 155 mg/dL. Steroids are not indicated in TBI patients.

15. D) Blood pressure

Opioids can lower blood pressure, which in a TBI can lead to cerebral hypoperfusion and worsening of neurological outcomes. Constipation is also a complication of opioids but does not worsen neurological outcomes. Opioids may cause some pupillary changes and can affect neurological assessment, but do not necessarily worsen neurological outcomes. Serum sodium levels are not affected by opioids.

16. A) Loss of smell

Cranial nerve (CN) injuries can be associated with basilar skull fractures. CN I (olfactory or sense of smell) can be affected if the cribriform plate is fractured. Other long-term complications include effects to CN II (optic), with unilateral blindness and pupillary changes, and to CN VII (facial) with asymmetry of the face.

17. D) Antegrade

Antegrade amnesia is the inability to create new memories after the injury, even after the patient has regained consciousness. Retrograde amnesia is the loss of memories before the traumatic event. Posttraumatic amnesia is the loss of memory from the time of unconsciousness until the first memory after the event. Transient global amnesia is not associated with trauma.

18. C) 50

CPP is calculated by subtracting the ICP from the MAP. An MAP of 70 minus an ICP of 20 is a CPP of 50 mmHg. The goal is to maintain CPP at greater than 60 mmHg.

19. B) Hyperventilating to partial pressure of carbon dioxide between 30 and 35 mmHg

Hyperventilation is a second-tier intervention to lower ICP in patients refractory to first-line therapy (i.e., hyperosmolar therapy). It lowers ICP by causing cerebral vasoconstriction, thus reducing cerebral blood volume. It is not considered a first-line therapy because of the decreased cerebral blood flow that can result in hypoperfusion. Steroids, including high-dose steroids, are not indicated in TBI patients. Preventing hypotension and maintaining normal cerebral perfusion pressure is appropriate, but elevating systolic blood pressure to greater than 200 mmHg is not indicated and may worsen cerebral edema. Hyperosmolar therapy will probably continue, but other therapies should be added to manage refractory increased ICP.

20. **D) Placing the gastric tube orally**
Any gastric or endotracheal tube requiring placement should be placed orally, never by the nasal route. During nasal insertion, the tube can enter the cribriform fracture and end up in the brain. If rhinorrhea is present, place gauze below the nose to determine the amount of drainage, but never pack the nose in patients with cerebrospinal fluid leaks. Bilevel positive airway pressure should be avoided in patients with basilar skull fractures because air could be forced up into the cranium (i.e., pneumocephalus).

21. **B) Corneal abrasion**
Corneal abrasion is a type of ocular injury that can be associated with a coup traumatic brain injury. Symptoms include ocular pain, a feeling that there is something in the eye, tearing, redness, sensitivity to light, blurred vision or loss of vision, and headache. Subconjunctival hemorrhage is a broken blood vessel in the eye that causes the area to appear bloody. This is not one of the patient's presenting symptoms. Choroidal hemorrhage is bleeding into the suprachoroidal space or within the choroid and is caused by the rupture of choroidal vessels. Choroidal hemorrhage and retinal necrosis present with a red, bloody eye; periorbital pain; decreased vision or decreased color vision; and reports of the appearance of "floaters."

22. **A) Tube cannulation for 3 to 6 months**
A dacryocystorhinostomy involves a silastic tube used to cannulate and repair a lacrimal duct injury. It typically remains in place for 3 to 6 months after injury. Disruption of the lacrimal duct leads to epiphora, or tear overflow, and usually requires repair. Removal of the duct is not recommended. Bypass is not a procedure used for parotid ductal repair, and parotid duct injury is not typically self-limiting.

23. **A) A light semi-pressure dressing is applied to the eye.**
Patients with corneal abrasions should have a light, semi-pressure dressing applied. The dressing should not compress the eye too firmly, just enough to keep the eyelid from blinking. Too much pressure on the eye causes central retinal artery occlusion. The dressing should be taped from the forehead to the cheeks. Some abrasions require instillation of antibiotic eye drops to prevent infection of the epithelium, but treatment does not typically involve oral antibiotics for 14 days.

24. **B) Base**
Bases (alkali) penetrate deeper and cause more injuries than acids. Acids can cause denaturation and precipitation of proteins within the cornea and sclera. This type of injury rarely penetrates the anterior chamber. Neutrals should not cause injury as acids and bases do, and corrosives are not recognized as causing a type of chemical burn.

25. **C) CT**
CT scans have replaced plain films as the gold standard because they are capable of three-dimensional reconstruction capabilities of axial sections. Angiography is considered with evaluation of massive facial trauma if there is suspicion of an injury to a major vessel at the base of the skull, lateral pharyngeal space, and cavernous sinus. It is not a gold standard for all facial injuries. Oral contrast studies are used to identify injuries to the pharynx and the esophagus, not facial fractures and injuries.

26. **A) Open-globe injury**
Assessing for extraocular eye movements should be avoided in an open-globe injury. Motility of the eye and any pressure applied to the globe can result in the loss of vision. These injuries are serious and frequently require emergency ocular surgery. Hyphema (accumulation of blood in the eye), chemical burns to the eye, and orbital fractures all require a full ocular assessment, including eye motility.

27. **D) Forceps used to grab the rectus muscle and rotate the globe in all directions**
Forced duction tests may be used to evaluate the presence of ocular muscle entrapment. This is done to distinguish between a muscle paralysis and a mechanical restriction. The procedural steps include instilling a local anesthetic, using forceps to grab the inferior rectus muscle, and then rotating the globe in all directions to assess motion. Oral antibiotics and nasal decongestants are frequently administered after orbital fracture reconstruction. Orbital fractures typically require reconstruction of the orbital floor and medial wall with titanium mesh, synthetic orbital plate constructs, or bony grafting. Needle decompression of the ocular muscle is not an appropriate assessment or treatment of this injury.

28. **B) Corneal infection**
Corneal infection is a complication of corneal injury or abrasions. Symptoms are increased eye pain and an enlargement of the gray area on the corneal surface. If a foreign body is left in the eye and not removed, it becomes a nidus of infection. Conjunctivitis and conjunctival infection are bacterial or viral infections in the eye, usually presenting with symptoms of pink eye. Corneal abrasion is most likely involved with this injury, and the patient is complaining of pain, which is a symptom of a corneal abrasion, but the symptom of a gray area on the corneal surface indicates corneal infection.

29. **D) Naso-orbital-ethmoid injury**
Naso-orbital-ethmoid injury presents with a depressed-nose profile and a widened, flattened, frontal view of the nose. *Telecanthus* is the term used for the illusion of the eyes being farther apart. This is typically seen with a naso-orbital-ethmoid injury, but it is a symptom of injury rather than an actual type of injury. Nasal fractures usually present with a deformity that is not as distinguished as in a naso-orbital-ethmoid injury. An ethmoid fracture is part of this injury, but the symptoms this patient presents with demonstrate the involvement of the nasal and orbital bones as well.

30. **B) Orbital blowout fracture**
An orbital blowout fracture is a fracture of the orbital walls without associated fractures of the orbital rims; it can cause entrapment of the inferior or medial rectus muscle, thereby restricting extraocular movements. A zygomatic fracture will have periorbital ecchymosis, but extraocular eye movements are not usually affected. A LeFort I fracture is a horizontal fracture through the maxillary body; it does not affect extraocular movements.

31. **A) Arteriogram**
An arteriogram should be considered following fracture of ribs one through three because the force of impact and the vascular structures underlying those ribs can result in significant arterial injuries, including damage to the subclavian artery or vein. Coronary arteries are less likely to be injured, and a CT coronary angiogram would not be routinely ordered. Barium swallow and bronchoscopy would not be indicated for this patient.

32. B) Hyphema

A hyphema is a pooling or collection of blood inside the anterior chamber of the eye. Opacification of the globe is commonly a result of an alkali chemical injury to the eye and is not associated with ocular fractures. Opacification can occur with traumatic exposure but is not associated with orbital fractures. Vitreous hemorrhage is the extravasation of blood into the areas in and around the clear gel that fills the space between the lens and the retina of the eye (i.e., the vitreous). The blood may cover most or all of the iris and the pupil, blocking vision partially or completely. It is usually painful. Optic nerve injury does not involve appearance of blood in the eye.

33. A) Aortic dissection

Fracture of the sternum requires a great force of impact and is associated with significant intrathoracic injuries, such as myocardial contusion and aortic dissection. The trauma nurse should be aware of the correlation between the sternal fracture and significant intrathoracic injuries, which may be life-threatening. Rib fractures can cause splenic or liver laceration, but this is not considered a thoracic injury. Diaphragm injury can be associated with blunt chest trauma but is not as life-threatening as an aortic dissection.

34. C) Level of the isthmus

The most common mechanism of injury for a thoracic aortic transection is a sudden deceleration mechanism of injury. The ligamentum arteriosum secures the aorta near the aortic arch, called the *level of the isthmus.* During a sudden deceleration, the aorta moves except at the point of the ligament, causing a transection at that level.

35. A) Persistent pneumothorax

Injury above the level of the carina can result in a delayed presentation, such as unresolved or persistent pneumothorax, even after placement of a thoracostomy tube. Hemothorax and decreased lung compliance are not signs of bronchial injury. Management of bronchial injuries may require intubation past the site of injury and is not typically recognized due to a cuff leak on an endotracheal tube.

36. B) Widened mediastinum

Widened mediastinum, loss of aortic knob, and presence of left apical cap are common findings indicating the presence of aortic transection. Hemothorax can be caused by injury to other vessels besides the aorta. Enlarged cardiac silhouette would be more indicative of pericardial tamponade. Kerley B lines are found in pulmonary edema.

37. B) Bronchoscopy

An injury above the level of the carina may not demonstrate mediastinal air on chest radiograph. The most definitive diagnosis is with a bronchoscopy. Sputum culture or tracheal pressures would not assist with the diagnosis of bronchial injury.

38. D) The left side is more commonly injured.

The majority of diaphragm injuries from blunt trauma occur on the left side. The most common blunt injury is large posterior lateral tears on the left diaphragm. The right diaphragm may be more protected by the liver and requires a greater force of impact to injure, thus resulting in higher mortality. Penetrating injuries can occur but are less common than blunt injuries. Presentation may be delayed with gradual herniation of stomach or intestines over weeks after the injury. It does not result in immediate loss of diaphragm movement.

39. D) Internal mammary artery
Hemothorax is most commonly caused by lung parenchymal lacerations, injuries to intercostal vessels, and injuries to the internal mammary artery and pulmonary arteries. Aortic and subclavian arterial injuries can cause hemothorax but are not as common a cause as internal mammary arterial injury. Coronary artery laceration is less likely to result in hemothorax.

40. C) CT
The most prominent feature found on a chest radiograph is elevation of the hemidiaphragm and potentially a bowel pattern in the chest. Chest x-ray and ultrasonography may identify large diaphragmatic injuries but frequently miss smaller defects. CT or MRI are more sensitive in evaluating for injuries or obtaining better visualization of the anatomy of the thoracic structures.

41. C) Cardiogenic
Myocardial contractility is affected following blunt chest trauma and cardiac contusions. There is a decrease in myocardial contractility with compensatory tachycardia similar to cardiogenic shock. Even though it is a contusion of the myocardium, the amount of blood loss is not significant enough to cause hemorrhagic shock.

42. B) 1,500-mL chest tube output after insertion
A hemothorax with greater than 1,000 to 1,500 mL of blood on the initial insertion of a chest tube or greater than 200 mL/hr of blood for 4 hours after insertion indicates the need for a thoracotomy. A tension pneumothorax requires emergency placement of a thoracostomy tube. Patients with blunt chest injuries presenting with cardiac arrest are not likely to survive, even with a thoracotomy. Sternal fractures do not require emergency thoracotomy.

43. C) Spleen
Common organs injured by blunt mechanism are the solid organs such as the spleen, liver, and pancreas. Hollow organs, such as the colon, stomach, and small bowel, are able to collapse during the increased pressure, which reduces the risk of injury.

44. B) Shortness of breath
A missed occult injury to the diaphragm may have a delayed presentation of shortness of breath due to herniated stomach or bowel into the thoracic cavity. Delayed diaphragmatic symptoms do not present as hemorrhage; a delayed splenic injury will. Pulseless electrical activity can be a result of hypovolemia or pericardial tamponade. It is not due to diaphragmatic injury. Elevated lipase and amylase levels lead more often to the diagnosis of pancreas injury.

45. A) Stomach laceration
The stomach is a hollow organ, and lacerations will cause air to be introduced into the abdomen. The liver and spleen are solid organs. Laceration of either of these organs results in the presence of blood in the peritoneal cavity. Aortic transections occur most often in the thoracic cavity and would not result in air in the abdominal cavity.

46. **D) "We might have to place a temporary drain in the area of the pancreas."**
A drain is usually placed for 8 to 10 days until the patient can tolerate feeding without an increase in pancreatic fluid. Pancreatectomies are hardly ever performed. It is possible to survive without a pancreas, but patients are then insulin dependent and require digestive enzymes. Debridement is avoided unless infected necrosis is present because it can potentially induce hemorrhage. Vaccinations are important for splenectomy patients but not for patients with pancreatic injuries.

47. **A) Esmolol (Brevibloc)**
Esmolol (Brevibloc) is a beta blocker that will lower the patient's blood pressure and slow the heart rate. This will lower the risk of the aorta rupturing. Sodium nitroprusside (Nipride) is an alpha blocker. It will lower the blood pressure but can cause tachycardia. The patient is already tachycardic, which can increase risk of aortic rupture. Fluids are not indicated. This patient is hypertensive, not hypotensive. Diltiazem (Cardizem) is used more often as an antiarrhythmic rather than as an antihypertensive.

48. **B) Liver**
The driver's seat belt crosses from the left to the right and buckles across the right upper quadrant where the liver is located. At the time of impact, the seat belt can cause injury to the liver. The passenger is more likely to sustain splenic injury from the seat belt. The bladder is most commonly injured by the lap belt. The pancreas is located in the retroperitoneal area and is less likely to sustain a sea tbelt injury.

49. **A) Shortness of breath**
Bowel can herniate through a diaphragm injury, which can lead to bowel herniation into the thoracic cavity. This leads initially to presentation of shortness of breath. Symptoms of bloody diarrhea, vomiting of blood, and constipation are not early signs of diaphragm injury with herniated bowel.

50. **C) "Two hundred mL of dextrose should be instilled into the bladder before a pressure reading is obtained."**
Always insert an indwelling bladder catheter using sterile technique. The transducer is leveled at the symphysis pubis. The patient should be in a supine position during measurement in order to reproduce and compare readings. Sterilely instill 35 to 100 mL of normal saline before obtaining the reading. Too much water causes bladder distention and an inaccurate reading. A normal bladder pressure reading is between 12 and 15 mmHg, and a reading greater than 20 mmHg may require decompression of the abdomen.

51. **B) Leukocytosis**
Pancreatic trauma is difficult to recognize because of coexisting injuries to other intraabdominal organs and the retroperitoneal location of the pancreas, which makes signs and symptoms less obvious. The triad symptoms of pancreatic injury include midepigastric abdominal pain, leukocytosis, and elevated serum amylase levels. Lactate levels and platelets would not be elevated due to a pancreatic injury.

52. A) Enoxaparin sodium (Lovenox)
Following a splenectomy, the platelet count is typically elevated and can cause a thrombotic event such as a myocardial infarction or deep vein thrombosis. Postsplenectomy patients should be placed on a venous thromboembolism prophylaxis medication such as enoxaparin sodium (Lovenox). Aspirin is considered an antiplatelet, but it is not a therapeutic anticoagulant. Pegfilgrastim (Neulasta) is a medication that would increase the number of WBCs. This would be inappropriate because postsplenectomy patients typically have leukocytosis. For treatment of anemia, a daily dose of folic acid is generally used, but this patient is not anemic.

53. B) Focused assessment sonography for trauma (FAST)
The FAST examination would be the test of choice in pediatric patients with suspected intraabdominal trauma because it provides a rapid evaluation of the abdomen for the presence of fluid. Abdominal distention in a pediatric patient may not always be accurate, especially in a crying patient, because children tend to swallow large amounts of air when crying. CT remains the imaging device of choice to evaluate suspected injuries in pediatric patients, but the FAST examination should be used first to evaluate whether further imaging may be warranted. Peritoneal lavage is not commonly performed in children. A KUB x-ray could be useful, but a CT is preferred if further diagnostic testing is required.

54. C) Carbon monoxide poisoning
Smoke inhalation during pregnancy can cause carbon monoxide poisoning, which can be fatal to the fetus. Carbon monoxide poisoning is most commonly associated with house fires. Maternal burns do not necessarily place the fetus at risk; it depends on the size and nature of the burn.

55. D) Tilt to left side
If a pregnant patient in the third trimester is lying supine, the enlarged uterus compresses the vena cava and aorta, impeding venous return and cardiac output. The pregnant trauma patient should be tilted to the left side while maintaining spine precautions.

56. C) Thoracostomy tube placement is higher than in nonpregnant trauma patients.
Thoracostomy tubes should be placed 1 to 2 intercostal spaces higher than in a nonpregnant patient. This is due to the uterus being an abdominal organ that is compressing the diaphragm upward. Vasopressors actually decrease fetal perfusion. Positioning should be titled left lateral. Airway management is more difficult in pregnant trauma patients and should be secured early.

57. B) Liver injury
A forceful injury may result in injury to underlying organs without any evidence of rib fracture because in children the chest wall is more pliable, and the liver lies more anteriorly with less protection by the ribcage. Cardiac injury and renal injury are unlikely based on where the child was struck. However, renal injuries in children are common because of the lack of fat protection around the organs. A lung contusion is possible, but the liver is more likely to be damaged in this particular situation.

58. **A) Positive Saegesser's sign**
A positive Saegesser's sign presents with left upper quadrant abdominal pain and radiation to the neck caused by irritation of the phrenic nerve. It is commonly found following splenic injury. This is a serious finding and can indicate a life-threatening hemorrhage. A positive Kehr's sign is pain in the left shoulder while in the supine position after a splenic injury. *Cervicalgia* is a term for neck pain, but in this case the pain is originating in the abdomen, and the nurse should take into consideration the diagnosis of the patient. Kernig's sign is severe stiffness of the hamstrings and an inability to straighten the leg when the hip is flexed to 90 degrees. This is usually seen in patients with meningeal irritation and meningitis.

59. **A) Compensated respiratory alkalosis**
Pregnant patients commonly have partial pressure of carbon dioxide levels of 25 to 30 mmHg with chronically compensated respiratory alkalosis because of chronic hyperventilation. This must be taken into account when interpreting the arterial blood gas. The patient has hyperoxia, not hypoxia. Pregnant patients do not typically experience metabolic acidosis.

60. **B) Fetal heart tones**
Fetal heart tones are used to evaluate the status of the fetus. Abnormal fetal heart tones indicate fetal distress. Pain has been called *the fifth vital sign*, but in pregnant trauma patients, fetal heart tones are the vital signs of the fetus and thus would be considered the fifth vital sign in this situation. Pulse oximetry and capnography may be indicated in individual trauma patients but are not considered a fifth vital sign.

61. **A) Preeclampsia**
Preeclampsia is a pregnancy complication usually beginning after 20 weeks' gestation and characterized by high blood pressure in a patient whose blood pressure had been previously normal. Patients commonly complain of headache, blurred vision, and epistaxis. Eclampsia is the onset of seizures in a patient with preeclampsia. Pregnant patients are usually hypervolemic because blood volumes increase by week 10 of pregnancy; this does not account for the symptoms this patient has developed. HELLP (Hemolysis, Elevated Liver enzymes, and Low Platelets) syndrome involves elevated liver enzymes and thrombocytopenia.

62. **A) Kleihauer–Betke (KB) test**
The KB test is important for this particular patient because the patient is Rh negative. The KB test detects fetal red blood cells in maternal circulation; the need for Rh immune globulin therapy is imperative. A beta HCG test is not important because the trauma team already knows that the patient is 32 weeks' pregnant. PT and PTT and hemoglobin and hematocrit are significant in a bleeding patient and should be drawn as well, but because the patient is Rh negative, the KB test is indicated for accurate treatment.

63. **B) Open-book pelvic fracture**
Open-book pelvic injury occurs when the front of the pelvis opens like a book; this injury results in damage to pelvic ligaments that hold the pelvic bones together. Subtrochanteric fracture is a fracture of the proximal femur, which is categorized as a hip fracture, not a pelvic fracture. A straddle injury is an injury to the bilateral pubic rami that occurs when a person falls while straddling an object. It is associated with urethral and bladder injuries. Vertical shear pelvis injury occurs when one half of the pelvis shifts upward.

64. A) Productive cough with coarse crackles

A patient with a fat embolus presents with a productive cough and coarse crackles because of the inflammation and the fluid leakage into the alveoli, which cause the alveoli to fill with fluid. A dry cough with scattered rhonchi would indicate a patient with asthma, bronchitis, or pneumonia. Productive cough with diminished breath sounds could belong to multiple diagnoses, including pneumonia. Dry cough with inspiratory wheezes is usually identified in asthma patients.

65. A) Pain

Pain is the most sensitive indicator of compartment syndrome because it is known to be reported as out of proportion to the injury and is not relieved with analgesic medication administration. Paresthesia would be the second most sensitive sign, followed by pulselessness and paralysis together, which are strong indications for compartment syndrome.

66. B) Reperfusion injury

Reperfusion injuries to muscle occur when there is an increased blood flow to the muscle following a period of ischemia, resulting in the washout of lipid-soluble intracellular metabolites. These metabolites can cause further injury called *reperfusion injury*. Inadequate decompression is a complication of a fasciotomy. Volkmann's contracture is a complication of untreated compartment syndrome. Hypoperfusion occurs during compartment syndrome but is not associated with an increased blood flow.

67. A) At the level of the greater trochanters

To provide adequate stabilization of the pelvic binder, it should be placed at the level of the greater trochanters. The binder should not be placed over the iliac crest or the abdomen. Application of a pelvic binder above the level of the greater trochanters is an inadequate method of reducing pelvic fractures and is likely to delay cardiovascular recovery.

68. D) Acute respiratory distress syndrome (ARDS)

Fat emboli occur when fat globules are filtered out of the pulmonary system and obstruct at the pulmonary capillary level. This causes release of oxygen free radicals, increased capillary permeability, vasodilation, and pulmonary interstitial edema, which leads to ARDS. ARDS is inflammation that occurs throughout the lungs. In the lung tissue, tiny blood vessels leak fluid, and alveoli collapse or fill with fluid, which prevents adequate oxygen exchange. The development of pneumonia would require an infectious source, such as bacteria. COPD is a progressive respiratory disease that makes it harder to breathe over time. Sepsis would need a source of infection and by itself does not result in pulmonary edema.

69. B) Petechiae

Appearance of petechiae usually occurs on the upper trunk, axilla, chest, conjunctiva, and mucous membranes. This is because the embolization of small dermal capillaries leads to extravasation of erythrocytes, which produces a petechial rash in these areas. Petechiae do not commonly appear on the upper extremities with fat emboli. Hives, purpura, and rash are not commonly found with fat emboli.

70. A) "We need to elevate the extremity."
Elevating the extremity would decrease perfusion and would not promote adequate circulation to the extremity with compartment syndrome. Instead, it is important to maintain the extremity in a neutral position and remove constricting clothing, casts, or dressings that may be present to correct management of an extremity with suspected compartment syndrome.

71. B) Wrap in penicillin-moistened sterile gauze.
Initial emergency care for an amputated body part in the ED includes rinsing with isotonic solution, wrapping in sterile gauze or moistening with aqueous penicillin, wrapping in a moist sterile towel, placing in a plastic bag, and then placing on crushed ice. Do not freeze the part by directly placing it on ice or adding coolants like dry ice. Never float the part in a bag of solution, and do not use antiseptics, hydrogen peroxide, or iodine.

72. B) Avulsion
An avulsion injury is a result of a forceful stretching, twisting, or tearing away of tissue and bone, resulting in an amputation. A cut or guillotine type of amputation has well-defined edges. A crush amputation involves more soft-tissue damage of the amputated part.

73. B) Fingers are good candidates for reimplantation.
Choices between amputation and reimplantation are usually based on clinical presentation and the limb involved. Fingers have less muscle and more tendon, which is less susceptible to ischemia and results in better reimplantation outcomes. Fingers are good candidates for reimplantation and are more commonly reimplanted than hands. Clinical variables include the extent of tissue damage, duration of limb ischemia, hypotension, age (older victims tend to not do well), preservation of protective sensation, and potential of limb length discrepancy and vascular injury.

74. B) Thumb
The occupational and functional value of the digit or extremity is a part of the decision-making for reimplantation. The thumb is important as an opposing digit to allow for activities of daily living. Bilateral hands, multiple digits, dominant hand, and amputation proximal to the most distal interphalangeal are associated with a high occupational value and should be considered for reimplantation.

75. A) 7,000 mL
The nurse should administer half of the total needed fluid in the first 8 hours. The remainder should then be administered over 16 hours. If 14,000 mL are required, 7,000 mL are administered in the first 8 hours and then 7,000 mL should be infused over 16 hours.

76. A) Keep the urine output at 75 to 100 mL/hr.
Urine output should be maintained between 75 and 100 mL/hr with electrical burn patients. If the pigment of the urine darkens as a result of the presence of myoglobin or hemoglobin, this can lead to renal dysfunction and possible renal failure. If the urine does turn dark, then intravenous fluids are typically increased to increase the urine output and flush the toxins.

77. **C) Place the amputated portion on ice.**
Partial amputation occurs when bone, muscle, or ligament remain attached to the body. Partial amputations should be treated as if fully intact and eligible for reimplantation. Partial amputations are managed by splinting the attached part, applying a saline-moistened sterile dressing, applying pressure to control bleeding, and placing oximetry on a distal part to monitor oxygen saturation. A complete amputation would be placed on crushed ice after being adequately wrapped.

78. **B) Significant tissue loss due to vascular injury may prevent the reimplantation of the lower extremity.**
When the continuity of major vessels, such as the sciatic or posterior tibial artery, is damaged, reimplantation becomes less of an option. Lower extremities are not typical candidates for reimplantation because of the risk of two different leg lengths, which would adversely affect the ability to ambulate. The loss of sensation to the sole of the foot because of nerve injury can make the reimplanted foot unable to be used for ambulation.

79. **B) Medicinal leech therapy**
The patient is presenting with a complication of venous congestion following reimplantation of the extremity. The reimplanted extremity appears blue and cool to the touch with brisk capillary refill, and skin turgor is tense. External bloodletting with leeches is a common treatment for venous congestion. Lowering the extremity will increase edema and venous congestion. Revascularization is the therapy for arterial insufficiency, not venous congestion. Antiplatelet medication is the treatment used to decrease arterial blood, not venous congestion.

80. **C) Administer sodium nitrate.**
Management would include using a cyanide kit, which contains amyl nitrate, sodium nitrate, and sodium thiosulfate, not sulfur nitrate. Sulfur nitrate is not indicated. This patient may require intubation but is not at the point requiring a high level of positive end-expiratory pressure. Bilevel positive airway pressure may not be enough ventilatory support for this patient.

81. **C) Administering fluid to maintain a urine output of 75 to 100 mL/hr**
Fluid resuscitation measurements cannot be calculated correctly in electrical burn patients because there is internal damage and equations using the total body surface area burned to calculate fluid administration volume are inaccurate. The fluids should be set at a rate that maintains urinary output of 75 to 100 mL/hr. Administering fluids at "to keep open" rate would result in significant hypovolemia.

82. **C) 0.5 to 1 mL/kg/hr**
After initial stabilization, it is recommended that the urine output in an electrical burn patient, with absence of dark pigmentation, be maintained at 0.5 to 1 mL/kg/hr. For example, a patient who weighs 77 kg should have a urine output of 39 to 77 mL/hr.

83. **B) 720 mL of lactated Ringer's along with 5% dextrose at 45 mL/hr**
Infants and young children should receive crystalloid solution fluid resuscitation using the formula in addition to 5% dextrose at an infusion maintenance rate. Pediatric patients have limited glycogen storage, which is quickly exhausted during early postburn stages; therefore, they require more blood sugar stability than adult burn patients.

84. **C) Increasing the room temperature to 86°F**
Burn patients typically develop poikilothermia, in which they pick up the temperature of the environment. The skin injury results in a loss of heat, so maintaining a room temperature of 86°F assists with the control of normal temperature for the patient. Applying ice to burn wounds is not recommended. Applying a cool dressing to the site within 10 minutes of the burn may be effective because it reduces the heat content and depth of the burn and relieves pain, but it does not aid in temperature regulation of the patient. Topical lidocaine is not recommended on burn wounds.

85. **B) Chemical exposure**
Chemical exposure usually causes an inhalation injury below the level of the glottis as opposed to a thermal injury. Thermal injuries are usually limited to the upper airway. Superheated air causes laryngospasm, which closes the glottis and protects the lungs. Steam inhalation poses greater damage to the upper airway because steam has a greater heat-carrying capacity.

86. **B) Blood urea nitrogen**
Patients with phenol contamination should be treated with copious amounts of irrigation to the site. Absorption of this substance can cause renal damage, so blood urea nitrogen and creatinine levels should be tested. Myoglobin and serum bicarbonate levels are usually monitored in patients with electrical burns. Serum calcium is depleted by hydrofluoric acid chemical burns and is monitored in those exposures.

87. **B) Pulmonary edema**
Pulmonary edema is a complication of burns because of inhalation injury and fluid resuscitation. Hyperkalemia (not hypokalemia) and hyponatremia (not hypernatremia) are common complications because of the fluid shift and capillary leakage. Hypothermia, not hyperthermia, commonly occurs because of the large portion of skin injured, resulting in loss of body heat.

88. **A) The water heater at home should be set below 120°F.**
Setting the water heater at 120°F or below is recommended to avoid burns. Instructing the parents to test the water before the child gets into the tub and to place a thermometer in the water are positive suggestions, but setting the water heater is a safety feature that can prevent additional burns that may be acquired by other water sources in the home. The parents should aim for bath water at around 100°F for children. By prohibiting manipulation of the hot water, safety features for the water faucet only mask the core problem.

89. **B) Position the patient in reverse Trendelenburg position.**
Patients with an alteration in capillary permeability have a fluid volume deficit, so replacing their circulating volume with crystalloid solutions and blood products is warranted. The patient can be positioned with the legs elevated to determine responsiveness to fluid. Placing the patient in reverse Trendelenburg position will decrease venous return and may worsen the hemodynamic status.

90. **B) An alternating-current injury is more dangerous than a direct-current injury.**
An alternating current is more dangerous because it does not travel in one straight direction but can periodically reverse direction, causing the victim's grip to tighten, strengthening the electrical source and lengthening the exposure to the current. The injury was caused by alternating current, not direct current.

91. A) This is a step toward acceptance.
Allowing the patient to reconstruct the event in a trauma situation and to talk to multiple people about the event is part of the movement toward acceptance. Anger is a stage of grief, but it is not expressed in this manner. The reconstructing of the event and telling of the story are done not to get sympathy or to tell their side but to desensitize the event to allow acceptance. The patient may repeat the story or talk about the event repeatedly, and the nurse should listen attentively each time.

92. A) Intravenous fluids should be warmed before administration.
Fluids should be warmed to avoid hypothermia when the capillary leak has been stabilized. Peripheral access is the route preferred over central-line access because of the time requirements and the increased risk of bleeding caused by coagulopathy of a burn patient. Burn patients require fluid resuscitation and should not have limited fluids. Initial resuscitation is typically with crystalloids, not colloid solutions.

93. C) The family member performs bathing and skin care only.
The *hands-off* phase is first. This is when the family is afraid of the environment, such as intravenous lines and monitors. The next phase is *pitching in*, when the family feels comfortable with performing some tasks without the nurse, like applying lotion to skin. Lastly, the *fitting in* stage happens when the family begins to know the nurse, they pick up on the culture of the unit, they assume some of the nurse's tasks, and they bring the nurses treats. Suctioning may be more invasive and would not typically occur until long-term care is needed.

94. B) Physiologic considerations
The four criteria used to make decisions prehospital are mechanism of injury and physiologic, anatomical, and special considerations. Physiologic considerations include BP and RR. This patient's BP was less than 90 mmHg, and the RR was greater than 29 breaths per minute, which meet the criteria to transport the patient to a higher level of trauma care.

95. C) Fractures
Patients with burns, amputations, brain injuries, or spinal cord injuries and specialty populations, such as pediatric or pregnant patients, would all be appropriate candidates for transfer agreements. Fractures can usually be treated at any facility and should not require transfer.

96. B) Spontaneous motor movement can occur in patients with brain death.
Spontaneous motor movement and false triggering of the ventilator can occur in patients with brain death. One of the determinants of brain death is a loss of papillary reaction and reflexes. Initiation of conversations regarding organ donation should be done by the organ procurement agency, not the bedside nurse. An electroencephalogram cannot replace a bedside examination of the patient when declaring brain death.

97. B) Information

The need for information is the number one identified need of the family following a trauma or hospitalization. Asking about labs and vital signs is a frequent occurrence. The nurse should keep the family informed of the patient's status and what is "normal" for the injury. Learning comes with the family being well-informed. Vigilance is also frequently experienced by the family but is not expressed as a need. Family members want to ensure that what is "said" is being done is "actually" what is being done. Hope is something that many families hold onto during a traumatic event, but the top need remains the need for information.

98. B) Ineffective coping

People who have ineffective coping frequently pace, talk fast, exemplify frustration, and are unable to make decisions. They may also have a difficult time using resources and become withdrawn. Stages of grief include denial, anger, bargaining, depression, and acceptance. Crisis intervention is emergency psychological care that occurs in a traumatic situation. The stress responses are the alarm, resistance, and exhaustion phases.

99. D) Penetrating injury to abdomen

Intravenous (IV) fluids should be limited or withheld in the prehospital setting for patients with penetrating trauma to the torso, chest, and abdomen. Administration of IV fluids before definitive treatment of the injuries may increase the blood loss, and the patient may require more blood transfusions. Limiting fluid intake until active bleeding is controlled is recommended. IV fluids in the prehospital setting should be titrated for palpable radial pulse using small boluses of fluid (250 mL). Aggressive rapid fluid resuscitation should not be used in the prehospital setting.

100. A) Medical screening examination

Any patient who comes to the ED seeking medical assistance must be provided with an appropriate medical screening examination to determine whether the patient is suffering from an emergency medical condition. Not all facilities are able to perform the necessary surgeries required to stabilize patients and may need to transfer patients to a higher level of care. Certain radiographs may be obtained prior to transfer to higher level of care but should not delay the transfer. The transferring hospital stabilizes the patient as well as possible within its limits. Case management may assist with the transfer but is not required to initiate transition of care.

101. D) PT primarily works with the legs and OT primarily works with the arms.

PT works with gait and ambulation, whereas OT works with upper extremities, fine motor control, and activities of daily living. Both therapies work as a team, but that response alone does not answer the family's question. Both therapies are very important to the rehabilitation of the patient.

102. C) Diabetes insipidus (DI)

A patient with brain death does not produce antidiuretic hormone (ADH), which results in development of DI. DI results in excessive diuresis from a lack of ADH. Patients with brain death do not release hormones. Patients with SIADH produce too much ADH and would not have brain death. CSWS is more common in patients with subarachnoid hemorrhage. Cushing's syndrome results in overproduction of corticosteroids or adrenocorticotropic hormone, which is not produced by the brain after brain death.

103. B) To identify improvement processes

The American College of Surgeons TQIP works to elevate the quality of care for trauma patients. The goal is to improve the quality of trauma care. TQIP accomplishes its work by collecting data from trauma centers, providing feedback, and identifying opportunities for improvement. The program provides education and training, establishes national comparisons, and facilitates the sharing of best practice. It does improve processes but does not necessarily focus on individual clinicians' care.

104. B) Quantitative

Quantitative research seeks to understand the causal relationship or correlation between variables through testing of a hypothesis. It uses experimental and control groups in the research design. Qualitative research seeks to understand situations within real-world contexts through use of interviews and observation. It does not use a hypothesis or control and experimental groups. Retrospective studies look backward and review situations that have already occurred. This method typically uses chart reviews of large sample populations. Case studies are more often retrospective without the control of a quantitative study.

105. B) Use the critical incident stress management (CISM) team.

The CISM team is beneficial in aiding trauma staff in stress incidents such as mass casualties. This team is usually composed of a mental health professional and peer support personnel. The CISM team is more effective than a support group or turning to other peers for support after a mass casualty event. This team is readily available at the time of the event, whereas consulting a mental health professional would not be an immediate intervention.

106. C) Performing decontamination strategies before providing care

Decontamination of potentially contaminated victims should be a priority before care can be initiated, even though this may delay interventions such as obtaining an airway, applying bandages, or obtaining intravenous access.

107. A) To regain independence and maximal recovery

The primary goal of all trauma patients is to regain independence and to obtain maximal recovery. Following a traumatic injury, the patient may not always return to their prior level of function or become productive, so these are not primary goals of rehabilitation. Rehabilitation's purpose is to improve quality of life, not lengthen life expectancy.

108. B) Trauma Registry

The purpose of the Trauma Registry is to obtain, code, and sort information on trauma events for analysis and to report individual and aggregate results. Registry data is used for performance improvement, medical research, statistical analysis, critical pathways, care coordination, epidemiology, and injury prevention. Registry data then goes to the National Trauma Data Bank and is compiled annually and disseminated in the form of hospital benchmark reports, data-quality reports, and research data sets. Action Registry is a quality-improvement program that focuses on high-risk ST-elevation myocardial infarction and non-ST segment elevation myocardial infarction patients for clinical guideline recommendations. Impact Registry assesses the prevalence, demographics, management, and outcomes of pediatric and adult congenital heart disease patients who undergo diagnostic catheterizations and catheter-based interventions.

109. A) Retrospective

Retrospective studies look backward and review situations that have already occurred. This method typically uses chart reviews of large sample populations. Biases are more common in retrospective than in prospective studies. *Quasi-experimental* and *experimental* are terms for two different types of prospective studies.

110. B) Closed-loop

Once the team leader requests a procedure or action to be performed, the team member should acknowledge the request and confirm once it is completed. This is called *closed-loop communication*. Closed-loop communication allows the team leader to know that their requests have been heard and allows for any clarification by team members.

111. A) Handoff

Handoff is the communication that occurs when one team is handing the patient over to another team for continued treatment. The team leader should listen to the EMS crew to receive information regarding mechanism of injury and prehospital assessment before starting to care for the patient. Airway is a priority but should be established before the handoff. Relationships and positive reinforcement to the EMS team are essential but are not the most important tasks when the EMS crew arrives with a trauma patient.

112. B) Disaster planning

Disaster planning should include plans to care for unusually high numbers of patients in the event of an unexpected surge in volume. Crisis planning is typically directed more toward individual patient management. Community planning is not related to disaster management. Hurricanes are one type of disaster for which a relief center is established to care for those without homes, food, or water.

113. C) Ethical dilemmas exist when two or more unattractive courses are possible but neither is the overwhelmingly rational choice.

Ethical dilemmas exist when two or more unattractive courses of action are possible but neither is the overwhelmingly rational choice. The alternatives are equally compelling, and a moral argument can be made for and against each alternative. Lack of understanding of medical conditions by the patient's family and healthcare clinicians' egos are not the only reasons that ethical dilemmas exist. There are many different ethical dilemmas in healthcare, not just end-of-life decisions.

114. C) The nurse may receive guidance from and be influenced by peers.

Nurses frequently are influenced by and receive guidance from their peers when formulating their ethical beliefs. There are many influences on ethical belief systems and development of personal beliefs, including peers, religion, and family. Physicians may also influence nurses, but not because they are the decision makers.

115. C) Central

Central herniation is a downward displacement of the brain stem that affects respiratory pattern and level of consciousness. Bilateral pupils will enlarge and become nonreactive. Uncal herniation would include ipsilateral dilation of the pupil. Patients with subfalcine herniation complain of a headache and contralateral leg weakness. Tonsillar herniation patients present with headache, stiff neck, and flaccid paralysis.

116. B) Ensure that the wrench is taped to the vest.
Making sure that the wrench is taped to the halo vest is very important to ensure that it can be removed in case of an emergency for chest compressions. A halo device does not involve traction and does not involve weights. Patient hair should be kept short to reduce the risk of its getting caught in the pin sites, and a fleece liner should be in place, but these are not the most important priority when caring for these patients.

117. D) Say something to the physician before the drug is administered.
Speaking up is essential when a team member is concerned or believes an error is about to occur. This ability to speak up without repercussions creates an environment of safety. There are many ways to handle the situation. Stopping the resuscitation could place the patient's life at risk. Continuing one's role and not saying anything also jeopardizes the patient. Distracting the team and administering a different dosage than ordered is practicing outside of the nurse's scope of practice.

118. A) Moral distress
Moral distress is caused when the ethically appropriate action is known but cannot be acted upon. To act against one's own conscience causes feelings of shame or guilt and violates one's sense of wholeness and integrity. These are not signs of posttraumatic stress disorder or depression. The nurse may be grieving for the patient, but moral distress rather than grief is the best and most complete description of the nurse's feelings.

119. A) Collect data.
Data collection includes the gathering of medical facts, including the prognosis, alternatives, and assessment of patient/family knowledge. It is considered the first step in an ethical dilemma. Identifying the conflict involves looking at the values and determining where they conflict or agree and determining who is involved in the conflict. This occurs after the data is collected. Defining the goals of the outcome and identifying the ethical principles to be used are all part of the process but follow data collection.

120. C) Anterior body
A fracture of the anterior vertebral body and posterior dislocation is commonly caused by hyperflexion mechanism of injury. A simple fracture is caused by acceleration or deceleration forces. Spinal cord compression usually occurs as a linear fracture of the spinous or transverse process. Compression fractures occur because of anterior or lateral flexion, hyperflexion, or vertebral body compression. A burst fracture occurs with axial loading and will result in a comminuted fracture of the vertebral body, which can result in a spinal cord injury.

121. D) Rollover vehicle crash
DAI is typically the result of a rollover vehicle crash. This injury results from the brain rotating in the skull, causing a shearing of the axons. Automobile crashes, sports-related injuries, falls, and shaken baby syndrome are other common causes of DAI. A direct blow to the head and flexion injury are less likely to cause DAI. Penetrating injury to the head does not result in DAI.

122. C) Halo immobilization

Halo immobilization is the expected treatment modality to promote healing of the odontoid fracture by limiting C1–C2 rotation. Soft-collar application is not used for an unstable fracture and would not assist in stabilizing a C1–C2 fracture. C1–C2 surgical fusion is necessary in some cases in which nonunion occurs, but halo immobilization is the first-line treatment. Paralysis and, in some cases, death occur in unstable dens fractures with cord involvement. Although a type II fracture is considered unstable, there is no cord involvement.

123. A) Central cord

Central cord syndrome is caused by injuries that result from stretching of the cord and swelling at the central portion of the cord. The mechanism of injury is frequently hyperextension. Anterior cord syndrome usually results from anterior cord compression or disruption of the anterior spinal artery. Posterior cord syndrome also occurs with hyperextension, but this is the rarest of the syndromes. Brown–Sequard syndrome occurs with transverse hemisection of the cord and usually is caused by a penetrating injury.

124. B) Chance of injury is greater in males because the urethra is longer and fixed by a ligament.

Urethral damage is less common in female patients because the urethra is short, mobile, and protected by the symphysis pubis. There is a greater chance of injury in male patients because the urethra is longer and fixed by a ligament. Blunt mechanism of injury most commonly results in posterior, not anterior, urethral injury. Urethral injuries are more often the result of blunt mechanism of injury. Diagnostic evaluation of the urethra after trauma is best performed with retrograde urethrogram.

125. D) Intraperitoneal bladder

MVCs are the most common cause of a ruptured bladder and are associated with full bladders and seat belt use. Compression of a full bladder by the lap belt during a sudden deceleration impact causes the dome of the bladder to rupture into the intraperitoneal, not extraperitoneal, space. Anterior and posterior portions of the bladder are less likely to rupture.

126. A) Pedicle injury

Avulsion of the renal artery and complete loss of blood flow to the kidney is called a *pedicle injury.* The term *extraperitoneal injury* commonly refers to a bladder rupture. Greenstick injuries involve bone fractures, not renal injuries. A dissection is a type of renal artery injury but is not a complete avulsion.

127. C) MRI

MRI has the capability of revealing ligamentous injury, spinal cord injury, and instability, and it provides prognostic information regarding long-term neurological outcomes in patients with SCIWORA. CT does not identify cord injury like MRI does and would not be the test of choice. Myelography and angiography have no defined role in the evaluation of SCIWORA.

128. C) Straddle injuries

Blunt trauma with the mechanism of a straddle injury, which occurs when the bulbous urethra is compressed against the symphysis pubis, is the most common mechanism of injury for urethral trauma. Common causes are motorcycle collision, horseback-riding injuries, and bicycle injuries. Penetrating mechanisms can cause urethral injury, but they are not the most common cause. Penetrating mechanisms include gunshot wounds, stab wounds, self-instrumentation, and perineal impalement after falls.

129. C) Pelvic x-rays

Posterior urethral injuries may accompany pelvic fractures. Blood at the meatus would be a significant red flag for the presence of urethral injury, and pelvic x-rays may be obtained to look for pelvic fracture. Abdominal injuries may be associated with genitourinary injuries, but abdominal CT would be preferred for evaluation over KUB x-ray. Chest injuries and femur fractures are not commonly associated with urethral injuries.

130. B) Cystogram

The majority of extraperitoneal bladder ruptures occur with pelvic fractures. A cystogram is recommended in patients with pelvic fractures because of the high association with bladder injuries. IVP best evaluates the kidneys. Urethrogram evaluates the urethra. KUB x-ray is not the recommended diagnostic radiographic test to evaluate bladder injuries.

131. B) CT scan

A CT scan is the gold standard for evaluating the kidneys following blunt trauma. Abdominal ultrasound has not been found to be accurate in identifying injuries of the renal system. Cystogram is used to evaluate the bladder, not the kidneys. KUB x-ray is not as specific for kidney injury as CT scan.

132. D) Gross hematuria

Gross hematuria is a cardinal sign of kidney and bladder injuries. Microscopic hematuria is not as concerning unless it occurs with the presence of hemodynamic instability. Pain on urination and anuria are more indicative of lower renal injuries.

133. D) Obtain retrograde urethrogram.

Blood at the meatus and a high-riding prostate are commonly associated with urethral injury. The best evaluation of urethral injury is a retrograde urethrogram. Insertion of a Foley catheter is contraindicated when there is blood at the meatus. MRI of the abdomen will not identify urethral injury. Insertion of a suprapubic catheter is a possible later intervention, but it would not be performed at this time. The diagnosis of an actual urethral injury is the first priority.

134. C) Extraperitoneal bladder rupture

The most common management of extraperitoneal bladder rupture is the placement of suprapubic catheter in the acute period. A suprapubic catheter is placed to drain urine and allow the bladder to heal. Intraperitoneal bladder ruptures and kidney injury may require surgical repair.

135. A) Elevated diaphragm

A patient with obesity may have an elevated diaphragm due to abdominal fat pressing up against the diaphragm when the patient is in a supine position. This contributes to increased work of breathing. Patients with obesity may have hypercapnia or chronic hypoxia, but neither of these is the most common contributing factor for increased work of breathing. A pneumothorax may be suspected following an MVC, but elevated diaphragm should be the first suspicion for this patient.

136. B) Obstructive sleep apnea

Obstructive sleep apnea is common in patients with obesity due to oropharyngeal adiposity. It is a risk factor for difficult airway in patients with obesity. Aspiration pneumonia, acute respiratory distress syndrome, and pulmonary contusions can occur in trauma patients with obesity but are not more commonly associated pulmonary complications.

137. A) Ureteral injury

IVP is a diagnostic study used to view the kidneys, ureters, and bladder. Contrast dye is administered intravenously, and consecutive x-rays are obtained to evaluate renal function, including identification of extravasation of dye from the ureteral injury. Urethral injury is evaluated with retrograde urethrogram. IVP is not used to evaluate duodenal or scrotal injuries.

138. B) Transureteroureterostomy

If large segments of the ureters are damaged, a transureteroureterostomy can be performed, in which one ureter is anastomosed to the other. A stent is placed in ureters to maintain alignment, ensure patency during healing, ensure tension-free anastomosis, and prevent urinary extravasation, but it is not indicated if large segments of the ureter are damaged. Bed rest is not indicated for this injury. Placement of a suprapubic catheter may be indicated, but it is not part of the most immediate care.

139. C) Class II obesity

A BMI of 35 to 39.9 kg/m^2 is considered class II obesity. A BMI of 25 to 29.9 kg/m^2 is classified as overweight. Class I obesity is a BMI of 30 to 34.9 kg/m^2, and class III obesity is a BMI of 40 kg/m^2 or more.

140. D) Abdominal stab wounds are typically less serious in patients with obesity.

The anterior fat in a patient with obesity protects the internal organs from injury with stab wounds to the abdomen and lowers the rates of exploratory laparotomies. The weight carried by the patient with obesity may affect gait and stability, leading to increased risk of falls. Lower extremity fractures, not facial fractures, are more commonly associated with patients with obesity.

141. B) Evidence should be preserved and collected for all trauma patients.

All trauma cases are potential forensic cases until ruled out. All nonvehicular trauma should also be considered abuse until ruled out. Both the victims and the perpetrators of violent crimes or accidental injuries should have evidence collected in the ED. In any trauma death, whether the patient is deceased upon arrival or dies in the ED or hospital, the patient's belongings, except for valuables, should not be returned to the family in case the death may require the medical examiner.

142. C) Spinal cord injuries without radiographic abnormalities
Spinal cord injuries without radiographic abnormalities, such as vertebral fractures, are more common in pediatric patients due to size of the head, increased flexibility between the C1 and C2 vertebrae, and poor musculoskeletal support. C-spine x-rays identify vertebral fractures but do not visualize ligaments or cord. Anterior cord, central cord, and Brown–Sequard cord syndromes are not more commonly seen in pediatric patients than in adult patients.

143. A) Bacteremia
Bacteremia is the viable presence of bacteria in the bloodstream, as determined by blood cultures that are positive for bacteria. Fungemia is the presence of a fungus in the bloodstream. An infection, including bacteremia, initiates the inflammatory response and the onset of sepsis. Sepsis presents with clinical signs of an infection. *Septic shock* refers to the presence of hypotension and hypoperfusion despite adequate fluid resuscitation.

144. C) Greater than 65 mmHg
Hypotension in septic shock is defined as an MAP of less than 65 mmHg. The goal in resuscitation of a septic shock patient is to maintain the MAP at greater than 65 mmHg.

145. B) A patient experiencing a second episode of infection after being on antibiotics
Fungal infections are found to cause a second episode of infection. This is due to use of antibiotics in treating the first infection, which alters the normal flora, thereby allowing opportunistic infections to develop. Patients with traumatic brain injuries are not at a higher risk for a fungal infection. Patients with bowel rupture following abdominal injury and geriatric patients with fractures are at a higher risk for bacterial infection, not fungal infection.

146. A) Bands
Bands are immature WBCs. When more than 10% of the circulating WBCs are bands, an overwhelming infection and sepsis are indicated. Kupffer cells are located in the liver. Megakaryocytes are large bone marrow cells. *Monoclonal* refers to antibodies, not WBCs.

147. D) Rubber-tipped forceps
Rubber-tipped forceps are used to handle a bullet in a trauma patient. The use of metal forceps can alter the markings on the outside of the bullet, thereby damaging evidence. Once removed, the bullet should be wrapped in gauze and secured in a container. Minimizing the handling of the evidence also helps prevent contamination of the evidence; even gloved hands can contaminate the bullet.

148. B) Sepsis
Sepsis is the inflammatory response to a known infection and presents with tachycardia, tachypnea, fever, and elevated white blood cells. Hypovolemia presents with tachycardia but not high fever. Pulmonary embolism can present with tachypnea and low-grade fever, but not typically high fever. Pulmonary contusions typically do not present with fevers.

149. C) Acute respiratory distress syndrome (ARDS)

Septic shock can lead to organ failure. Injury to the lungs may result in ARDS. Increased ICP is a complication of traumatic brain injury. Abdominal compartment syndrome is a complication of trauma and third-spacing but not necessarily septic shock. Cardiogenic shock is not associated with septic shock.

150. B) Decreased ejection fraction

Sepsis has a negative contractility effect on the myocardium and results in a decrease in ejection fraction. The cardiac output is usually high in sepsis because systemic vasodilation lowers the vascular resistance. A dilated, not hypertrophied, cardiomyopathy may occur with the decreased ejection fraction. Mitral valve insufficiency is not an effect of sepsis.

151. B) Accurate intake and output in a critically ill patient

Removing the indwelling catheter as soon as possible lowers the incidence of CAUTIs. There are certain circumstances in which an indwelling catheter may be beneficial, including the requirement of accurate intake and outputs in critically ill patients. They may be required for accurate fluid management. External devices can be used if the patient is incontinent. Diuretic therapy does increase urination, but if the patient is awake, they should be able to participate with the use of a bedpan or external device. Not all postsurgical patients require an indwelling catheter, and if the patient comes out of the operating room with one, the goal is to remove it within 24 hours.

152. D) Procalcitonin level

Procalcitonin levels may be beneficial in determining when to discontinue antibiotics, but they are not recommended to be used to determine when to start antibiotics. Plasma C-reactive proteins and prolactin are biomarkers for diagnosis of infection. They may be used as additional information but are not shown to distinguish from infection and other causes of inflammation and are not necessarily used to determine discontinuation of antibiotics. Calcium levels are not used to determine the presence of infection.

153. C) Initiation of massive transfusion protocol

Massive transfusion protocol has been found to decrease mortality and overall use of blood products. The protocol should be available as a written document to all members of the trauma team. The content should be based on the principle of damage control. Older protocols used a 4:1 ratio for PRBC:FFP platelets, but current blood product administration is now recommended at a 1:1 ratio. Delayed resuscitation has been studied, but permissive hypotension is the current recommended practice. Use of artificial intelligence is not a recommended practice at this time for hemorrhagic shock in trauma patients.

154. C) Third-spacing

Large volumes of crystalloids contribute to third-spacing and volume overload complications. Administering universal blood products is the initial resuscitation recommended in massive transfusion protocol over crystalloids, and colloid fluids may decrease the risk of volume overload. Hypokalemia and hypophosphatemia are not commonly associated with volume resuscitation. Hypernatremia can be associated with large volumes of normal saline increasing sodium, but normal saline is not identified as the fluid in this case.

155. A) O positive
O Rh negative is the universally compatible blood type used in transfusions when the patient is not stable enough to wait for the type and crossmatch. O Rh positive can also be used as universal donor blood, except in female patients of child-bearing age, and should be used in male trauma patients. Crossmatched blood should be administered as soon as available. The ideal universal plasma donor is AB.

156. B) Rate of acceleration
Force is mass multiplied by the rate of acceleration or deceleration. A mechanism of injury is the transfer of energy from an external source to the human body. Body weight and size can be considered *mass* in the equation. The size of the impact surface can affect the severity of injury but is not included in the equation for force. *Kinetics* refers to motion and is studied in mechanisms of injury but is not part of the equation.

157. C) Oral decontamination
Oropharyngeal decontamination with chlorhexidine gluconate is a nursing intervention recommended to lower the incidence of VAP. Saline boluses into the endotracheal tube prior to suctioning and routine suctioning have actually been found to increase the risk of VAPs. Intubation is not a nursing intervention.

158. A) Transfusion-associated circulatory overload
Exposure to blood products can place the patient at risk for volume overload and for all blood transfusion complications. One of the most common complications of massive transfusions is volume overload or transfusion-associated circulatory overload. Febrile nonhemolytic transfusion reactions, transfusion-related sepsis, and transfusion-related hypokalemia are complications of MTP but are not as common as transfusion-associated circulatory overload.

159. C) After major bleeding is controlled
Massive transfusion protocol should be continued as long as the patient has an ongoing blood loss. Once the bleeding is controlled or patient is hemodynamically stable, the transfusion process may be changed to one determined by the patient's lab values. During resuscitation, infusion is continued to stabilize the patient hemodynamically. When the patient presents as hemodynamically unstable in hemorrhagic shock, resuscitation should not be delayed while awaiting lab results. Once the patient is stabilized, labs are used to guide resuscitation.

160. D) Identification of risks for trauma
When risks for trauma or injury are identified, then prediction of an injury and prevention are possible. Injuries follow patterns; therefore, they are frequently preventable. Analysis of risk factors leads toward identifying steps that may be used to prevent the injury.

161. B) Intramural trauma education
Intramural education involves continuing education for trauma nurses and is a required metric at all levels of trauma centers. This includes real-time debriefing following a trauma case. Extramural education and trauma outreach involve education in the community for trauma prevention. Real-time debriefing after a high-profile trauma is not an example of quality improvement.

162. C) Human factor

The *human factor* refers to the person's drinking alcohol before driving a motor vehicle. There are several risk factors to be considered for an injury, including the human factor. This is usually the behavior that needs to be modified to prevent an injury. Other risk factors include environmental factors, agents involved in injury, and social factors.

163. B) Prevention of head injuries with helmets

Injury prevention outreach programs should be specific to the community for which they are intended. This community has a large population of children in grade school to junior high school. This age group has a higher risk of traumatic brain injuries from use of bicycles and other activities. This group is older than the age requiring car seats. Fall prevention is typically focused on older adult populations. Driver's education is focused more on those in high school.

164. D) Angioedema

Angioedema can cause the loss of airway from edema and is the most life-threatening symptom of anaphylaxis. Urticaria is a common associated symptom. Sudden loss of consciousness and hypotension can be initial signs of anaphylaxis but are not as life-threatening as angioedema.

165. A) Insect stings

Food sensitivities, insect stings, and use of antibiotics are the most common causes of an IgE-mediated anaphylaxis reaction. Use of contrast media, ACE inhibitors, and NSAIDs may cause nonimmunological hypersensitivities.

166. D) Epinephrine

If hypotension is severe, epinephrine should be administered via continuous infusion. It is an alpha and beta agonist, but it will also decrease the release of mast cells. Antihypertensives and calcium channel blockers are not indicated in anaphylaxis. Patients will be hypotensive, not hypertensive. Corticosteroids are used but would not be the priority medication over epinephrine in severe cases.

167. D) It is based on data analysis of trauma in the community.

Data and quality improvement drive community education. Injury prevention should be specific to the community based on the community's needs and high-frequency trauma. The local government and emergency medical services may assist with providing some of the data to the trauma center, but the data itself should determine the needs of the community for specific trauma prevention programs; the focus of the program should not be based on the preference of the trauma center.

168. C) Trauma support group

A monthly support group for trauma survivors is a form of outreach frequently provided by trauma centers. These support groups provide a place for open communication between trauma survivors to share their struggles and solutions. Support groups would typically be an early offering for the trauma survivor before psychiatric support. Educational outreach programs on trauma prevention would not assist the trauma survivor with learning to deal with a traumatic event. Clinic follow-up appointments are typically done but are not geared toward being emotional support for a trauma survivor.

169. C) Mast cells releasing chemical mediators
Mast cells are activated in both anaphylaxis and anaphylactoid reactions, releasing several chemical mediators. Overall, the mediators increase capillary permeability and cause peripheral vasodilation. The increased capillary permeability can cause airway swelling and angioedema. Catecholamines released as a stress response would cause hypertension and tachycardia, not airway edema. TNF has been found to cause sepsis and septic shock but is not the primary cause of angioedema. Triggering of the RAS will result in vasoconstriction and fluid reabsorption in the kidneys.

170. B) Airway protection
These symptoms would indicate that the patient is probably experiencing anaphylaxis. The most life-threatening complication is loss of airway in anaphylaxis. Hypotension requiring blood pressure management is important, but airway protection is the highest priority. Patients with anaphylaxis do not require isolation. The patient's current symptoms do not indicate the need for transferring the patient to a higher level of care.

171. A) Myocardial ischemia
Myocardial ischemia is the primary cause of cardiogenic shock. Myocardial contusions, pulmonary embolism, and cardiac tamponade can also be traumatic causes of cardiogenic shock but are not the most common cause overall.

172. C) Pretreat with corticosteroids and antihistamines.
Pretreatment can be performed with steroids and antihistamines prior to giving contrast dye to a sensitive patient requiring a diagnostic procedure. Some diagnostic studies can be performed without contrast but may not be as effective in diagnosing traumatic injuries. Even though pretreatment does not guarantee the patient will not have a hypersensitive reaction, it does lower the incidence and severity. Diagnostic studies may be required to identify severe or life-threatening complications and should not be held if needed. Interventional radiology can be used for vascular studies but still use contrast medium for the study.

173. B) Increased myocardial demand
Inotropic agents are frequently needed to increase cardiac index and reduce filling pressures in the right and left ventricles, but they can increase the oxygen demand in the heart with limited oxygen supply in cardiogenic shock. Tachycardia and arrhythmias can be adverse reactions and concerns for the management of the patient, but they are not the most significant concern with cardiogenic shock patients. Hypotension is not a common complication of inotrope use in managing cardiogenic shock.

174. B) Low cardiac index
Cardiogenic shock demonstrates persistent hypotension with severe reduction in cardiac index. This is the most prominent feature of cardiogenic shock. Compensatory mechanisms for low cardiac index include vasoconstriction, which elevates systemic vascular resistance, and tachycardia, which actually worsen the cardiac index because of the high resistance and increased workload of the heart. Tachypnea typically accompanies shock states but is not considered the most prominent symptom in cardiogenic shock. Fevers are not commonly associated with cardiogenic shock.

175. D) Renin–angiotensin system (RAS)
During periods of hypovolemia and hypoperfusion, the kidneys release renin, which converts angiotensin I to angiotensin II. Angiotensin II is a potent vasoconstrictor that shunts blood away from nonvital organs. Angiotensin II stimulates the release of aldosterone, which results in sodium and water reabsorption. This decreases the urine output while increasing vascular volume. The SNS is another compensatory system activated during hypovolemic shock. It results in tachycardia, increased myocardial contractility, and vasoconstriction, but it does not improve circulating blood volume. BNP blocks the RAS and increases urine, thus decreasing circulating blood volume. TSH is not affected by hypovolemic shock.

Bibliography

CLINICAL PRACTICE: HEAD AND NECK

Chen, M., Wang, Z., Fan, Y., Wan, N., Zhang, N., Lin, Q., & Chen, W. (2020). Nursing care of a patient with cervical spinal cord injury without fracture and dislocation: A case report. *American Journal of Nursing Science, 9*(5), 347–353. https://doi.org/10.11648/j.ajns.20200905.16

Compton, E., Smallheer, B., Thomason, N., Norris, M., Nordness, M., Smith, M., & Patel, M. (2020). Minimal risk traumatic brain injury management without neurosurgical consultation. *Journal of Neurocritical Care, 13*(2), 80–85. https://doi.org/10.18700/jnc.200011

Hills, T. (2020). Caring for patients with traumatic spinal cord injury. *Nurse, 50*(12), 30–40. https://doi.org/10.1097/01.NURSE.0000721724.96678.5a

Kamar, N., Choudary, R. S., Malhorta, K., & Kathariy, R. (2020). Maxillofacial nursing: Assessing the knowledge and awareness of nurses handling maxillofacial injuries through comprehensive survey. *Journal of Oral and Maxillofacial Surgery, 19*(1), 136–142. https://doi.org/10.1007/s12663-019-01240-x

Konar, S., Maurya, I., Shukla, D., Prakash, M., Deivasigamani, B., Dikshit, P., Mishra, R., & Agrawal, A. (2022). Intensive care unit management of traumatic brain injury patients. *Journal of Neurointensive Care, 5*(1), 1–8. https://doi.org/10.32587/jnic.2022.00486

Kord, Z., Alimohammadi, N., Mianaei, S., Riazi, A., & Zarasvand, B. (2020). Clinical guidelines for nursing care of children with head trauma: Study protocol for a sequential exploratory mixed-method study. *Pediatric Health, Medicine and Therapeutics, 11*, 69–75. https://doi.org/10.2147/PHMT.S260720

Kovacs, G., & Sowers, N. (2018). Airway management in trauma. *Emergency Medicine Clinics of North America, 36*, 61–84. https://doi.org/10.1016/j.emc.2017.08.006

Li, L., Dilley, M., Carson, A., Twelftree, J., Hutchinson, P., Belli, A., Betteridge, S., Cooper, P., Griffin, C., Jenkins, P., Liu, C., Sharp, D., Sylvester, R., Wilson, M., Turner, M., & Greenwood, R. (2021, March). Management of traumatic brain injury (TBI), a cinical neuroscience led pathway for NHS. *Clinical Medicine Journal, 21*(2), e198–e205. https://doi.org/10.7861/clinmed.2020-0336

Liu, F., Halsey, J., & Oleck, N. (2019). Facial fractues as a result of falls in the elderly: Concomitant injuries and management strategies. *Craniomaxillofacial Trauma and Reconstruction, 12*(1), 45–53. https://doi.org/10.1055/s-0038-1642034

Nowicki, J., Stew, B., & Oi, E. (2018). Penetrating neck injuries: A guide to valuation and management. *Annals of the Royal College of Surgeons of England, 100*(1), 6–11. https://doi.org/10.1308/rcsann.2017.0191

Pan, Y., & Hou, L. (2022). Epidemiological analysis and emergency nursing care of oral and craniomaxillofacial trauma: A narrative review. *Annals of Palliative Medicine, 11*(4), 1518–1525. https://doi.org/10.21037/apm-21-2995

Rutland-Brown, W., Wallace, L., Faul, M., & Langlois, A. (2018). Health disparities and TBI. *Journal of Head Trauma Rehabilitation*, *33*(3), E40–E50.

Simpson, C., Tucker, H., & Hudson, A. (2021). Pre-hospital management of penetrating neck injuries: A scoping review of current evidence and guidance. *Scandinavian Journal of Trauma, Resuscitation and Emergency Medicine*, *29*, 137. https://doi.org/10.1186/s13049-021-00949-4

Tominaga, G., Dandan, I., Schaffer, K., Nasrallah, F., Gawlik, M., & Kraus, J. (2017). Trauma resource designation: An innovative approach to improving trauma system overtriage. *Trauma Surgery and Acute Care Open*, *2*(1), e000102. https://doi.org/10.1136/tsaco-2017-000102

Wang, S., Hong, S., & Tan, J. (2022). Five different lives after suffering from spinal cord injury: The experience of nurses who take care of spinal cord injury patients. *International Journal of Environmental Research and Public Health*, *19*(3), 1058. https://doi.org/10.3390/ijerph19031058

Zrelak, P., Eigsti, J., Fetzick, A., Gebhardt, A., Moran, C., Moyer, M., & Yahya, G. (2020). Evidence based review: Nursing care of adults with severe brain injury. *Clinical Practice Guidelines*, *21*, 684–697. https://aann.org/uploads/Publications/CPGs/AANN20_sTBI_EBR.pdf

CLINICAL PRACTICE: TRUNK

Blank-Reed, C. (2022). Abdominal trauma: Dealing with the damage. *Nursing*, *34*(9), 42. https://doi.org/10.1097/00152193-200409000-00037

Bourke, M. M., & Silverberg, J. Z. (2019, November). Acute scrotal emergencies. *Emergency Medicine Clinics of North America*, *37*(4), 593–610. https://doi.org/10.1016/j.emc.2019.07.002

Canelli, R., Leo, M., Mizelle, J., Shrestha, G., Patel, N., & Ortega, R. (2022). Use of eFAST in patients with injury to the thorax or abdomen. *The New England Journal of Medicine*, *386*(10), e23. https://doi.org/10.1056/NEJMvcm2107283

Jahanshir, A., Moghari, S. M., & Ahmadi, A. (2020). Value of point-of-care ultrasonography compared with computed tomography scan in detecting potential life-threatening conditions in blunt chest trauma patients. *Ultrasound Journal*, *12*(1), 36. https://doi.org/10.1186/s13089-020-00183-6

Jung, P. Y., Chung, J. S., Youn, Y., Kim, C. W., Park, I. H., Kim, O. H., & Byun, C. S. (2022). Characteristics of pediatric thoracic trauma: In view of before and after the establishment of a regional trauma center. *European Journal of Trauma and Emergency Surgery*, *48*, 195–204. https://doi.org/10.1007/s00068-021-01658-4

Lee, R., Gallagher, J., Ejike, J., & Hunt, L. (2020). Intraabdominal hypertension and open abdomen. *Critical Care Nurse*, *40*(1), 13–26. https://doi.org/10.4037/ccn2020772

Ludwig, C., & Koryllos, A. (2017, April). Management of chest trauma. *Journal of Thoracic Disease*, *9*(Suppl. 3), S172–S177. https://doi.org/10.21037/jtd.2017.03.52

Manjunath, A. S., & Hofer, M. D. (2018, March). Urologic emergencies. *Medical Clinics of North America*, *102*(2), 373–385. https://doi.org/10.1016/j.mcna.2017.10.013

Morey, A. F., Brandes, S., Dugi, D. D., III, Armstrong, J. H., Breyer, B. N., Broghammer, J. A., Erickson, B. A., Holzbeierlein, J., Hudak, S. J., Pruitt, J. H., Reston, J. T., Santucci, R. A., Smith, T. G., III, & Wessells, H. (2014). Urotrauma: AUA guideline. *Journal of Urology*, *192*, 327–335. https://www.auanet.org/guidelines-and-quality/guidelines/urotrauma-guideline

Nelson, Q., Leslie, S. W., & Baker, J. (2020). Urethral injury. *StatPearls*. StatPearls Publishing. Retrieved January 2020 from https://www.ncbi.nlm.nih.gov/books/NBK554575/#:~:text=Urethral%20injury%20is%20a%20relatively,bruising%2C%20laceration%2C%20and%20transection

Ntundu, S. H., Herman, A. M., Kishe, A., Babu, H., Jahanpour, O. F., Msuya, D., Chugulu, S. G., & Chilonga, K. (2019). Patterns and outcomes of patients with abdominal trauma on operative management from northern Tanzania: A prospective single centre observational study. *BMC Surgery*, *19*(1), 69. https://doi.org/10.1186/s12893-019-0530-8

Quencer, K. B., & Smith, T. A. (2019). Review of proximal splenic artery embolization in blunt abdominal trauma. *CVIR Endovascular*, *2*, 11. https://doi.org/10.1186/s42155-019-0055-3

Rajkumar, P., Kumar, K., & Deepak, G. (2018). Challenges in management of blunt abdominal trauma: A prospective study. *International Surgery Journal*, *5*(10), 3298–3304. https://doi.org/10.18203/2349-2902.isj20184078

Shimizu, T., Umemura, T., Fujiwara, N., & Nakama, T. (2019). Review of pediatric abdominal trauma: Operative and nonoperative treatment in combined adult and pediatric trauma center. *Acute Medicine and Surgery*, *6*(4), 358–364. https://doi.org/10.1002/ams2.421

Tasneem, B., Fox, D., & Akhter, S. (2021, July 28). Blunt abdominal trauma in the third trimester: Eight departments, two patients, one survivor. *Cureus*, *13*(7), e16688. https://doi.org/10.7759/cureus.16688

Zahran, M. R., Elwahab, A. A. E. M. A., El Nasr, M. M. A., & El Heniedy, M. A. (2020). Evaluation of the predictive value of thorax trauma severity score (TTSS) in thoracic-traumatized patients. *Cardiothoracic Surgeon*, *28*, 3. https://doi.org/10.1186/s43057-020-0015-7

Zimmerman, W., Baylor, A. E., Hall Zimmerman, L., Dolman, H., Ciullo, J. R., Dornbush, J., Isaacson, A. R., Mansour, R., Wilson, R. F., & Tyburski, J. G. (2020, January 31). Impact of genitourinary injuries on patients requiring an emergency laparotomy for trauma. *Cureus*, *12*(1), e6826. https://doi.org/10.7759/cureus.6826

CLINICAL PRACTICE: EXTREMITY AND WOUND

Bettencourt, A., McHugh, M., Sloane, D., & Aiken, L. (2020). Nursing staffing, the clinical work environment and burn patient mortality. *Journal of Burn Care & Research*, *41*(4), 796–802. https://doi.org/10.1093/jbcr/iraa061

Butowicz, C., Dearth, C., & Hendershot, D. (2017). Impact of traumatic lower extremity injuries beyond acute care: Movement-based considerations for resultant longer term secondary health conditions. *Advances in Wound Care*, *6*(8), 269–278. https://doi.org/10.1089/wound.2016.0714

Carey, M., Valcin, E. K., Lent, D., & White, M. (2021). Nursing care for the initial resuscitation of burn patients. *Critical Care Nursing Clinics*, *33*(3), 275–285. https://doi.org/10.1016/j.cnc.2021.05.004

Dolan, C. P., Valerio, M. S., Lee Childers, W., Goldman, S. M., & Dearth, C. L. (2021). Prolonged field care for traumatic extremity injuries: Defining a role for biologically focused technologies. *NPJ Regenerative Medicine*, *6*, 6. https://doi.org/10.1038/s41536-020-00117-9

Feliciano, D. V. (2017, December). For the patient-evolution in the management of vascular trauma. *The Journal of Trauma and Acute Care Surgery*, *83*(6), 1205–1212. https://doi.org/10.1097/TA.0000000000001689

Huber, G. H., & Manna, B. (2021). Vascular extremity trauma. *StatPearls*. StatPearls Publishing. https://www.ncbi.nlm.nih.gov/books/NBK536925/

Jeschke, M., van Baar, M., Choudhry, M., Chung, K., Gibran, N., & Logsetty, S. (2020). Burn injury. *Nature Reviews Disease Primers, 6*(1), 11. https://doi.org/10.1038/s41572-020-0145-5

Kim, M. J., Yang, K. M., Hahn, H. M., Lim, H., & Lee, I. J. (2022). Impact of establishing a level-1 trauma center for lower extremity trauma: A 4-year experience. *BMC Emergency Medicine, 22*, 123. https://doi.org/10.1186/s12873-022-00682-w

Markiewicz-Gospodarek, A., Koziol, M., Tobiasz, M., Bak, J., Radzikowska-Buchner, E., & Przekora, A. (2021). Burn wound healing: Clinical complications, medical care, treatment and dressing typres: The current state of knowledge for clinical practice. *International Journal of Environmental Research and Public Health, 19*(3), 1338. https://doi.org/10.3390/ijerph19031338

Zeelanberg, M., Hartog, D., Halvchzdeh, S., Pape, H., Verhofstad, M., & Lieshout, M. (2022). The impact of upper extremity injuries on polytrauma patients at a level 1 trauma center. *Journal of Shoulder and Elbow Trauma, 31*(5), 914–922. https://doi.org/10.1016/j.jse.2021.10.005

CLINICAL PRACTICE: SPECIAL CONSIDERATIONS

Braasch, M., Turco, L., Cole, E., Karim, B., & Winfield, R. (2020). The evolution of initial-hemostatic resuscitation and the void of posthemostatic resuscitation. *The Journal of Trauma and Acute Care Surgery, 89*(3), 597–601. https://doi.org/10.1097/TA.0000000000002576

Brown, C. (2021). Emergency airway management in the morbidly obese patient. *UpToDate*. https://www.uptodate.com/contents/emergency-airway-management-in-the-morbidly-obese-patient

Caldwell, N., Mithun, S., Garcia-Choudary, T., & Van Fossen, C. (2020). Trauma related hemorrhagic shock: A clinical review. *American Journal of Nursing, 120*(9), 36–43. https://doi.org/10.1097/01.NAJ.0000697640.04470.21

Cap, A. P., Gurney, J. M., & Meledeo, M. A. (2020). Hemostatic resuscitation. In P. Spinella (Ed.), *Damage control resuscitation*. Springer Publishing Company. https://doi.org/10.1007/978-3-030-20820-2_7

Cortez, R. (2018). Geriatric trauma protocol. *Journal of Trauma Nursing, 25*(4), 218–227. https://doi.org/10.1097/JTN.0000000000000376

Cowell, C. (2021). Geriatric trauma: Initial evaluation and management. *UpToDate*. https://www.uptodate.com/contents/geriatric-trauma-initial-evaluation-and-management?search=Geriatric%20trauma:%20Initial%20evaluation%20and%20management&source=search_result&selectedTitle=1~150&usage_type=default&display_rank=1

Dugar, S., Choudhary, C., & Duggal, A. (2020). Sepsis and septic shock: Guideline-based management. *Cleveland Clinic Journal of Medicine, 87*(1), 53–641. https://doi.org/10.3949/ccjm.87a.18143

Evans, L., Rhodes, A., Alhazzani, W., Antonelli, M., Coopersmith, C. M., French, C., Machado, F. R., Mcintyre, L., Ostermann, M., Prescott, H. C., Schorr, C., Simpson, S., Wiersinga, W. J., Alshamsi, F., Angus, D. C., Arabi, Y., Azevedo, L., Beale, R., Beilman, G., . . . Levy, M. (2021, November). Surviving sepsis campaign: International guidelines for management of sepsis and septic shock, critical care medicine. *Critical Care Medicine, 49*(11), e1063–e1143. https://doi.org/10.1097/CCM.0000000000005337

Goddard, A., Janecek, E., & Etcger, L. (2021). Trauma-informed care for the pediatric nurse. *Journal of Pediatric Nursing, 62*, 1–9. https://doi.org/10.1016/j.pedn.2021.11.003

Llompart-Pou, J., Perez-Barcena, J., Chico-Fernandez, M., Sanchez-Casado, M., & Raurich, J. (2017). Severe trauma in geriatric population. *World Journal of Critical Care Medicine, 6*(2), 99–106. https://doi.org/10.5492/wjccm.v6.i2.99

Muacevic, A., Adler, J., Gray, S., & Dieudonne, B. (2018). Optimizing care for trauma patients with obesity. *Cureus, 10*(7), e3021. https://doi.org/10.7759%2Fcureus.3021

Napolitano, L. (2020). Hemostatic defects in massive transfusion: An update and treatment recommendations. *Expert Review of Hematology, 14*(2), 219–239. https://doi.org/10.1080/17474086.2021.1858788

Ntourakis, D., & Liasis, L. (2020, October). Damage control resuscitation in patients with major trauma: Prospects and challenges. *Journal of Emergency and Critical Care Medicine, 4*, 20–24. https://doi.org/10.21037/jeccm-20-24

Papazian, L., Aubron, C., Brochard, L., Chiche, J.-D., Combes, A., Dreyfuss, D., Forel, J.-M., Guérin, C., Jaber, S., Mekontso-Dessap, A., Mercat, A., Richard, J.-C., Roux, D., Vieillard-Baron, A., & Faure, H. (2019). Formal guidelines: Management of acute respiratory distress syndrome. *Annals of Intensive Care, 9*, 69. https://doi.org/10.1186/s13613-019-0540-9

Roney, L., & Bautista-urand, M. (2019). Pediatric trauma. *Journal of Trauma Nursing, 26*(2), 66. https://doi.org/10.1097/JTN.0000000000000422

Saguil, A., & Fargo, M. (2020). Acute respiratory distress syndrome: Diagnosis and management. *American Family Physician, 101*(12), 730–738. https://www.aafp.org/pubs/afp/issues/2020/0615/p730.html

Simko, L. (2022). Cardiogenic shock and use of percutaneous mechanical assist devices. *Critical Care Nurse, 42*(1), 56–67. https://doi.org/10.4037/ccn2022140

CONTINUUM OF CARE FOR TRAUMA

Alharbi, R., Lewis, V., Shrestha, S., & Miller, C. (2021). Effectiveness of trauma care systems at different stages of development in reducing mortality: A systematic review and meta-analysis protocol. *BMJ Open, 11*(6), e047439. https://doi.org/10.1136/bmjopen-2020-047439

Bardes, J., Khan, U., Cornell, N., & Wilson, A. (2017). A team approach to effectively discharge trauma patients. *Journal of Surgical Research, 1*(213), 1–5. https://doi.org/10.1016/j.jss.2017.02.018

Blaževičienė, A., Laurs, L., & Newland, J. A. (2020). Attitudes of registered nurses about the end-of-life care in multi-profile hospitals: A cross sectional survey. *BMC Palliative Care, 19*(1), 131. https://doi.org/10.1186/s12904-020-00637-7

DuBois, E., Schmidt, A., & Albert, L. (2021). Location of trauma care resources with inter-facility patient transfers. *Operations Research Perspectives, 8*. https://doi.org/10.1016/j.orp.2021.100206

Fatuki, T., Zvonarev, V., & Rodas, A. (2020). Prevention of traumatic brain injury in the United States: Significant, new findings and practical applications. *Cureus, 12*(10), e11225. https://doi.org/10.7759/cureus.11225

Follette, C., Halimeh, B., Chapparro, A., Shi, A., & Winfield, R. (2021). Futile trauma transfers: An infrequent but costly component of regionalized trauma care. *Journal of Trauma and Acute Care Surgery, 91*(1), 72–76. https://doi.org/10.1097/TA.0000000000003139

Frostick, E., & Johnson, C. (2018). Prehospital emergency medicine and trauma intensive care unit. *Journal of the Intensive Care Society, 20*(3), 242–247. https://doi.org/10.1177/1751143718783601

Graham, M., Parikh, P., Hipara, S., McCarthy, M., Haut, E., & Parikh, P. (2020). Predicting discharge disposition in trauma patients: Development, validation and generalization of a model using the national trauma data bank. *American Surgeon, 86*(12), 1703–1709. https://doi.org/10.1177/0003134820949523

Griffiths, I. (2019). What are the challenges for nurses prviding end-of-life care in intensive care units? *British Journal of Nursing, 28*(16), 1047–1052. https://doi.org/10.12968/bjon.2019.28.16.1047

Nicolas, C., Renard, A., & Meyran, D. (2020). In response to: Early and prehospital trauma deaths: Emergency physicians should not be alone to win the game. *Journal of Trauma and Acute Care Surgery, 89*(4), e117. https://doi.org/10.1097/TA.0000000000002814

Safavi, K. C., Gaitanidis, A., Breen, K., Seelen, M., Raja, A., Velmahos, G. C., & Dunn, P. F. (2020). Direct admission to improve timely access to care for patients requiring transfer to a level 1 trauma center. *Trauma Surgery & Acute Care Open, 5*, e000607. https://doi.org/10.1136/tsaco-2020-000607

Shellito, A., Sareh, S., Hayley, H., Keeley, J., Tung, C., Neville, A., Putnam, B., & Kim, D. (2020). Trauma patients returning to the emergency department after discharge. *American Journal of Surgery, 220*(6), 1492–1497. https://doi.org/10.1016/j.amjsurg.2020.08.021

Stenehiem, J., Roise, O., Nordseth, T., Clausen, T., Natvig, B., Skurtveit, S., Eken, T., Kristiansen, T., Gran, J., & Rosseland, L. (2021). Injury prevention and long-term outcomes following trauma-the IPOT project: A protocol for prospective nationwide registry-based studies in Norway. *BMJ Open, 11*(5), e046954. https://doi.org/10.1136/bmjopen-2020-046954

PROFESSIONAL ISSUES

American College of Surgeons. (n.d.). *Part 5: The time is now: Creating and sustaining a unified, learning trauma system*. https://www.facs.org/quality-programs/trauma/tqp/systems-programs/traumaseries/part-v

Bruce, M., Kassam-Adams, N., Rogers, M., Anderson, K., Sluys, K., & Richmond, P. (2018). Trauma providers' knowledge, views and practice of trauma-informed care. *Journal of Trauma Nursing, 25*(2), 131–138. https://doi.org/10.1097/JTN.0000000000000356

Frieri, M., Kumar, K., & Boutin, A. (2017). Nursing education, trauma and care in the intensive care. *International Archives of Nursing and Health Care, 3*(3). https://doi.org/10.23937/2469-5823/1510076

Gosnell, J., & Slivinski. (2021). The building blocks to a highly effective trauma program. *Journal of Trauma Nursing, 28*(2), 126–134. https://doi.org/10.1097/JTN.0000000000000570

Gregory, J. S., Walker, C., Young, K., & Ralchenko, A. (2018). Essential processes of successful trauma systems: Template for analysis of trauma systems. *Journal of Emergency and Critical Care Medicine, 2*, 22. https://doi.org/10.21037/jeccm.2018.02.05

Hamilton, A. R. L., Södergård, B., & Liverani, M. (2020). The role of emergency medical teams in disaster response: A summary of the literature. *Natural Hazards, 110*, 1417–1426. https://doi.org/10.1007/s11069-021-05031-x

Jillson, I. A., Clarke, M., Allen, C., Koehlmoos, T., Mumford, W., Jansen, J., McKay, K., & Trant, A. (2019). Improving the science and evidence base of disaster response: A policy research study. *BMC Health Services Research, 19*. https://doi.org/10.1186/s12913-019-4102-5

Linder, F., Holmberg, L., Eklöf, H., Björck, M., Claes, J., & Mani, K. (2019). Better compliance with triage criteria in trauma would reduce costs with maintained patient safety. *European Journal of Emergency Medicine*, *26*(4), 283–288. https://doi.org/10.1097/MEJ.0000000000000544

Lupton, J., Davis-O'Reilly, R., Newgard, C., Fallat, M., Brown, J., Mann, C., Jurkovich, G., Bulger, E., Gestring, M., Lerner, B., Chou, R., & Totten, A. (2022). Under-triage and over-triage using the field triage guidelines for injured patients: A systematic review. *Prehospital Emergency Care*, 1–8. Advance online publication. https://doi.org/10.1080/10903127.2022.2043963

Tominaga, G., Dandan, I., Schaffer, K., Nasrallah, F., Gawlik, M., & Kraus, J. (2017). Trauma resource designation: An innovative approach to improving trauma system overtriage. *Trauma Surgery and Acute Care Open*, 2(1), 1–5. https://doi.org/10.1136/tsaco-2017-000102

Index